Thinner This Year

A *Younger Next Year®* Book

Thinner This Year

....

A *Younger Next Year®* Book

....

Chris Crowley &
Jen Sacheck, Ph.D.

Bill Fabrocini, P.T., C.S.C.S., Strength Training
Riggs Klika, Ph.D., Aerobic Training

WORKMAN PUBLISHING • NEW YORK

Library of Congress Cataloging-in-Publication Data

Crowley, Chris.
    Thinner this year : a younger next year book / by Chris Crowley and
    Jen Sacheck.
        p. cm.
    ISBN 978-0-7611-6800-3 (alk. paper)
    1. Weight loss--Physiological aspects. 2. Nutrition. 3. Exercise.
    4. Self-care, Health. I. Sacheck, Jen. II. Title.
    RM222.2.C76 2012
    613.2'5--dc23
                        2012027353

Design by Sarah Smith
Illustrations by Susan Hunt Yule
Front cover images: Scale by Joachim Angeltun/iStockphoto; jogger by Melissa Lucier
Photos on chapter openers and back cover by Lucy Schaeffer
Images on page 28 used with the permission of Dr. Miriam Nelson, Tufts University

Workman books are available at special discounts when purchased in bulk for premiums and
sales promotions as well as for fund-raising or educational use. Special editions or book
excerpts can also be created to specification. For details, contact the Special Sales Director
at the address below, or send an email to specialmarkets@workman.com.

Workman Publishing Company, Inc.
225 Varick Street
New York, NY 10014-4381
workman.com

WORKMAN is a registered trademark of Workman Publishing Co., Inc.

Printed in the United States of America
First printing November 2012

10 9 8 7 6 5 4 3

....

The program of diet and exercise in *Thinner This Year* is safe and scientifically structured.
Nevertheless, consult your doctor before beginning this or any exercise program—particularly if
you have ever had a heart attack or been diagnosed with cardiovascular or coronary heart disease,
have frequent chest pains or often feel faint or dizzy upon physical exertion, have high blood
pressure or high cholesterol levels, diabetes, liver or kidney disease, are female and more than three
months pregnant or less than three months postpartum, or are under eighteen years of age. In
addition, ask your doctor's advice if you have muscle, joint, or bone problems that might be
aggravated by exercise. And for Pete's sake, if you don't feel well or if something hurts, stop.

To Hilary Cooper, David Bliss, Ranie Pearce,
S. Hazard Gillespie (1910–2011), and the
committed readers of *Younger Next Year*

—C. C.

To my husband, Chris Ward,
and my spunky kids, Tess and Austin

—J. S.

Acknowledgments

start with Jennifer. One simply could not ask for a wiser, steadier, or more sweet-tempered colleague, teacher, and friend. We have tried to cover some difficult ground in this book. We hope it doesn't show too much, but the science of nutrition ain't beanbag. Jen's leadership has been sure-footed and even-tempered throughout. And she's been great fun *all* the time. How good is that?

Our colleagues, Bill Fabrocini and Riggs Klika, have been wonderful. They too are profound students of extremely complex fields and have led you and me through the complexities with good judgement and good humor. Bill in particular has done nothing less than attempt to convey the creative work of a lifetime—a book, really—in his chapters. I am endlessly indebted to them both. And special thanks to Sam Fabrocini, eighty-seven, who taught Bill everything about hard work and caring for others . . . traits that shone like fire during the years I worked with Bill.

The list of our friends at Workman is long and important. Peter Workman, Bob Miller, and especially Suzie Bolotin—editor of the *Younger Next Year* books—"got it" from the earliest days. Suzie has been unstinting in helping to shape and give focus to a potentially diffuse book. She got me to change direction in a couple of important places (and getting me to change direction is not for the fainthearted). Bruce Tracy, our editor, has been smart, tough, and wonderfully understanding. His ear for language has been a blessing. Our original draft had to be reduced by a third, an agonizing process; we have trusted him at every turn.

The "visuals" in the book have been terrific. Ann Kerman and Sarah Smith have worked like crazy and have made some complex material accessible. Bill Fabrocini deserves special thanks in this area, too. He made the pictures "right."

On the promotion side, we have been lucky in the help of Selina Meere, Courtney Greenhalgh, Jessica Wiener, Molly Kay Frandson, Lindsey Kline, Page Edmunds and, always, the wonderful Jenny Mandel. They are all *such* a pleasure to work with. To a remarkable extent, Workman continues to be a family . . . a happy and pleasant one, at that. And doing a book with Workman is an intimate *partnership*. Jen and I were lucky to be in their hands, and we knew it.

Karen Kelly came into this process, late, to give Jen an important editorial hand. She was very good indeed and a pleasure to work with.

Carol Mann, our agent, did all kinds of things, including finding Karen, promoting the book to Workman, and holding Jen's and my hands. Our thanks to her.

One of the solid bits of advice in the book is "make new friends" in the Third Act. I have followed that advice with exquisite luck in the case of David Bliss, one of my very closest friends these days. He came into our lives first as a lunatic fan of *Younger Next Year* (it *really* changed his life) and participant in the first *six* Aspen Total Immersion Weeks. He got this whole business moving when he insisted that I read Caldwell B. Esselstyn, M.D. (*Prevent and Reverse Heart Disease*) and Colin E. Campbell, Ph.D. (*The China Study*). Creative geniuses both, they were my introduction to and inspiration in the world of nutrition and its extraordinary perils and opportunities. When I decided to do the book, David simply *found* Jennifer, as a result of his work on the Childhood Obesity 180 Project at Tufts. During the long process of writing this book, he read *every single iteration* of every chapter, *hundreds* of them. And he did so with intense interest and great advice every time. We talked on the phone almost daily. He is listed as a dedicatee of the book; it would not have been amiss to list him as a coauthor.

Caldwell B. Esselstyn, M.D., ("Essy") deserves my special thanks. I'm not sure what he'll make of them: One of his chapters is captioned, "Moderation Kills," and I'm sure that Jen and I are way too moderate for his tastes. I spent a great weekend with Essy and his wife, Ann, and have taken my fundamental orientation in this field from him ever since. Jen and I don't agree with him about everything, Lord knows. But I think he is one of the authentic heroes and creative thinkers in the field. He was brave as a lion, thirty years ago (when the idea that the Western Diet caused the Western Diseases was heresy), and he is still fundamentally *right* in his orientation. Read him. And if someone ever tries to put a nonemergency stent in your body, run straight to Cleveland, find Essy, and follow his All Plant-Based diet to the letter.

S. Hazard Gillespie died at the age of one hundred, before this book was finished. He is, quite simply, the model of the good life to me and has been for fifty years. Not everyone gets a mentor, but I got a beauty. For me, he invented the idea that *really* hard work and serious achievement are the highest form of *fun* in a good life. He was fit, slender, and he had fun, all the way out. He bought a new exercise machine in his hundredth year. He lights the way.

My daughter, Ranie, is a dedicatee because she—and her extraordinary achievement of swimming the English Channel last summer—have been *such* an inspiration. She is amazing. Her brothers, Chris and Tim, too, Lord knows. But this year Ranie stands alone on the little podium we lug around.

In the matter of guiding one into the good life—and fun at the high end—Don Pillsbury and Jack Tigue—both lost to life—are with me *all* the time. There are others too numerous to mention but several stand out. Terry Considine, Marnie Pillsbury, Blake Cabot, Jimmy Benkard, Bobo and Bobby Devens, Tony Robinson, Joan Crowley, Rob Bettigole, Michael Fox and Alana Appleby. They count for a lot.

My beloved friend Harry Lodge chose not to do this book. Broke my heart at the time, but he was right. One of his great gifts, as one of the best internists in the country, is knowing when to call in a specialist.

He is not answerable for anything in the book, but he has always been ready with wise, "contextual" advice. And his close friendship is a rock in my life.

Awestruck thanks to the thousands of new friends who have read *Younger Next Year*, fundamentally changed their lives and told me about it, on the road and on the Web. *More than anything else*, their warmth and the astonishing example of their lives persuaded me to do this book. They are another "family"; it's big, and it's a beauty! I could not be prouder to be part of it and them.

Finally, profound thanks to Hilary. Talk about making everything worthwhile. In recent years we have become closer, which I would not have thought possible. And the reason is that she has made the writing of this book and the running of our writing-and-speaking lives her job too, along with her portraiture. She has impeccable judgment about all kinds of things, especially including *people*. I am sometimes rash, impatient, and wrong; she never. As with my life, she made all the difference.

—C. C.

First, I must acknowledge my hilarious and endlessly enthusiastic coauthor, Chris Crowley. Thank you for making the trip to Boston and walking into my office that one summer's day. You not only believed in my skills as a nutrition scientist, but also in our relationship potential almost immediately. Thank you for digesting lots of science, for your patience with my impatience in having to explain certain scientific details nine times before it made sense to you, and for making a tremendous effort to synthesize it all into exciting news for this book. *Thinner* also would not have completely gelled without the stellar support of Karen Kelly, a wonderful science editor, who kept me sane during the editorial process and helped me stay true to myself. To Whitney Evans, M.S., R.D., who knows the good foods cold, as only a smart dietitian can. And to Suzie Bolotin for her careful guidance and to Bruce Tracy, our patient and thoughtful editor at Workman—I still can't figure out how he does it all without screaming.

To all of the scientists who helped shape my scientific perspective and who have been so supportive of my endeavors—in research and teaching—over the years. I would especially like to acknowledge my two closest colleagues and mentors at Tufts—Drs. Miriam "Mim" Nelson and Christina Economos. Mim is responsible for connecting Chris and me, and she had faith that I could actually write this book even while juggling an ever increasingly busy academic job and a young family. She has truly inspired me with her ability to write ten of her own popular books, and still maintain a strong research and leadership role at Tufts. And to Christina, another "Chris," who helped infuse a sense of undying scientific rigor and ethics into the work that I choose to do. Her national leadership in obesity prevention is making *change* possible. Both are truly amazing role models. Of course, to every student who asked "*why . . . ?*" and made me a better teacher, scientist, and mentor—thank you.

Finally, and most important, to my family. To my husband, Chris, my partner in life who has supported me through the years as an athlete, student, scientist, academic, and mother. To my little peanuts, Austin and Tess, who let me squeeze in my exercise whenever possible and also eat their vegetables when their mother asks. Thank you for dealing with Mommy while she was "always working on a big chapter book." You two truly keep me going. And finally, to my biggest fan, Charlotte Wilson, lovingly known as Oma, who is not only a mother to me, but a constant source of support and inspiration. She is a *Younger* poster child.

—J. S.

Foreword

The biology of lifestyle is endlessly fascinating to me. Every day, science unveils more about the mechanisms driving the great biological choices in our bodies—between growth and decay, between health and illness, and between lives that are spiritually and emotionally enriched or impoverished.

When Chris and I wrote the *Younger Next Year* books we thought we had covered the waterfront on the subject, and in some very important ways we had. People who read the books wrote in with remarkable stories of success: dramatic leaps upward in fitness, joy, energy, and quality of life, and also dramatic reductions in weight, blood pressure, cholesterol, blood sugar, and all the other medical markers of the toxic lifestyle we have somehow embraced as normal. As people shared their stories they also asked in-depth questions about specific road maps to better fitness, better nutrition, better health, and better lives.

I was reluctant to take on a book about diet and the deeper details of exercise for a couple of reasons: The first was my deep conviction that diets don't work, and that diet books that don't provide a comprehensive education in nutrition are not only useless but also border on fraudulent. The second was my keen awareness that, as an internist, my expertise in nutrition was more at the level of competence than mastery, and the same held true for my knowledge of the specific details of formal exercise programs. The job of an internist is to recognize patterns, make diagnoses, help people with the biological context of their lives, and, critically, refer them to the best possible experts when a situation needs deep and thorough investigation and treatment.

Chris, never known for resting on his laurels or taking no for an answer, made the compelling case that this wasn't going to be a diet book—it was going to be a nutrition book, an exercise manual, and a detailed road map for taking charge of the *Younger Next Year* biologies.

He has found truly outstanding experts. Jen, whom you will meet in the book, is one of the world's outstanding nutritional scientists, and has a passion for passing on her knowledge. Her credentials are the kind you get only through intellectual rigor and hard-core, bedrock, honest science. Billy and Riggs have devoted their lives to understanding the way the body moves and the deeper aspects of fitness. They are impressive enough on their own, but then they got to play in the intellectual sandbox with Chris. Which is where his unassuming talent for bringing out the best in people worked its magic.

Chris is a delightful companion, a gifted writer, and a wonderful raconteur. What you can miss if you are enjoying the ride is what a powerful critical intellect he has, and what a gift he has for bringing out the intellectual best in extraordinarily smart people. It is in many ways a stiffer challenge to write a book about the details than a book about the concepts, as we did, but Chris, Jen, Billy, and Riggs have done it. They have written the road map to your being younger next year.

If you read *Thinner This Year*, and more important, live it, you will be changing your life. If you give it to your friends and family, and they pass it on, you will be part of changing America as well, which is the urgent task for us all.

Henry S. Lodge M.D., F.A.C.P.
Associate Clinical Professor of Medicine
Columbia University College of Physicians and Surgeons
Columbia University Medical Center
The New York–Presbyterian Hospital

Contents

• *Living More Than One Life* • *The Other Side of Your Brain* • *Get Over Yourself, At Least Your False Self* • *Take Control* • *The Gifts of Women* • *Get Your Lines Out Early* • *Keeping Your Lines Out All Your Life* • *Ranie and the Great Kedge* • *Full House* • *The Old Girl on 57th Street with the Four-Footed Cane* • *The Recap: The Three-Legged Stool*

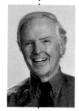

CHAPTER ONE

The Third Act

isten, you're not *fat*. That is *not* what this is all about. You are a
bright, accomplished man. A focused, attractive woman. You've
led a useful, successful, high-energy life, and you're ready for
more. And you are *not* fat because you are not the type. It's as simple
as that. What you are is—I don't know the exact word. *Confused*, perhaps? You were confused about the fact that—by shoveling just a little
too much slop into your pretty little mowser, day after day, year after
year, for, oh, twenty years (while turning bone idle)—you could become, well, a little different from what you were. Different from your
old self. *That's* the word, *different*. There.

Okay, let's have just a moment of candor: You *are* a hair overweight. Possibly two hairs. Because you didn't know how much it
mattered. In the heat of your very busy and important life you felt free
to do a little extra chewing, a little extra swallowing, a little less movement, and you put on a pound or two, on your upper thighs, just under
your butt. And around your middle. Also a little on your upper arms.
Not your biceps, I'm afraid—the triceps. The old tricep *area*, anyway.
Which flutters just the least bit when you wave. "Ta-ta, Janes" they are

called. Because they move ever so slightly when you wave good-bye. "Ta-ta, Jane!" Flutter, flutter. As if your whole arm was saying good-bye to Jane; kind of sweet in a way.

And, men, you have put on just the gentlest pot belly that surely cannot matter because it does not even stick out really. It just pooches out your shirtfronts sometimes when you forget to suck it up. Also the sides. Which you cannot suck up. Hey, no matter; happens all the time. To *everyone*. Now that we're forty or fifty or sixty. But not *fat*, my sweet petunia. Not you. Because *you* are not the type.

"Fat" is some square-butted honey down at the All-You-Can-Eat Café. "Fat" is some guy in forty-four-inch bib overalls down at the feed store. "Fat" is someone *else*, for God's sake. Look, you may be ten or fifteen pounds overweight, period. Which is *extremely* common at your age, in our nation. Almost mandatory. Well, twenty or twenty-five pounds overweight during the winter. I don't know: forty pounds overweight. Call it fifty somewhere in there. Sixty.

Sixty pounds! My God, you are fat, aren't you? *You're fat as butter, and you've been lying to yourself, your family, and your dog for twenty dreadful years! Until today, when you are hideously, shamefully, ravenously, steam-risingly* fat! *That's disgusting, isn't it? Maybe that's the word I was looking for.* Disgusting, *sir!* Disgusting, *madam! Yuckko!* You poor devil, I am *so* sorry! *Fat!*

Hey, hey, hey! Relax I'm just kidding. Mostly. You are not steam-risingly fat, whatever that may mean. You do not have a square butt or forty-four-inch bibs, and you're in much better shape than most people your age in this country. But you have put on some weight. Maybe twenty-five pounds. Just like me, until recently. Just like everyone in this sometimes-ridiculous country. (That's the average per capita gain here in the last twenty-five years: twenty-five pounds apiece, for *everyone*.) Maybe more, maybe less. But listen: You were drop-dead wonderful as a young man, as a young woman. And it is surprisingly realistic—and a great idea—for you to get back to your wonderful self. Your self at, say, thirty-two, or whenever you last looked and felt right. That sounds like a wildly aggressive idea, but you really, really can. And it would be a great idea, for your health, your optimism, your energy, your looks . . . everything. And we believe we can really help a bunch of you do it. Not all, but an awful lot. And we can do it *fast* . . . before you even stop sobbing. Get you back to *you*, by heaven! Where you surely *belong*! You have gotten to us and this little book in the *nick of time*. And we can *fix* this thing, with your serious help. We really, really can.

Here's why: For bright, responsible people like you, being overweight (and idle) really *is*, at the core, a misunderstanding. You did not begin to understand (and certainly nobody said) how rotten the Great American Diet is for you . . . how fat it was making you. And how damn near suicidal it is for you to be carrying stored fat like that. Nor did you begin to understand how utterly dependent you are on regular, serious exercise to survive, as yourself. *Movement, all the time*, you are about to learn, is the single, great key to keeping your miraculous body from going completely to hell after age thirty or forty or fifty. Which it is *absolutely guaranteed to do*, in idleness. A *horror* out there waiting for you, if you don't do something. A life-ruining horror, believe me.

But you're smart, thank God, and once you understand how your body really works, when it comes to this stuff, you can unwind the misunderstanding and get back to being yourself. Not *totally* easy, but obvious, once you get it. And not that hard, either, once you understand a little something about the interplay of nutrition and exercise. It is the business of this book to make sure you do understand. And then to give you a detailed road map . . . to show you *how to do it*. This is a "how-to" book, kids. The manual for The Great Third Act. Out of confusion, denial, and sloth . . . and into the Good Life. Oh boy.

The Promise: Plan A

This is a longish book, and it's full of complex information. But here's a little promise, right up front, to keep it simple: On your side, you have to do three things: (1) You have to read the whole book, (2) You have to make up your mind, and (3) You have to change the way you eat and the way you move, in profound but pleasing ways that we'll talk about.

And then our side: Do that, and you will lose twenty-five pounds in the next six months (less if you need to lose less). Lose it in the first six months and *lock it in* over the next six months. And then, by heaven, you will be radically thinner, *radically* healthier, more energetic, cuter, and way more fun for the rest of your sweet, sweet life! *Thinner and fit, this year and forever.* That's the deal.

Did you like that? I thought you might. And it's true, too, which is nice. But, uh, there's a little caveat. That is the deal if you're interested. That is the deal, if you really make up your mind and go for it. Which, of course, may not happen. There is a tremendous temptation at your age to say, "Hey, thanks for the offer, buddy, but no thanks. I am a hair overweight, but so what? That's the real deal at my age. Everyone puts on some weight. We all look like this. It's part of getting older, and I say the hell with it."

That is a perfectly reasonable response. Indeed, it was my response for a long time. A *long* time. I was a hair overweight—sometimes two hairs—but it was surprisingly hard for me to do anything about it, even though I was in great shape and exercised a lot. And surprisingly hard to care; it didn't seem to matter that much. So I said the hell with it. Just as you may be tempted to say.

But here is what I have learned in the course of writing this book, and what you'll learn, reading it: That was a deeply mistaken idea. Not dumb, you know, because so many people share it. But deeply wrong. I have been slogging along on this project for a couple of years now and I have learned, with great personal sadness, that being a hair or two overweight at our age is not okay. It is the opposite of okay. It is rotten for our health. Rotten for our mobility. Rotten for our joints. Rotten for everything! Stored fat makes you ugly and sick. Ugly is too bad, but sick is serious business. And eventually, stored fat makes you sick. It makes a ton of sense to go to a lot of trouble to get rid of it. A pity, but true. Jen and I are slow to urge you to lose ugly fat because it is so damn hard, and so many will fail. But we do it anyway—passionately—because it is so damn important. But do remember this: Even if you cannot, in the end, lose a ton of weight, doing the exercise and eating sanely will *still* transform your life. So go for it!

And now is the *perfect* time for it. Just as you are wheeling the great ship of your life around and heading into open water. Heading into your all-important Third Act. You want to be in decent shape for the Third Act. Third Acts are tricky because the range of possibilities, for good or ill, is so broad. The Third Act can be much better than you had dared to hope. *Much* better. But it can be a horror too if you get it wrong. That's what this book is really all about: We want you to lose some weight and whatnot. But mostly we want your Third Act to be terrific, and we want the part of You to be played by *you*. The *real* you, not some fat, ridiculous imposter. That will make all the difference.

The Promise: Plan B

There are going to be sane people out there who simply do not like the sound of this "Twenty-five Pounds in Six Months" business. Sounds too gung ho. Too popular. Too some-damn-thing. Fine. It's not the only way. For you there is Plan B, which may work almost as well, and it won't make you crazy.

It goes like this. You do everything in Plan A: Read the book, make up your mind, really do the exercise regimen and change the way you eat. But do not sign on for the six-month commitment. You get where you're going when you get there. The *Promise* is softer, but it is still pretty sweet. The promise is that—if you're serious (that's the soft part)—then, in a surprisingly short time, you will see profound changes in health, fitness, energy, and general youthfulness. Profound and wonderful changes.

The weight loss is less clear for you, but there is a good chance that you'll get that, too. Because the food and nutrition messages embedded in the text are so powerful that they will work, regardless of what you consciously decide to do. Give it some thought and then come aboard. It will radically change your life, however much you lose. That is a promise.

Key Point: Eat Less!

Listen, we are going to talk an awful lot about exercise in this book. And about swapping out rotten food for good. We'll stress how hugely important both are for weight loss, and the good life in general. But in the end you still have to *eat less*. About 20 percent if you exercise hard, more otherwise. There are *three* keys to permanent weight loss and a great life: exercise like crazy, eat right, and eat less. Gotta do all three. If you do only the first two, you will have a much better life. But do all three and it will be radically better.

"Up the Revolution!"

Gee, you may be thinking, that's quite a bit to absorb in the first few pages of what I took to be a simple diet book. What's going on here? And who are you people?

Fair questions. Start with the first one: What's going on here? The answer is "Quite a lot." First and most important, there is this flat-out revolution in aging going on. It has been unfolding for a while, but it is still under the radar for most people. Despite the fact that it may well turn out to be the most important thing in your life. How come? If it's as important as all that?

Well, there's no dough in it for one thing. It's behavior, not drugs or gadgets, so no ads on TV. And historically, medical schools don't teach it, insurance companies don't insure for it, and great corporations haven't figured out how to sell stuff for it. Despite all that, the impact of the revolution is so great that word is slowly getting out. And changing lives in profound and important ways.

How important? Try this: Make some of the behavioral changes we are going to be talking about in this book—and in its predecessor, *Younger Next Year*, where these numbers first appeared—and you can put off 70 percent of "normal aging" until the very end of life. That is a wild claim, and it probably understates the case. Make those same changes, and you can avoid, forever, more than 50 percent of the serious illness and accidents that the other kids are going to have between the time they turn thirty and the day they die. Not put 'em off till the end—avoid them forever, with all the pain and misery and lost joy and expense that go with them. That's how important.

Younger Next Year

The revolution is based on a developing understanding of how the body ages—and how it does *not* age—at the molecular/biological/ evolutionary level. It is the subject of the *Younger Next Year* books, which some of you may have read and a lot have not. They were written by my friend, the drop-dead-brilliant doctor, Henry S. Lodge, M.D., ("Harry" after this) and me awhile back, and they have changed a bunch of lives. A *bunch* of them.

This book is intended to expand on—and go a little deeper into—the themes developed in the *Younger* books. It has been written by the drop-dead-brilliant nutrition and exercise professor, Jennifer Sacheck, Ph.D., and me. Just as Harry was the brain behind the *Younger* books, Jen is the brain behind this one. And an elegant brain she is, too.

The *Younger* books were "Why to" books that gave a broad, strategic overview of the revolution. This one is designed to be more focused and *tactical*. We see this one as The How-To Book of the Revolution: A Tactical Guide to Living the Great Life.

This book is not built on *Younger Next Year*, but, for it to make sense, it helps to have some idea of the basic message of the *Younger* books. The basic message is that there is this amazing (and only recently understood) signaling system inside our bodies, billions and billions of signals all day going to every cell. The system is exquisitely complex, but the signals are simple. It's always one of two things: grow or atrophy, grow or decay. That's the message to the cells, all day long, throughout your life. When you are young, the *default* signal is to grow. And every day you get a little stronger, more coordinated, smarter, more sexual, more fun. All the good things. That default signal sets up the *tide of youth* inside your body. Nice.

Then, suddenly, when you're about thirty-two, the default signal flips over to *decay*. A *tragic* change for individuals, believe me. Fine for the "survival of the species," maybe, but not so great for us. Every year, for the rest of your life, you get a bit weaker, less coordinated, sicker, more pain-wracked, less sexual, grumpier, and so on. A tide of aging sets up in your body, and eventually it sweeps you up on the rocks of decline and decay, where the gulls and the crabs are waiting to eat your big fat gut. Nasty. That tide of aging seems irresistible because it is so steady, so relentless. But here is the great news: The tide is not that strong. If you consciously send some *grow* signals over the same signaling system, you can overcome the tide of aging to an astonishing degree. In particular, you can be about the same man or woman you were at, say, forty-five or fifty until you are eighty and beyond. Not exactly the same, to be sure, but about 70 percent the same. Pretty good. Stunning, in fact. Profoundly important news for all of us. I'd know, by the way; I am almost there, and I gotta tell you: This stuff works.

The master signal for growth is movement. Exercise, in fact, because "movement" has gone out of most of our day-to-day lives. Thus the first and most important of what we called "Harry's rules": Exercise, six days a week, for the rest of your life. "Eek," you say. And I don't blame you. But the consequences are so terrific and so obvious that there really is no rational alternative. It will take awhile for that notion to sink in, but it will.

The next great rule is to change the way (*and how much*) you eat. "Quit eating crap!" as we elegantly put it. Eating good food and being a reasonable weight sends good signals all around your body, much the way exercise does. Not *exactly* the same way but fundamentally similar. Eating Bad Stuff and being overweight sends bad signals. Very bad signals. In *Younger*, nutrition was given rather scant treatment, and readers have been asking for more in this area ever since. We go a lot deeper here. Two thirds of the book is about nutrition and weight management, and exercise as it bears on those things. The remaining third—also new and important stuff—is about the "how-to" of actual exercise.

The third great rule can be summarized like this: Care, connect, and commit to others. It has to do with our fundamental "limbic" or mammalian character, which is the need to be *emotionally connected* with and caring of others. Mammals, including us, have a whole separate brain, the limbic brain, which only sends and receives emotions. As a result we are hardwired to be connected, to live in herds and packs and families . . . and we get isolated at our peril. It sounds funny but this is a signaling matter, too. Isolation sends bad signals. Connection sends good ones.

Finding Jen

A couple of years after Harry and I published *Younger Next Year*, I wanted to do a how-to book, but Harry had to go back to his day job, saving lives and whatnot. I confess I had two motives, one public and noble, the other, private and selfish. The public one was to promote the revolution and give readers the detail they demanded. The private one was that I wouldn't mind dropping a pound or two myself, and I was deeply curious to learn how. The *Younger* books were all that a host of people needed on that front: We got a lot of success stories from folks who had changed their lives and dropped twenty or thirty or seventy pounds along the way. Good for them: It didn't work for me. I changed my life in amazing and satisfying ways by adopting the exercise side of the old book. But I was still a hair overweight. Maybe two hairs. Like you, perhaps, I needed a little more to move me along on that difficult front. I needed this book. And Jen.

I did get the exercise and limbic lessons in *Younger Next Year* and—as a result—fundamentally changed my life. I am about a hundred years old now (okay, seventy-eight, which is close enough), I am in remarkably good shape, and my life is sweet. I have the energy of a golden retriever and the aerobic base of, say, Jennifer Sacheck. Well, that's a lie. Jen is thirty-nine and a onetime all-American rower. She is a different species altogether. *But* I did take this dreadful test in Aspen a couple of years ago, the "VO_2 max test" (maximal oxygen uptake), which is the gold standard for assessing aerobic fitness. And—listen to this—I was in the top 10 percent of men aged forty to forty-nine! That's a *miracle*. I am still a wretched athlete but a wonderfully fit one. Unlike most of the athletic pals of my youth, I am still skiing the double black diamonds in Aspen and riding up to a hundred miles a day on my bike over the Rockies. And I am bubbling over with optimism and drive and Lord knows whatall. Goody. Hooray for me.

But I was fat.

So I really wanted to do the next book, and I cared intensely about finding a wise guide who could help *me* while helping everyone else. I went looking and—clever chap that I am—found Jen. Which was a life-altering break.

Jen is Associate Professor at the Friedman School of Nutrition at Tufts—widely thought of as the best nutrition program in the country —where she does research, advises graduate students, and lectures on nutrient biochemistry and metabolism along with exercise physiology. It's very heavy stuff. Along with these obligations, she does community-based research focused on obesity prevention; runs a multimillion-dollar clinical trial; and has served on numerous committees promoting physical activity and sound nutrition, including an Institute of Medicine committee on Fitness Measures and Health Outcomes in Youth. She also works with a handful of collegiate athletes and aspiring Olympians on proper sports nutrition for the sheer love of it. (As an undergraduate at Syracuse, Jen was captain of the crew and competed nationally and internationally.) She has her master's degree in exercise science and got her Ph.D. at Tufts, and then spent four years in postdoctoral study at Harvard Medical School. She is, quite simply, a rock star.

Cut to our first meeting. We are in Jen's office at Tufts on a pleasant summer morning. Not an impressive office, to tell the truth. But Jen was plenty impressive. She was 5' 10", a bit of a beauty, and in superb shape. She looked for all the world like the serious masters rower, runner, and athlete she still is. No one is healthier or better looking than a serious rower; it is a superb sport. And it was obvious in about ten seconds that—as I had already been told—she was cracklingly smart and knew her field in dazzling depth. She was much too busy doing all kinds of professional things (and raising a young family) to take on a project like mine. But she agreed on the spot because she thought it was important. And because we liked each other. Simple as that. Jen may have regretted it a time or two since, when her life was particularly crazy, but it has been an unmixed blessing for me. Because she is so damn smart. And hardworking. And fun. And she knows this stuff cold.

"How Come I'm Fat?"

"So, look," I said at one point that morning, "how come I'm fat?" She didn't say anything for a minute. Then, "Stand up," she said. Oh, Lord! I did. Turned around, too, as if I were trying on a suit for her.

Nothing for a long minute. Then, "You're fine," she said. And I heaved a huge, silent sigh of relief. But before I could settle into relaxation, she said, "Fifteen pounds." Oh, no! "That will do it. And that will be easy." Pause. "Fine," she said, as if agreeing with herself. "You'll be fine."

"Yeah?" I said, a little warily; I thought she had been looking a little scary when she asked me to stand up. "What do I have to do?"

She shrugged, as if surprised at how easy this was going to be. "There's no magic and it really is pretty easy. There are just three things." Do you notice how there are always three things when people are handing out heavy advice? Harry had three things, too, God bless him. And they weren't easy either.

"First, exercise, which you already have in hand. That is a *huge* advantage and a major difficulty for some people. Exercise alone won't do it. But it really is the *flywheel* of weight loss, weight management, and almost everything else that's good in life.

"Second, you simply have to eat less. No place to hide on that one. As a nation, Americans are some 20 percent fatter now than they were thirty years ago. And, sure enough, we eat about 20 percent more than we used to. There are some tricks but, in the end, weight loss is mostly a matter of calories in (what you eat), over calories out (the amount you burn), running your body, exercising, and so on. Exercise is the biggest variable on the burn side. And food, of course, is the *only* variable on the fuel or intake side. You have to eat less, probably 25–33 percent less, depending. It's partly a matter of simple portion control. Less on your plate, no matter what. But the *real* difference is in *what* you eat.

"That's the third thing, *what* you eat. In this country and in the West generally, we eat a stunning amount of what I call Dead Food, which is food high in caloric density and almost useless or inert, as far as nutrients go. Nutrients are the vitamins and minerals that you get in good food—vegetables, whole grains, and fruit—and none of in Dead Food. Nutrients, which almost no one understands, have a huge role in making your body run right. Your body will not run right on Dead Food. On average, in America, we get more than half our calories from Dead Food, mostly refined white flour and rice and sugar and solid fats. And listen to this: We get 35 percent of our total intake of calories from 'added sugars and solid fats' that food processors *inject* into their products to make them more addictive and give them a bit more shelf life. If you want your body to work right *and* if you want to lose weight, quit eating Dead Food, and replace it mostly with vegetables, fruit, and whole grains. About half of what you put on your plate—half by volume, not calories—ought to be vegetables and fruit. Up to a quarter can be whole grains. Swap out Dead Food for vegetables and whole grains. Fish and a little meat and a very little dairy make up the rest. Cut back radically on meat, especially red meat, which should become a relatively rare treat. Pork and poultry, almost as much. Animal-based food should be cut back radically. There is a drumbeat of persuasive studies showing a clear correlation between eating animal-based food and sickness . . . between animal-based food and mortality. I do not go the all-veg route. Too extreme for me: We have been carnivores for millions of years, and there are some wonderful things about animal proteins. But I sure have cut back. *Way* back.

"Here's the payoff: Good foods—vegetables and fruits, whole grains, and lean proteins like beans and fish—are chock full of nutrients and fiber. *But* they are very low in calories. So they are superb for your health *and* they make it much easier to lose weight. Some portion control still counts, but swapping good food for bad will take care of a lot of the reduction in calories that is so essential. It is an amazing 'two for one.' That swap and maybe cranking up your exercise a bit more, if you like—that'll do it." Then that lovely grin and she just looked at me.

"Easy-peasy," I said, although in fact I was plenty skeptical.

"Easy-peasy," she grinned. "Just make up your mind and off you go."

She was looking very pleasant and wonderfully confident . . . inspirational, you could say. But there was something a little bit sly, too. As if I were not being told everything. "There's more, isn't there," I said.

"A little bit," she said. And there was. A lot. But that's the rest of the book.

"Who Are You People?"

Okay, on to the second big question, from about ten pages ago: Who are we? You now have some idea who Jen is. Let me introduce myself briefly. Most of my life I was a Wall Street lawyer, litigating big cases for mighty corporations. I quit at fifty-six because I wanted to live more than one life. Which eventually led me to doing the *Younger* books with Harry, lecturing on the subject all over the place, and now writing this one with Jen.

Jen's role is obvious: She is the brains of the outfit, and she is going to give you the knowledge that may make all the difference. My job is much simpler. I am here to tell you a little about my experience, my journey, with Jen and the revolution and trying to follow Jen's lead on nutrition and everything else. I am basically Jen's project (and my own) in all this. The notion is that my experience may throw a little light on yours, if you decide to try it yourself.

I am not your role model, by the way; I am your companion. I shine the light on the path, and we struggle along together.

Does This Really Matter?

I n that capacity, as fellow learner, let me tell you briefly about the other big topic we covered that morning at Tufts. I asked Jen what you might have asked me at this point: "Does this stuff really matter that much, Jen? I'm in awfully good shape. My life is mostly a pleasure. And I don't look hideous, by the standards of our society. We say this is going to be easy-peasy, but I *know* that is not true. Is it worth it, when I'm only fifteen pounds overweight and in good shape? Should I bother?"

"Yes."

I waited. "That's it? 'Yes'? Could you put a little meat on that bone?"

"Sure. You ride a bike, right?" I do. "And you paid a fortune for one that weighs what?"

"Under fifteen pounds," I said with childish pride. "And it did cost a fortune, for every ounce of weight reduction. And worth every penny because it's a rocket ship and a joy."

"I'm sure. Now think about this: Suppose you could take *another fifteen pounds* off your bike. You couldn't, of course, but think of it that way. If you dropped just fifteen pounds, it would be a revelation, a miraculous change in your bike riding. I'm not a cyclist but I am an athlete, and I know. It would revolutionize your bike riding. *And* your walking around. And your climbing a hill. Your *whole* life. You would not be a different person, but you'd be a deeply *changed* one.

"And think about this," she went on. "Are your joints beginning to hurt a little?" They were. Not terrible but serious. And a little bit scary because the trend was wrong. And exercise alone was not solving it.

"Take fifteen pounds off your hip joints, off your knees and your ankles, your metatarsals, almost your whole skeleton. And it will mean that your joints will last much, much longer, without pain. It is not a lot of pounds, but fat is different from muscle: Lugging it around is very hard on your body. If you are twenty-five pounds overweight—to say nothing of fifty or sixty—it is much, much worse, of course. But even at fifteen, there will be a big difference. And it will count a lot, in the general pleasure of your life."

Jen swung her chair around and rolled it closer: She was getting into it. "But here's the big one. You said that Harry told you that your numbers, from your physical, were a little off, right?" I had.

"Makes perfect sense. Your numbers are off because fat is a killer. Fat harms your health, even a relatively little of it, like the fifteen you're packing. Eating 'crap,' to quote your book, is much, much worse for your health than almost anyone in this country imagines. Getting fat is a real health hazard."

"But I exercise like crazy," I whined.

"Yes, you do. You exercise more than 99 percent of the people in the country, so you have overcome the way you eat by quite a lot. And it is still making you a little bit fat. And a little bit sick. Gaining fifteen pounds after forty is not a free shot. It is not something that just happens that you can ignore. It is bad for you, and you ought to fix it. You really should."

"You're mean," I said, with a fake pout.

"You bet I'm mean." She didn't care one bit. "When the rowers I train eat slop, I am all over them. My girls want to go to the Olympics, some of them, and they're eating Dead Food? Uh-uh. I am all over 'em for that."

"And you're going to be all over me, if we do this book?" I asked, with a slight look of horror.

"No," she sat back. "No, that is *not* going to be my job. I'll keep track with you, if you like. But mostly I suggest that we do for you what we do for the people who read the book.

"I think we should explain—in more depth than anyone has explained before—how your body works when you eat good food in sane amounts. Describe the actual process, which is very complicated. Then we describe just what happens when they eat Dead Food and meat, especially when they eat much too much of it, day after day, year after year, the way so many do in this country. Which is plenty scary, believe me. Then they can do what they want. It is not our place to tell people how to eat, how to exercise. Our job, it seems to me, is to tell them what happens, in various scenarios. Then they pick. Just like you're going to."

The War Zone

Here is something that Jen did not say that day, perhaps because you need *some* background in her field (which you'll soon have) in order to really get it. But I don't care, I'm going to lay it on you right now. Because it is so profoundly important, and because it will cast a certain light on the rest of the book. Jen cautions that this is developing science and the contours may change a little. But not the basics. She has been studying this stuff all her professional life (it is her great passion) and she says that the premise is sound.

There is a war going on inside your body, a war of signals. A war between sickness and health, strength and weakness, optimism and despair . . . everything. And—"on the ground"—it is a war between stored fat (especially in your gut) and lean, active muscle mass. Stored fat (pat your gut) sends out a terrifying cascade of signals that promote inflammation and disease. Lean, active muscle mass (squeeze your thigh) sends out an overwhelming cascade of signals (especially when you're exercising) that fight inflammation and disease. Inflammation (and free radicals) are The Great Satan inside your body. They are the great progenitors of heart disease, many cancers, adult-onset diabetes, and lots of other dreadful things . . . the worst things in our lives. So, as you turn these sometimes daunting pages, bear in mind that there is almost nothing as important as understanding this War . . . and taking sides. Taking sides means fighting hard to shrink stored fat and fighting hard to grow (and use) lean muscle mass. We live in a War Zone, kids; we gotta pick sides. Quit eating garbage, start working out. We'll show you how.

I walked out and headed for my car that miraculously did not have a ticket. And affectionately I patted my stomach and "handles" as I walked along . . . reached up and twisted the wattle under my chin. "Good-bye, my dear friends," I said softly. "I have enjoyed growing you very much. But you are out of my life now. You are so *gone!*" Which—four months and a lot of work later—was mostly true. Not the wattle, actually. Wattles are forever.

A Program for You

Over the next months, Jen and I spent a lot of time together, and we mapped out a program for you, the same one that's summarized in The Promise. We want you to lose up to twenty-five pounds in the next six months while you're learning to move again. We are not all the same, and some of you will take longer . . . up to a year in some cases, but six months for most. That's a pound a week, which does not seem aggressive, but it is. Very. Or do it more sporadically, à la Plan B. But do it. It will change your life.

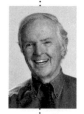

CHAPTER TWO

The Mountain of Slop and Despair

This is not a totally restful book, is it? Kind of fun, we hope, but slightly serious. Sorry about that. But look: We are changing lives here. And changing lives ain't beanbag. Think about the exercise piece, for example: Exercise six days a week until the day you die. Good grief! That sounds awful tough to some, downright impossible to others. But it's much easier than you might think. And it's the least you can sanely do, in the circumstances of your life.

Welcome to the Tar Pit

We were designed to exercise, and we are idle at our peril. The idleness most of us are living now is a tar pit . . . it is going to suck you down like a mastodon into a slow, dying Third Act that will be a horror to watch. And much worse to live. Feet just stuck in the tar! Screams every hour or two, when you have the strength, then terrified silence. For a sane, informed man or woman over forty, over fifty, idleness is insanity. Not just a "bad idea"; craziness. Exercise makes your body and your mind work. While it makes you thin. Exercise is at the core. Don't care for it? Tough; do it anyway. Skip it, and your feet get stuck in the tar. And you are just plain done.

As long as I've got the gloves off, let me add another, blunt word. Being fat all by itself is messing up the workings of our bodies. Stored fat is actually toxic. First it will sap your energy, your mood, and your strength as it interferes with the workings of your body. Then it will make you sick. Because stored fat is a dangerous font of inflammation and free radicals (those are the little guys that break your body down, bring on the heart attacks and cancers and such). And "visceral fat," that adorable potbelly, is much, much worse. It looks vaguely cute, right? Wrong! It's scary. Your potbelly is an open sewer inside your body. And at night, the rats come out. Don't want those suckers scurrying around, gnawing on your kidney and liver and whatnot. Gotta get 'em out of there! Gotta drop a couple of pounds and get rid of that puppy.

Okay, just thought I'd stress that up front . . . wake up the kids who had fallen asleep.

Back to You and *Your* Third Act

So weight loss counts. But we submit that the great question in your life these days is a little broader than weight loss. And it goes like this: What is your life going to be like, in this Third Act we're so hyped about? Is it going to be any fun? Or is it going to be long stretches of boredom and decline, punctuated with little pops of terror? Do you get to retire? Or do you work at the same damn thing till you drop, like the horses in Central Park? Is there going to be interesting stuff to do? Will you and your spouse weather the changes that are coming at you at about a hundred miles an hour? Or will you blow apart like dry leaves when the autumnal gales begin to blow? And—as important as anything—are you going to be able to *move* or not? And *do* stuff. And *care*? And have some *energy* and *optimism*? And be decent company? Are you going to be yourself all the way out? That's the big one, believe me: Are you going to be yourself, all the way out? Or are you going to turn into a grumpy old loser who sits in the corner of a darkened room, watching daytime TV and eating crap, drinking bourbon out of a jelly jar? While the real world goes whizzing by without you 'cause you're no fun anymore.

Look, the choices are not quite that stark. But they are broadly along those lines. And for a scary number of people, the dark side is a good deal worse. Take a look at The Old Woman of Bogota. She's not from Bogota, she's from Maryland, but Bogota is where I heard about her. And it was scary.

The Old Woman of Bogota

gave a talk in Bogota recently, and there was a terrific gerontologist, a doctor for the elderly from Johns Hopkins, on the program right after me. She projected on the screen the photo of a gaunt old woman in her eighties and listed, under her picture, all her diseases and disabilities (about *fifty* of them, literally) and all her meds. The poor woman's life was a horror. She was dazed and in serious pain when she wasn't out of it altogether. She was taking a huge number of pills that she often got messed up, with serious consequences. She was often in tears. Often terrified. Talk about the mastodon in the tar pit. Scariest part of the story: The young gerontologist said that this woman was a typical patient in her excellent facility. Typical "frail old" as they are called. This was the future for a lot of Americans.

But what struck me, as a lifestyle guy, was that almost all the stuff she suffered from seemed so unnecessary. I asked the doc, who had just heard my talk about behavioral change, "Couldn't she have avoided some 80 percent of her ailments if she'd worked out and eaten right and stayed in touch with others?"

"Oh, of course she could," the doc said. "*More* than 80 percent. That's the horror. Our medicine does not address the basics of behavior. That's up to us."

The Upside

Okay, that's the downside. What about the upside?

The *upside* in the Third Act can be awfully damn good. You can, if you like, be your own sweet self, almost all the way out to the waterfall. Step out onto a broad sunlit upland of energy, optimism, and grace whose very existence you did not begin to suspect until now. Interesting woman, interesting man, good company, good time, *doing new stuff*, more or less forever. Cause you *care* so damn much and because you *feel good* and can. *More* fun, if anything, than you are now. More energetic. Younger, you could say. And as part of the whole business *thinner*, too. There's a surprise for most of us: seriously *thinner* in your fifties and sixties. Who knew?

The Context of Your Effort

W e wander in a dark wood when it comes to nutrition because so many of the popular writers on the subject are simply delusional. Others are charlatans, or close to it. And plenty of authoritative-sounding souls simply do not have the least idea what they are talking about. They use this scientific-sounding lingo with great panache. They are absolutely sure of themselves and of what we should do. And they are nitwits. Hint: If there are a lot of details about just how miraculously fifty different supplements work magic inside your body—or if they say you can get in great shape working out four minutes a week—the author is a nitwit.

Finally and most dangerous, there are great armies of special pleaders—brilliant and persuasive men and women, with unlimited budgets and no morals, who work for the powerful growers of, say, corn, beef, milk, and cheese (of which we eat twice as much as we did thirty years ago)—and the producers of the best-known processed foods that take up 80 percent of the space in the middle of the supermarket. The processed foods that are injected with all these solid fats and added sugars. And for the good people who own and market the fast-food places. The "gastro-pedophiles" who hand out little toys to get the boys and girls to come and play under the Golden Arches and eat in the Gingerbread House. Which is not a safe place. The economic stakes for them and their masters are very high indeed. And these hired hands will say any damned thing charmingly, alluringly, irresistibly to get us to eat more processed slop—and more Dead Food.

Against that grim background, it is critically important to have a scientifically conservative and solid academic, like Jen, to tell us what is what. Jen sets the baloney to one side and shines a bright light on what the best people in the field *know* is right. Jen is sound. Jen's Rules are sound. There is no magical thinking, no nonsense, and no easy fixes. Jen is one of the good guys, in a field where there are not enough.

Speaking of the good guys, permit me to say that most of this book is annoyingly balanced, fair, and restrained. Jen will not say extreme things, no matter how I goad her. So many times, her message is that you must strike a sane *balance* of this food and that—a "balanced diet" of good foods. Yawn. But I submit that she is just what you want to guide you through a subject where there is so much hype and downright baloney. Jen is a scientist, through and through. She is incapable of overstatement. Hell, she is incapable of *emphasis*.

But I am not. I believe there are fundamental issues of right and wrong at play in all this, and that we should see them in that light. This stuff *matters*. Not to get too hot about it, but this really is nothing less than a struggle for the soul and well-being of the country and of each of us. This is a *revolution* we are talking about. This is a fight, and the stakes are enormous. Let's slip off the gloves again, for just a few minutes here and tell it exactly as it is. Get ready for tear gas, kids. Here come some home truths.

The Mountain of Slop and Despair

We live, most of us in the West, on the lower slopes of the Mountain of Slop and Despair where an infinitely appealing bounty of poisonous food is grown for us by dark and powerful forces. Which we eat, even though it makes us fat. And eat some more, even though it makes us sick. As if a dark miasma were being floated down from the crater at the top to blind us to all reason—lotus eaters in the fog. We are a brilliant and successful people here in America, but we are heedless of the horror at the center of our lives. Two thirds of us are overweight, and half of that number, a *third of us,* are clinically obese. A third of our precious children are either overweight or obese, too. It is sick. And so are we. It is ruining our lives and may bankrupt the country because health care can't keep up. *No system* can keep up with this level of madness. It is not more *medicine* that we need. It is less madness.

But some morning soon, my friends, a great wave of revulsion is going to rise up in this country and sweep away the Mountain of Slop and Despair that has been built in the last thirty years: the mountain of fast food, dead animals, and processed junk where we all go to feed, obscenely, two and three and four times a day. Until we get so fat we can barely walk. And we get so sick we can barely work. And where, *shamefully*, we train our young to feed as well. As if we were blind to the stench, blind to the disease, blind to the ugliness of our big, fat selves.

When we are stuffed, we wipe ourselves off and waddle along to lie down under the Tree of Lies, in the Arbor of Forgetfulness, until our bloated bodies, which can no longer tell the truth about these things, *twitch* that we are hungry again. And we stumble to our feet, blink our eyes, and go back to our filth. We've got to raise the waters, my friends. Got to tear that Mountain down. Tear ourselves away from it, one by one, to start. Then the children. Then tear down the whole damned mountain! And become thinner, healthier, happier, and, by heaven, *cuter. Cute as buttons*, you darlings. You've been ugly *lo-o-ong* enough!

Remember the lines from the great spiritual? "Moses stood on the Red Sea shore / Strokin' that water with a four by four. And Pharaoh's army got drowned-ed / Oh, Mary, don't you weep." Pharaoh's army is *real*, children. It is the cruel phalanx of greedy agribusiness, cynical marketers, and corrupt politicians. Pharaoh's army is *real*, and it is driving us into a Red Sea of obesity and disease where we will all be drowned-ed, if we do not rise up and turn the waters back. Leaders are starting to show up, but it has to be all of us, I'm afraid. Because the enemy is so many and so strong. Because the government and our leaders have been bought, plain and simple, by lobbyists and agribusiness billions and the power of those who make their living selling us slop.

So we have to go down to the Red Sea shore by ourselves. One by one and in small groups. Pick up some four by fours. And begin. In a few months, I hope there will be thousands of us, standing up to our waists in the waters of ignorance, sloth, and greed. And slowly—but with tremendous resolve—strokin' that water with a four by four. To raise the waves and *wash that Mountain down.*

You may think, in places, that we are a bit extreme on both diet and exercise. Well, *of course we are*! The *problem* is extreme! It is *crazy* extreme. Just look again at those obesity numbers and think of the consequences. There is a raging *epidemic* of adult-onset diabetes, for instance. Victims are having their legs *amputated*, for God's sake, to halt its spread. We're cutting off our arms and legs because we're so *fat*! And there is *no need for it whatsoever*! You get that kind of diabetes only by living on the Mountain. You get it only by getting *fat*.

And that most assuredly is not all. Living on the Mountain, you also get a bunch of cancers and heart disease—and good old Alzheimer's, which I sometimes forget. They aren't so great either. Think about heart attacks and strokes. In a rational country, heart disease would be a rare sickness and the treatment of heart disease a minor specialty in medicine. In our country, it kills more than half of us. And there are huge, billion-dollar buildings, all over the place, full of expensive doctors and technicians, devoted just to heart disease. Not to cures, by the way. With all the billions we have spent, we have not found any cures. Those huge buildings are devoted just to temporary *fixes*. Stents and bypasses and mechanical hearts—neat (indeed miraculous) patch-up jobs that cost a fortune and don't work very well. Or for very long. Or give you much of a life.

You know how you *do* cure those things? Or avoid 'em? With lifestyle changes, that's how. With the stuff in this book.

So, yeah, we're a bit extreme in places. And you better be, too. Because this is *serious business*. We've got to get our muzzles out of the trough. We've got to *move. We've got to tear that Mountain down!*

CHAPTER THREE

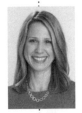

Where I'm Coming From and Where You're Going

As you may have figured out by now, Chris and I make a slightly odd couple but maybe an effective one. He beats the drum and sounds the trumpet . . . gets everyone marching. And I provide you with the scientific road map for where we're going. In the end, Chris and I both believe that it is the actual *knowing* of what's going on inside your body with food and exercise that you'll find the most motivational. Once you *understand* why healthy practices are so beneficial, the logic of making profound changes to your lifestyle becomes obvious.

So despite a crazy schedule of teaching and research, not to mention motherhood mayhem, I took on this project for three important reasons. First, if I can inspire you to move more and fuel your body with great food, it will be a small but important step in reversing our tendency to accept our ever-expanding waistlines. We see overweight men, women, and children everywhere because we live lives that promote weight gain. This environment creates a sense of complacency, as if to say, "Yeah, I am a bit overweight and not happy about it, but look, I'm in good company." While there's a lot of talk about obesity these days, including from the government, we still seem oddly detached from it, strangely lacking a sense of both collective purpose and individual responsibility. The solutions have yet to fully penetrate our daily lives. The work that needs to be done has only just begun. We have to get to the root of the problem: Stop making terrible food choices and change the fact that we simply don't walk, run, or get off our behinds enough.

Second, the levels of nonsense and downright deception about diet and exercise that the average person in this country encounters are astonishing. At a time when there is such a desperate need for accuracy and truth there is so much baloney fed to Americans about nutrition and weight loss: do-nothing diet pills, "miracle" supplements, "eat everything" diets, "eat nothing" diets, four-minutes-a-week exercise regimes—easy "solutions" that are nothing of the sort. I have looked at a great many quick-fix big promise diet books, and for the most part, they are beyond aggravating. Many focus narrowly on unsustainable severe calorie or food-specific restrictions when the negative influences on our waistlines are more complicated than that. It's not only food but also exercise that make the difference between achieving a healthy body weight and yet another failed diet. I want to give you some home truths on the subjects of nutrition and exercise so those of you who are trying to do the right thing won't waste your time.

Third, I am fundamentally optimistic about the possibility that we can change the way we eat and move. We have to change, we are going to change, and I would like to be part of that because the way we live now is not sustainable. Here's some important news: I am absolutely certain that exercise is as important as food when it comes to weight loss and long-term weight maintenance, as well as being the single most important component for your overall health, energy, and wellness. We do both here, obviously—eat great food and exercise hard. But if you find yourself in a difficult food predicament, keep the exercise going. Regular exercise promotes a desire to fuel your body healthily in addition to keeping you on track with some nutritional leeway, meaning that occasional celebratory indulgences won't affect your bottom line as much as they would a sedentary person. Exercise really is the flywheel of the good life.

Why I'm So Passionate

As Chris mentioned, I was a serious rower in college. Oddly enough, I never thought once about nutrition during my early competitive rowing years. That changed when I started to work on my master's degree and was coaching Division I rowers. As it turned out, I coached the lightweight team (women had to be 130 pounds or less on race day), but many happened to weigh closer to 140. They were in superb shape, didn't have much body fat, and wanted to stay healthy while still dropping ten pounds apiece. Exercise more? Sure. But diet? I needed to learn more.

So I dug in and researched everything I could get my hands on about sports nutrition. I told the rowers what to eat. The regime also combined intense exercise and once-a-week weigh-ins—so they wouldn't go crazy worrying about minor day-to-day fluctuations. Two things happened: First, my athletes did lose the weight, and they did become division champions. Second, I became a serious student of nutrition and even did my thesis on the subject. It became very clear to me that nutrition is a key factor for both performance and healthy weight loss not only for athletes in training, but also everyone else. Exercise gets your machinery in great shape, but you need the right fuel to achieve truly amazing and sustained results.

Since then I've focused much of my academic career on how the response of our bodies to our environments becomes dysregulated with age and how nutrition and exercise strongly influence this process. You lose muscle mass as you age (the medical term for this is *sarcopenia*), and unless you take certain steps it decays precipitously. The wiring goes off, the muscle cells decay, and a serious decline follows if you don't do something about it. A sedentary lifestyle mixed with poor nutrition also contributes to a loss of the body's signaling capacity, which is key to coordination, balance, and, curiously, strength itself. When your body falls apart, your cognition declines, depression sets in, and you are less able to live life fully. It does not have to be that way. People who stay very active and eat rationally offset "normal" sarcopenia to a remarkable extent. Some of you have read that thesis in *Younger Next Year*; I saw it in the laboratory, and it is strikingly true.

Today, at Tufts, I focus mainly on obesity prevention, which may seem odd at first, but as it turns out muscle and fat have a lot do with each other. They have a dialogue of sorts which I'll talk about in more depth later. Much of my research focuses on how fitness mitigates health risks associated with being overweight. Being fit truly does wonders for your health. All my years of study, research, and practice have proven that good nutrition and serious exercise result in a good life for *everyone*. That is the foundation of my professional life and my message in this book.

Finally, I work hard to practice what I preach. I have a mildly sick passion for predawn exercise. And I need my kedges (see Chris on them later). I continue to train and always have at least my annual "big two"—typically one running and one rowing race. There's something invigorating about getting up before dawn and going down to the Charles River for an early row. I also love the challenge of running "hill repeats"—serious intervals that build aerobic capacity—to get in shape for the Mt. Washington road race, an excruciating race 7.6 miles straight up the famous New Hampshire mountain. I've been a marathoner (I've done seven) and I try to be a good yogi (for balance and body awareness). Pushing my kids around town in a double jogger—not yet an Olympic event, although it should be—is way tough, but likely my ultimate favorite. And it's efficient: I get my exercise in and I also get to be with my kids.

Who Are You?

As you can see, I ride the exercise-nutritious food range every day so I know it adds up to something good. But let's focus on you. In shaping my exercise and nutritional advice, I am assuming you're a typical man or woman, mid forties to mid sixties, probably at least twenty or thirty pounds overweight—someone who may work out a little, but nowhere close to six days a week and not very intensely. My advice works if you're younger or older, but if you're stronger or weaker, or heavier or thinner than my assumption, you're going to have to extrapolate a little. For people age thirty to forty who are not overweight and who already have a very substantial workout habit, the adjustment is going to be easy. You can whistle through the weight loss chapters without paying much attention. Just remember that maintaining proper weight gets more difficult as you get older. The exercise advice is worth a close look by everyone, including those of you who are already into the subject. Virtually everyone will learn important, new things in the exercise chapters.

For those at the other end of the scale—the truly "deconditioned" —the adjustments may be more extensive. If you are more than forty pounds overweight and have not exercised at all for a long time, or ever, we urge you to (1) See your doctor before you start an exercise program, and (2) Start slowly and proceed more gradually. The basic rules are the same and the journey is to the same place, but you stand to gain much more because you are traveling farther. If you have any anxiety and if you can possibly afford it, you might want to consult a registered dietitian and perhaps get the assistance of a good trainer. An exercise trainer, even if it is only to start with or once in a great while, is a great idea for newbies who need to learn proper form to avoid injury. A trainer offers moral support and keeps you motivated, too.

Why Exercise Is the Key Component for Weight Loss: The 101 Version

Before we address the mechanics of exercise in terms of weight loss, I want you to buy into the idea that exercise is a critical aspect of weight loss as well as overall longevity and health. Simply put, it is healthier to be "fat and fit" than to be "thin and in rotten shape." Razor-thin models who smoke while looking *soigné* but who have never broken a sweat are losers. Not just weight losers but losers in life. They may look good to the fashion editors, but they are seriously compromising their health to get into the pages of their magazines. It is far, far better to be a woman or a man packing an extra twenty pounds and in great shape than either a sickly underweight and out-of-shape model or someone who suffers from both excess weight and a sedentary lifestyle. To give this point some punch, here's a scary illustration of what failure to exercise can do to your body. Do no exercise after age thirty and you will lose about one percent of your muscle mass per year. That process speeds up a bit after sixty, and it looks something like this:

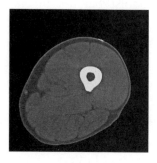 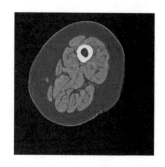

Young, active   **Older, sedentary**

This is an actual photograph of "normal American aging": a computed tomography (CT) of the cross-section of two women's thighs. The left-hand picture is that of a young active female; the one on the right is a picture of an older sedentary woman. The white circle in the middle of both legs is the femur (thigh bone). The outer dark circle is the layer of subcutaneous fat that lies just under the skin. On the young woman, the layer is very thin. On the older one, the layer is huge. The middle or gray portion is lean muscle mass. See how it has shrunk with age? In the young woman it is solid and takes up most of the thigh. In the older woman it is much smaller and marbled with fat. One of those legs works. Its owner can stand up out of a deep chair, ski, and walk up stairs easily. The other one does not work very well, and the owner cannot do most of those things. Whether you're male or female, this is what happens if you don't exercise, no matter what you eat. Does this scare the dickens out of you? It should.

It doesn't have to be that way. If you work out hard six days a week, including serious strength training, your leg will look much more like the one of the left, even when you're in your sixties or seventies. By "hard" I mean exercise that makes you sweat and raises your heart rate. Don't worry—we'll explain it in detail in the coming chapters, and

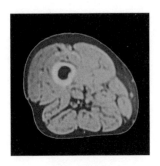

Chris's thigh

Chris shows you exactly what "hard" means, too. In the meantime, take a peek at the third photo. That is Chris's leg at age seventy-eight. There is some added fat, inevitably, but not much because he exercises hard. As a result, his legs *work*. He can still ski moguls, row, and ride a bike a hundred miles—activities he loves that most of his contemporaries gave up some time ago.

Another benefit of exercise is that the more you do, the more you naturally use up the fuel you feed your body by way of food. Expend more energy than you consume and you lose weight. Studies have shown that if you either moderately restrict calories or exercise to burn the same number of calories as the calorie restriction, you will lose the exact same amount of weight. No voodoo, no magic. There is also some very compelling evidence that when exercisers consume meals, they metabolize their calories differently and more efficiently than nonexercisers. For instance, exercisers tend to burn more stored fat during and after exercise, whereas nonexercisers are much better at burning carbohydrates. It takes much longer for a sedentary body to figure out how to use fat for energy so the fat stays put longer.

Regular exercise also has a profound effect on the structure and function of your muscles, which in turn affects weight loss. Muscle is inherently more metabolically active at rest than fat. Each pound of muscle burns approximately six calories per day, whereas fat burns about two calories per day per pound. Increase your muscle through exercise and weight training, and increase your resting metabolism. The differential in calorie burn between the two tissues is not mind-blowing, but these extra calories of burn a day add up over time.

What's Food Got to Do with It?

Plenty! Although exercise is crucial in weight loss and maintenance, there is no doubt that food, the kind you eat and how much of it you consume, also plays a crucial role in the weight loss equation.

Obviously, if you are obese, losing weight is your number-one priority: You have to start eating good food in more moderate quantities than you're used to. If you're "just" overweight, you risk becoming obese, and for that reason you have to nip the problem in the bud before your weight becomes a serious health issue. If you're exercising, and you should be even if you're overweight, you need nutrient-dense fuel to maintain health and stamina. Nutrients feed all sorts of important functions in the body, and many can stave off the effects of aging, too.

That said, let's consider food from three basic perspectives. The first is the most primal: the pleasure principle. That may be a surprise, coming from a scientist, but I seriously believe that eating and drinking are great delights that should be preserved and celebrated. It is both unrealistic and wrong to put forward a regimen that takes the fun out of eating. It won't work in the long run, and it shouldn't. That's why the foods we suggest in both the food list and the meal plan in Chapter 9 are whole healthy foods that also happen to be yummy. Chris has had some interesting and entertaining adventures with these foods, and I know his tales of trying new things will be a terrific source of encouragement, and certainly amusement.

Second, food has value over and above the way it tastes: its ability to deliver nutrition and optimal health. It is the critical business of eating enough of the right foods that makes our bodies function properly. It's hard to believe, but the notion that you need to eat certain kinds of food just to make your body work right is unfamiliar to a lot of otherwise educated people.

Nutrient-dense foods provide the wherewithal for building cells—go without them, and important internal tasks simply do not get done. And then you get sick. Junk food, the garbage on Chris's Mountain of Slop and Despair, is almost nutrient-free, an astonishing nonaccomplishment of the fast-food and processed food industries. You have to come down off the Mountain and combine nutrient-dense foods with exercise if you want truly spectacular health results.

Importantly, the Good Stuff is also much less calorie dense than junk food, so you can eat more of it in terms of volume than the alternative. Nutrient-dense vegetables and fruits and whole grains are slower to digest than the simple carbs found in white breads and pastas, and junk and processed foods, and these powerhouses keep you feeling fuller longer, a huge double blessing. If you learn to love the nutrient-dense stuff (and I know you can), you'll find it so much easier to lose weight and keep it off. Our taste preferences *can* change over time. If you make a job of dining heavily on nutrient-dense vegetables, fruits, and whole grains, before long they will become your first choice as a matter of taste and pleasure. This is not to say that you have to turn to an *all* plant-based diet, although many reputable researchers believe in it. I am not a vegetarian, but red meat and high-fat cheeses and other rich dairy products play minor parts in the diet we recommend here.

Finally, and this is the reason why many of you are here, food has an enormous impact on how we look, depending on what and how much we put in our mouths. The reason why so many of us embark on diet after diet is because we want to look good. Let's face it: Being paunchy or chubby is a *visible* problem. If it's vanity that helps you get on and stick to what we're suggesting, great! What you're doing for your outside appearance is also doing wonderful things to your insides.

Good Eating with Exercise

My prescription for weight loss is simple. To *maintain* your weight against the strong propensity to gain a pound or two a year after the age of thirty, cut your caloric intake by roughly 20 percent. To *lose weight*, you may have to cut your intake by as much as a third, depending on how much you're eating now. In addition, embark on or continue a serious exercise program, six days a week, at least forty-five minutes a day, for the rest of your life. No one loses serious weight and maintains the loss over time without a serious exercise habit. However, the opposite is also true: No one *loses* serious weight with exercise alone. Remember what I said about being "fit and fat." If you want to be fit and thin you have to work both ends, calories in and calories out, for the rest of your life. That's the deal.

There are a couple of ways to cut your food intake. The simplest and best way is to fill half of your plate with vegetables. At least another quarter should be whole grains and legumes. That shift, plus exercise, reduces calories enough so you can lose weight. The other way is to cut portion size. It's an unbeatable trifecta: better food in smaller portions than you're accustomed to, with a regular exercise practice. Good food, nutrient-dense food, has built-in appetite suppressors or "satiety bells" that junk foods don't have. Have you ever seen someone (maybe you) scarf down a super-sized serving of fries and a cheeseburger, and still have room for a soft serve ice cream? Then, two hours later, a craving for chips kicks in? In contrast, few people who dig into a plate of beets and greens, brown rice, and a piece of fish require extra food when they're done.

Junk Food Is Addictive

J unk food is literally addictive, like a habit-forming drug. If you find yourself having a little trouble breaking your junk food habit, don't be surprised. You're not just a fan; you're an addict. The solid fats and added sugars (the SoFAS) that are pumped into processed foods hook you like heroin. Sure enough, sugar and fat similarly trigger a rewiring of the brain's pleasure circuitry that amplifies desire for those foods. Addictive substances rewire your brain to increase cravings and drive you to satisfy them. There is every reason to believe that the manufacturers put SoFAS in food deliberately in abundance, for that very reason: to keep you coming back for more.

Interestingly, it looks as if aerobic exercise works on exactly the same centers and creates its own addiction. Only difference: One is great for you and the other is dreadful.

Setting a Realistic Weight Goal

A chieving an "ideal" weight or level of fitness may seem like a daunting goal—so big that it seems unreachable, unnecessarily depressing, and deeply *anti*motivational. Still, we have to start somewhere, and the body mass index (BMI) guide is as good a place as any because it gives you some perspective. It looks complicated but it's not. Just take a moment to find where you are and what numbers put you in the "normal" part of the chart. Don't go nuts looking at the numbers; this is just the beginning.

FIND YOUR BMI (BODY MASS INDEX)

HEIGHT IN FEET AND INCHES

	80	90	100	110	120	130	140	150	160	170	180	190	200	210	220	230	240	250	260
6'4"	10	11	12	13	15	16	17	18	19	21	22	23	24	26	27	28	29	30	32
6'3"	10	11	13	14	15	16	18	19	20	21	23	24	25	26	28	29	30	31	32
6'2"	10	12	13	14	15	17	18	19	21	22	23	24	26	27	28	30	31	32	33
6'1"	11	12	13	15	16	17	18	20	21	22	24	25	26	28	29	30	32	33	34
6'	11	12	14	15	16	18	19	20	22	23	24	26	27	28	30	31	33	34	35
5'11"	11	13	14	15	17	18	20	21	22	24	25	27	28	29	31	32	33	35	36
5'10"	11	13	14	16	17	19	20	21	23	24	26	27	29	30	32	33	34	36	37
5'9"	12	13	15	16	18	19	21	22	24	25	27	28	30	31	32	34	35	37	38
5'8"	12	14	15	17	18	20	21	23	24	26	27	29	30	32	33	35	36	38	40
5'7"	12	14	16	17	19	20	22	23	25	27	28	30	31	33	34	36	38	39	41
5'6"	13	14	16	18	19	21	23	24	26	27	29	31	32	34	35	37	39	40	42
5'5"	13	15	17	18	20	22	23	25	27	28	30	32	33	35	37	38	40	42	43
5'4"	14	15	17	19	21	22	24	26	27	29	31	33	34	36	38	39	41	43	45
5'3"	14	16	18	19	21	23	25	27	28	30	32	34	35	37	39	41	42	44	46
5'2"	15	16	18	20	22	24	26	27	29	31	33	35	37	38	40	42	44	46	48
5'1"	15	17	19	21	23	25	26	28	30	32	34	36	38	40	42	44	46	48	50
5'	16	18	20	21	23	25	27	29	31	33	35	37	39	41	43	45	47	49	51
4'11"	16	18	20	22	24	26	28	30	32	34	36	38	40	42	44	46	48	50	52
4'10"	17	19	21	23	25	27	29	31	33	36	38	40	42	44	46	48	50	52	54

WEIGHT IN POUNDS

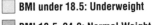

BMI under 18.5: Underweight BMI 30–34.9: Obese
BMI 18.5–24.9: Normal Weight BMI 35–39.9: Severe Obesity
BMI 25–29.9: Overweight BMI 40+: Extreme Obesity

How did you do? If you are in the "normal" range already, congratulations. That is anything but normal in this country today. But if you are in either the overweight or obese categories, join the crowd. The problem is, there's no safety in numbers—it's a bad crowd to be in. There is a sharp and undeniable correlation between a high BMI and bad health. Alarmingly, things start to get noticeably worse, especially in terms of diabetes and heart disease risk, as we creep over a BMI of 30, the threshold for obesity. Health starts to decline as one moves into the "overweight" area. And it climbs at a terrifying clip as you move into the "obese" range. Being obese is very dangerous indeed. Don't be scared: We're going to fix all this.

If you are in great shape and your numbers look illogical, they may be. This chart does not work for some serious athletes, with highly developed musculature. They can read as "overweight" when they are anything but. So while variations in fundamental body type can throw the numbers off (e.g., a short male with very large musculature), BMI is still a very good general guide to a goal worth shooting for.

Another customized way to come up with an "ideal" weight is simply to look back to what you actually weighed when you were twenty-two, or just getting out of college. You can't look at a twenty-two-year-old in your neighborhood these days as a guide; he or she may be shockingly overweight. The same wasn't true thirty years ago. Assuming you were in good shape in your twenties, that weight is a goal in the sense that your body is the same one you have today, just with a touch more padding.

A third and fairly accurate way to find your goal is to have a body-fat analysis done by a health or sports professional. That's the one where a professional uses calipers on specific areas of your body and compares the results to a set of standards. Many gyms offer this service, and I urge you to take advantage of it. It might be slightly embarrassing to have a stranger pinch and *measure* your fat, but the results are good for goal setting. Besides, the person doing it will do so privately, and he or she is a professional.

Here are some ballpark body-fat percentages to shoot for that correspond roughly to a BMI of 25. Twenty-five or below is what you want to aim for, so do the same here with the approximate corresponding body-fat percentages: Get *below* these numbers. In a way, they are kind of shocking, perhaps more so than simply knowing your BMI is hovering around 28.

Body Fat Percentages to Get Below

AGE	WOMEN	MEN
30–49 yr	36–38%	23–26%
50–84 yr	38–40%	26–28%

Adapted from *The American Journal of Clinical Nutrition* (Heo, Faith and Heymsfield)

We often hear about athletes with a body fat in the teens. Chris referred to one of his "success story" guys who had a body-fat percentage of 12. Super-low body fat percentages make sense for professional-level athletes, but most of us don't have to go that far to be healthy. We want you to run yourself healthy, not run yourself ragged.

The two charts should give you a sense of what your ideal weight range should be. If you are there today, congratulations. If you're not, there are compelling health reasons for you to try, *ultimately*, to get there. Reaching the goal won't happen today (or tomorrow) especially if you're thirty pounds or more over the recommended weight. Focus on the more realistic, saner goal of practicing a healthy eating and exercise regime that takes into account the pressures that brought you to this point in the first place and there's no reason why you cannot get back to your twenty-something range this year.

Where Does All the Energy Go?

As you orient yourself for a major effort at weight control, it may be good to get some idea of just where the calories you put into your body go in the normal course of things. Most of what you consume, about 60–70 percent of a *rational diet*, are burned just keeping the great machine of You running. That is your "resting metabolism" and amounts to around 1,200 calories per day. It has little to do with exercise, lifestyle, or anything else; it just goes on, night and day, 24/7, keeping your body alive. Your respiration, heartbeat, pumping blood; the circulation of food and oxygen out to the millions of little internal combustion engines in the muscles (those would be your mitochondria); the return trip to get rid of the muck, the metaphoric ashes after the fire, the waste, the carbon dioxide, the water; the maintenance of your vital organs—all that work is taken care of by this resting metabolism.

Oh, and let us not forget the brain, a real power hog. It weighs only three pounds—barely 1–2 percent of your body weight—but it consumes over 400 calories per day. It's the last organ to be shut off when things are bad. The largest consumers of this 60–70 percent of your *rational diet*, however, are your muscles. As I said earlier, the fitter you are and the larger your muscles, the more calories they burn, even when you are at rest. All of which goes to explain the variation in your metabolism and also the gender difference in caloric needs because men are typically taller and have more muscle mass.

Another 5–10 percent of the calories you take in (on top of the 60–70 percent that keeps your body running) go to the actual business of digesting the food we eat, which is called *thermogenesis*. The thermogenic effect is like a little discount off the "caloric cost" of what you eat. The harder the food is to digest, the more calories you use in the process. Protein-rich foods have the greatest thermic effect, with almost 30 percent of your calories from a protein source burned just from metabolizing it.

Fiber-rich carbs, like whole grains, beans, and produce, require work to digest, too. These foods have far fewer calories per ounce than other foods, *and* it takes work to digest them. And sure enough, they are nutrient dense, too. So, if we harp on broccoli, there's a reason for it. Win, win, win. And *kale*—well, you wouldn't believe it. If you can

Percent of Daily Caloric Intake
Burned by Different Bodily Activities

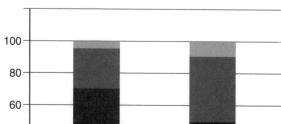

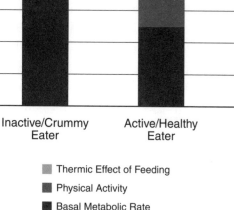

bear kale, knock yourself out. Here's a good one: It's not an old wives' tale that celery has negative calories—it *does* take more calories to digest a piece of celery than the stalk itself contains. Refined grains, like white flour, and sugar, are easily digested and have a low thermic effect. Fat basically has zero thermic effect; it takes *no calories* to digest. The same is true for most fast food.

What about the last 20 percent of calories? That is the great joker in the deck: physical activity. In the "normal" course, physical activity accounts for about 10–20 percent of the energy you burn every day. It can be less if you're a real slug. And it can be as much as 50 percent if you are an exercise maniac (see page 37). *None* of you should think in terms of burning 50 percent of your intake with exercise: That is Olympic or professional athlete territory. But 20 percent? You bet. Or even 25–30 percent for serious amateur athletes. You can readily burn an extra 300–500 calories a day in serious exercise, which makes it a *huge* part of weight loss!

By the way, that was a discussion of how a *rational* diet gets burned up. It does not address the possibility that you are eating 500 or 1,000 calories more a day than you should. Where do those calories go? That's easy: They become fat around your middle, packed all around your vital organs, all over the place—as dangerous, as we say, as an open sewer.

It's Worth It!

What we are offering is the only thing that works: a lifestyle regimen with a very key exercise component and a major nutrition piece. It is a *regimen* that works and is doable by a large number of people. By getting on board you can lead the way, set an example, and be a change maker. Besides, I think the regimen is kind of fun, to tell the truth. And *so* worth it. You'll feel good right away, and you'll feel amazing in the longer run.

CHAPTER FOUR

Going Deep

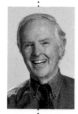

Over the next two years, after that first session in her office, Jen and I spent a lot of time together, most of it on the phone or "talking" by email. But a bunch of times I'd drive the three hours to Boston (I had more time, so I did the traveling) and get a suite at a hotel I like between Harvard Square and the Charles. We'd spend a day together, Jen teaching me stuff. Then I'd drive back to the Berkshires and try to digest what I'd learned.

Take a peek at one such session in Cambridge, after we'd been working together about six months: We put in a long afternoon yesterday and we're going to have another session this morning. I got up early today and went out for a walk in the rain, down past Weld Boathouse, where I used to row as a kid, and along the river. Nice. Always a poignant area for me, Harvard Square and the Charles. I was such a dope when I was an undergraduate; what a waste. But here's a nice thought: I'm not quite as much of a dope at seventy-seven as I was at twenty. *Much* happier, too. Hey, that's good; sometimes, it's the other way around.

We have been talking for two days about muscles and the metabolism of food in the muscle and—most urgently—the role of nutrients and other things from good food in the process. Jen is trying to persuade me—and you—to eat good food and cut back on crap because good food does hugely important (if invisible) things inside our bodies. Sends signals, foments reactions, opens and closes doors that are critical to life. Eat crap, she wants to say, and wildly complex and important things (of which you and I are totally ignorant) won't happen. We'll feel sluggish, dispirited, and slow. And if we are stupid enough for long enough, we'll eventually get sick and even die. So it's important.

Jen is a little more intense than usual this morning. Almost grumpy, to tell the truth, which is rare. Because, she says, of the pouring rain. She did not get to row before coming here. We had breakfast downstairs and she ate like a petulant child. French toast, maple syrup, butter. I couldn't believe it. *"Hey,"* she says, *"I missed my row. . . . I'm grumpy."* I reach over and take a piece of French toast. I had already eaten oatmeal and berries, for God's sake, just like I am supposed to. And now she gets French toast? This project is falling apart. Pretty good French toast, though. I pour a little more maple syrup on my plate. *"Can't be perfect,"* Jen says. I order a Diet Coke. Pretty soon, it's going to be Bloody Marys if we don't watch out.

Back in the suite, Jen describes muscle cells to me, and how they actually *contract* so that we can *move*. Movement is *the* fundamental gift of people and all other mammals and the reptiles and the fishes and the birds of the air. The thing that makes us different from plants. Or rocks, I guess. And from too many old people. So it matters. I have had brilliant people try to explain this to me for years, but I never really got it. This morning I am going to get it. Because Jen is so damn smart. And she has studied it so long. I have gotten stuck on something she has just said about electrolytes. I had heard the word *electrolytes* from sports drinks but had no idea. "Come here," she says, "let me show you some graphics." I pull my chair over, Jen turns on her computer, and some exquisitely detailed anatomical drawings come up.

"This," she says, "is a nerve cell, coming down from the brain."

"Oh," I say, mildly surprised that a signaling nerve is an actual *thing*, like a blood vessel. It's this long hollow tube, with stations along the way. And little chemical symbols, she later explains, on the inside and on the outside. The long nerve cell—and there are billions of them—runs from the brain to individual muscle cells, every one of them.

"Like almost all cells," Jen says, "this one has an 'electrical gradient' from positive to negative. The muscle cell has an electrical gradient, too. That is one of the ways the brain and the muscle talk to each other. The other is purely chemical. That," she points to a huge space on the drawing that dwarfs the nerve cell and a lot of other things in the little pictures, "is the muscle cell."

I give her a sheepish grin. "What?" she asks, worried that she's lost me already.

"Um it's big," I say. "And complicated, isn't it, the muscle cell?"

"Sure," she says, "Very. Why?"

"Um," sheepish grin again. "I sort of thought that all cells were tiny and simple, like small eggs with a shell, a yoke and goo, and nothing else." She just looks at me.

I take advantage of the pause to blurt out another confession: Until this very moment, I also had had no idea that cells *had* electrical properties or that it mattered. Or, come to that, that our bodies had such a frenzy of electrical connectivity. I vaguely understood that we were "wired" in some mysterious way, that there was this amazing signaling system. That was in the old book. And I had intuited that signaling was as important in nutrition. But *this*? I had no *notion*. You see things differently when you get into the details.

We started down this particular road when I asked her about sports drinks and are they any good or just a scam. And she said they were a bit of a scam for nonathletes and they have a shocking amount of sugar, which she says is close to being a poison. But they are useful for long rides or runs in that they have sugar for energy and electrolytes. "Oh," I say. "What are electrolytes?"

"Well," she says, "they maintain an electrical gradient across cells."

Did you hear that? I am sitting around with this attractive woman and she has just said to me, in utter seriousness, "They maintain an electrical gradient across cells." Are we still in Kansas, Toto?

I indicate that I am not quite following. "And," I say, a little defensively, "I am not a lot dumber than our average reader." Jen smiles that room-warming smile. "No, you are not," she says, comfortingly. "You certainly are not. It's just that there are things I take for granted that you don't know. Different educations is all.

"Okay," she goes on, "look at the nerve cell a second." I dutifully look. "See those little letter symbols? That one, on the outside of the nerve cell, is the symbol for sodium, and that one on the inside is the symbol for potassium. These minerals, or ions, and the amounts of them, inside and outside the cell, change the electrical gradient of the cell, change its electrical charge. Like a switch. That charge runs up and down these cells to and from the brain, to and from the muscle. And everyplace else. It is how the message is moved along, from the brain to the muscle, shifting masses of sodium and potassium in the nerve cell to change the electrical gradient. It is how muscles are told to do what they do—stand up, ski, whatever."

"Goody," I say. I am still reeling from the notion that we are so darned *wired*, so intensely *electrical*.

Jen shrugs me off. "Look," she says, "our readers do not have to understand how this signaling system works. But they should have some sense that it exists and that it is complicated. And—this is the critical point—that it depends significantly on these little shifts in the concentration of sodium and potassium. Those are *minerals*. Our people have to have some sense of all this. So that they will eat *some damned bananas* once in a while. For potassium."

Jen never swears. "Oh," I say.

"It's more than 'oh,'" she says. "It's important. There are millions and millions of places inside your body where critical transactions like this take place. And where the critical player is a *nutrient* or something else you ate: a vitamin, a mineral, an essential fatty acid. To get sodium, so the signaling system works, we do have to consume some salt. But ideally from unprocessed foods as part of the deal. To get potassium you have to eat a banana or something. Without them, or with too little of them, the basic signaling system slows down and maybe even stops. You don't work. Not eating crap goes deep. Eating Good Stuff goes deep!" She stops and just looks at me for a second. Bananas, I think, dutifully. Eat a banana.

"What happens next?" I ask.

"If crap like added solid fats and added sugar make up 35 percent of our diet today, and they do, where does the Good Stuff come from? And if a lot of people drink sodas and alcohol, too, so that the combined Dead Food intake, sodas and alcohol, is way over 50 percent of their intake, where does the Good Stuff come in? It just doesn't."

Long pause. I nod.

"Good food has 'nutrients.' That means vitamins, minerals, certain kinds of 'good fats' called 'essential fatty acids.' They make up wonderful things: hormones are messenger molecules made in your glands; cytokines are messenger molecules made in various tissues; enzymes are proteins that are catalysts that drive various chemical reactions. And then there are those electrolytes you asked about which are ions that regulate the fluid balance and, much more urgently, the electrical gradient, in a bunch of important cells. And lots and lots of other bioactive substances, not including the ones that scientists have not even identified yet.

"How important is this stuff?" she asks rhetorically. She pauses a minute, thinking how best to get at this. "Look," she says, "there are four fat-soluble vitamins: vitamin A, vitamin D, vitamin E, and vitamin K. Are they important? At Tufts alone there are a dozen researchers whose *whole life* is the study of *vitamin A alone*. And they are very able, highly motivated people. They are doing it—and federal funds are paying a fortune to have it done—because vitamin A (and understanding it better) is so important. There is a similar cadre of researchers studying D, E, and K. And all the water-soluble vitamins, too. And other enzymes and hormones, and on and on. It is huge. Far bigger than the smartest layperson begins to suspect.

"Laypeople know a little about vitamins," she goes on, "and what little they know makes vitamins sound minor. They know you get vitamin A from eating red and orange vegetables, among others. And it is good for your eyes. Fine. But that does not begin to convey their importance, even for sight alone. If you don't get enough Vitamin A, you go blind. There are children in Africa today with no night vision because they happen not to get enough vitamin A. They developed a whole new kind of rice, just to get them more of it. But that's a tiny hint at how important vitamin A is. A tiny hint. And not just vitamin A either, obviously. But all the other vitamins and minerals and on and on. There is an ocean of information and, taken together, it makes it clear that these things are very important indeed." I sit there, chastened.

"Back to the muscle metabolism story," she says. "Muscle cells are *not* like eggs," she says, not unkindly. "For example, they have maybe ten thousand mitochondria in each one. Those are the little engines that burn what you eat, to let you move. Inside they have intricate pathways of signals that convey messages. And on the surface, inside the cell wall, they have all kinds of things, including recessed receptors." She sketches them on a pad.

"Buttercups," I say. "They look like a field of buttercups."

She pauses a second. "Yes," she says, finally, as you might to a small, slightly dim child. "They do look like buttercups, don't they?"

She watches my face to see if anything is going on in there, in my poor head. She can't be sure, but she's going to take a chance. Going to keep moving.

"Here's another interesting thing," she says, "this time about exercise. Exercise up-regulates the buttercup response. The buttercups respond to exercise by being quicker to pop up, faster and with less insulin. One of the basic points of the book," she says, "is that exercise makes the body metabolize food or energy much more effectively because the buttercup/receptors pop up more readily. In this instance, your muscles are more efficient at scooping up blood sugar for muscle during exercise or for muscle glycogen storage following exercise. And this is all done with less insulin. People who are in good shape and exercise regularly also burn fat much more effectively for much more of the time. *They burn or lose fat faster and for more of the time.* So they can run or swim or bike much longer, because the whole process becomes so well-tuned. And they are thinner because they burn more fat than out-of-shape people. In that and other ways, exercise cleans out the system—cleans up extra sugar and fat and insulin in the blood, and makes it all work cleaner and better and with many fewer damaging side effects. Exercise, man!" She grins. Jen loves to talk about exercise. Believes in it with all her heart. Me, too. At least I get that.

"A little bit more?" she asks.

"Sure," I say. She has to leave to teach a class at noon, thank God.

"Okay. When the message gets to the muscle, telling it to contract, what actually happens is that the inside of the nerve cell becomes more positive. Tons of sodium floods in and tons of potassium floods out. The muscle cell gets both a chemical and an electrical signal to contract. But there are some mechanical changes. For example, when a muscle fiber contracts, what actually happens is that filaments inside of a fiber take a tight grip on one another and shorten. The *gripping* is a key part of it."

"I can imagine," I say, dubiously. Jen gives me a look and goes on. "But there are particular places—grooves—where the grippers *grip*."

"Just as I thought," I say, straight-faced.

She smiles. Then holds up a cautionary finger, as if to tell the grippers, "not so fast." "But those grooves normally have little *covers*, which must be peeled back for the gripping to occur and the contraction to take place. Now here's the point: Are you listening?" I nod. I certainly am. Jen goes on: "A *signal* has to be sent for the cover to retract. *Calcium*, a mineral, plays a critical part here. Calcium binds to a filament and *unblocks the site* so grabbing can occur. A critical step in all muscle contraction."

"I'll be damned," I say.

"Yup," Jen says, pleased. "It's a small but critical step in any muscle contraction. and you *must have calcium* to make it work. And you don't get calcium in French fries! Or Cokes. Or martinis, you silly bugger. You only get calcium eating a balanced diet!"

"Ta-dah!" I say.

"Ta-dah is right," Jen agrees. "If you only eat crap, lots of important little things don't work right. Because you don't get your nutrients."

"This is a little complicated," I say.

"You have no idea," Jen grins.

✱ ✱ ✱

Look, do you have to know all that stuff that Jen told me that morning? No. Not for one minute. But it would be an awfully good idea if you kept a few things in mind: (1) Your body in general, and your metabolism in particular, is dazzlingly complex. (2) It is deeply dependent on a massively complex signaling system. (3) What you eat is critical to the effective running of the signaling system. That is, eat food with a lot of nutrients and your signaling system and your body work like gangbusters. Eat crap and both get badly gummed up. Because signaling matters so very much.

CHAPTER FIVE

The Good Stuff: What Happens Inside When You Eat the Right "Mix"

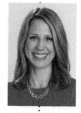

Now a bit more science. Specifically, the science of what happens inside your body when you're eating right. These are the rules that govern your body, and they are strictly enforced. We'll come to the grim consequences of eating too much junk in Chapter 7, "The Bad Stuff: What Happens When You Eat Junk." That's the gory part. But I insist on starting with the good news, because so many people don't have any idea how beautifully food and metabolism work in the normal course of eating well.

We buy into an astonishing number of diet books and programs in this country—the U.S. weight loss market is $60 billion a year. Yet most people still don't have a clue what our body does with food. There are two basic notions to consider: How our body turns a wide range of edibles into *fuel* for the engines in our body, on the one hand, and on the other, how it uses *nutrients* as catalysts, signalers or building blocks, handmaidens, which foment a million processes inside the body. Both are equally important and very different.

All *food* comes in three categories: carbohydrates, fat, and protein. Most foods are a mix of all three. They each have calories (energy) and therefore all provide fuel for the engine, our body. Carbs and fats provide the most energy, protein not as much because it has other important roles as I explain later. Carbs, fats, and protein are fundamentally different from each other at the molecular level. They also have very different "densities" of calories. Carbs and proteins yield about four calories per gram (written "4 kcal/gram") while fat yields a whopping 9 kcal/gram. As for *nutrients,* foods in all three categories provide them, although the amounts and types vary tremendously (more on that in Chapter 11).

How We Use Carbs and Fat

I t is a helpful simplification to think of our bodies as big, internal combustion engines. We eat carbs and fat for fuel. They are broken down into a burnable form (glucose from carbs, fatty acids from fat) and shuttled by the blood mostly to millions of microscopic engines, the mitochondria, in the muscles and elsewhere. There, they are burned with oxygen, which the blood also brings in, from the lungs. (Okay, mitochondria are not *quite* like engines. Rather, they make adenosine triphosphate or ATP, which is *really* the form of energy used by our cells.)

The circulatory system also takes away the exhaust products after the "combustion," the carbon dioxide and other "ashes." Our heart is a sophisticated pump, and our circulatory system is mostly a network of fuel pipes and exhaust pipes, to take fuel and oxygen to the mitochondria and to take away the exhaust, later on. This system works amazingly well all our life long, especially when we feed it properly.

Carbohydrates

T he first great category of food is carbohydrates, which should constitute about 50 percent of your total diet. Carbs encompass sugar in all of its forms and are present in all fruits, vegetables, grains, and legumes. Once eaten, they are broken down in your stomach and small intestine into simple sugars (mainly glucose) and this glucose is picked up by the blood and sent all over your body. Glucose is stored in limited supply and is so basic that if we don't eat enough carbs, our body goes searching for glucose and actually starts to pirate protein from our muscles and converts it into glucose for energy. Unfortunately we can't do that with fat. Our brain relies on glucose exclusively (you know how hard it is to move or think when your blood sugar is low). Less acknowledged and very important, without glucose, fats can't be burned.

Once in the circulation, glucose stimulates the pancreas to release insulin. Insulin is critical for "introducing" glucose into the muscle. Our muscles are super "glucose sinks." Muscle gobbles up circulating glucose but it needs help from insulin. Insulin signals an elaborate cascade of events within the muscle cell, enabling a receptor (Chris's buttercups) to come to the surface of the muscle cell and allows the glucose to enter. Glucose then goes through aerobic or anaerobic metabolism to produce ATP, which your muscles can then use to contract—end result, you move (we'll dive much deeper into this later). That's one reason why our muscles are such hounds for glucose.

If your muscles don't need glucose immediately, it is converted to glycogen, a storage form of glucose that is found and stored in the muscles and liver as a ready reserve. The glycogen storage capacity is limited, so once filled up, the insulin signals your fat cells to convert any excess glucose to fat and store it in your fat cells. Not as ready a reserve as glycogen, but there when you need it. An elegant system, and it works perfectly when you eat enough so-called "good" carbs, or what's known in scientific circles as low glycemic index foods.

Not all carbs are created equal. They come in two forms: simple and complex. Simple carbs are chemically made of one or two sugars (which includes most processed and "white" foods, table sugar, syrup, honey, and so on), and are broken down and absorbed quickly into the bloodstream. These foods have a "high glycemic index" because they produce a rapid increase in blood sugar. Some complex carbs, such as starchy potatoes and white rice, are also quickly absorbed and therefore high on the glycemic index.

Other complex and/or "good" carbs include vegetables, legumes, and whole grains. While fruit is technically considered to be a simple carb, because it offers so many nutrients and is high in water and fiber, it's considered a "good" carb. An apple, for example, it not as quickly absorbed into the bloodstream as cotton candy would be. These foods

A WORD ABOUT FIBER

Fibers are part of the carbohydrate family and come in both soluble and insoluble forms. The insoluble, as you may have guessed, goes undigested and passes right through you. The soluble fibers, like those found in many fruits, are digested but yield few calories. Both provide a great deal of satiety to foods, slow digestion, keep blood sugar levels steady, and prevent blood sugar spikes. They make you *feel full*. Soluble fiber inhibits dietary cholesterol absorption from our small intestine and reduces cholesterol synthesis in our liver. With all of these benefits, you can see why diets high in fiber have been linked to decreased risk of diabetes, cardiovascular disease, and cancer and lower obesity risk. Most Americans do not even come close to meeting fiber recommendations, which should be 28 grams or more on a 2,000 calorie per day diet. A fiber-rich diet should include a high percentage of vegetables, fruits, legumes, and whole grains—no surprise there.

move through the gastrointestinal tract more slowly and add sugar to the blood in a steadier, more orderly and stable manner. Simply put, eating "good" carbs makes you feel better over the long haul.

Fats

While fat is essential to health, I believe we should eat far less of it than we do. On average we get just over 35 percent of our total calorie intake from fats of all kinds, which is the top end of the U.S. Dietary Guidelines of 20–35 percent. That's too much in my view. Fat should constitute between 25 percent of our total caloric intake. If you follow the Eating Plan recommendations, you'll be in sync with this. However, I have to say that fat quantity is the first major area where responsible experts are still in substantial disagreement. For instance, there are other, credible views that put fat intake below 20 percent. Alarmed at the role of non–plant-based food in the creation of elevated cholesterol, heart disease, and other illnesses, some scientists urge that fat be cut to as little as 10 percent of our diet, and that all of it be non–animal-based. Other, less responsible viewpoints, including Atkins diet proponents and followers of the Paleo diet, suggest way more than 30 percent fat is acceptable, including animal fats. I am baffled by these fat fans who seem blind to the link between fat—especially saturated fat—consumption and heart disease, many cancers, adult onset diabetes, and other diseases.

I don't recommend a daily fat intake of less than 20 percent for several reasons. First, fat is one of the critical building blocks of the body. The walls of every cell are made of it. It is also an excellent fuel for exercise. It packs 9 kcals/gram, and it burns efficiently. To give you an idea, a molecule of glucose, or sugar, burns with oxygen to generate 36 ATPs or units of energy. A molecule of fat burns, with oxygen, to generate closer to 150–200 ATPs. The good news/bad news is that we store a lot of it.

In mass, fat gives us cushioning to let us sit down. It separates the organs and other body parts so they don't bounce around. And it plays an important part in the great world of *signaling* within the body, in particular with respect to regulating our immune function. Finally, fat allows us to absorb fat-soluble nutrients. Without fat, absorbing the essential vitamins A, D, E, and K from the foods is more difficult. Healthy fats, such as omega-3 fatty acids, prevent blood clots and keep blood pressure down. Cholesterol (a form of fat for simplification purposes) foments the creation of hormones such as estrogen and testosterone and other cool things like vitamin D. Fat is key in the development of our brains and maintenance of our nerve cells. Key immune system regulators are also by-products of certain fats.

Finally, fat is highly palatable, feels good in the mouth, and is satiating. Because of the complexities of fat in digestion, even though it has no thermic effect it takes time to digest and therefore makes you feel full for longer. There is also no impact on blood sugar swings; instead it may actually help moderate blood sugar depending on the food source.

My point here: Fat is essential, but like almost everything in nutrition should be consumed in its healthiest form and in moderation to enjoy its benefits. The best versions come from fish as well as vegetables and their oils. Avocados and olives, for example, are great sources of *good* fats. Even corn, broccoli, nectarines, peaches, and kiwis have some fat in them.

The bad ones are saturated, which tend to become solid at room temperature, like those found in butter and other dairy products, and in certain cuts of beef, pork, lamb, and chicken. Man-made trans fats, or "partially hydrogenated" fats and oils, are found abundantly in processed foods both sweet and savory. The trouble is, it's hard to know how much you're getting in packaged food. Labeling helps, but it's imperfect: FDA rules say that if one serving of food contains less than 0.5 grams of trans fat, food companies are allowed to say the food has "0" trans fats per serving. That means a serving size might actually contain 0.4999 grams of trans fats. If you ate two to four servings of this food, you'd eat about 1–2 grams of trans fat. Keep this in mind when reviewing labels for total fat, saturated fat, and trans fat content.

The Metabolism of Fats

Fat works a little differently in the body than carbs. The majority of the fat we eat (95 percent) comes in the form of something called triglycerides. Almost all the fat in your body (95 percent again) consists of triglycerides. Triglycerides are made up of a backbone (glycerol) with three fatty acids attached to it. It is the fatty acids we need to pay attention to as they confer the relative "healthiness" of the fat we eat. A fatty acid that is attached to the glycerol backbone can be one of four things: (1) Mono-unsaturated, (2) Poly-unsaturated, (3) Saturated, or (4) Trans-fatty-acid. The first two are healthy, and the last two aren't. The free fatty acids ("FFAs") serve as the main fuel source for metabolism. FFAs are basically chains of carbon atoms of varying lengths, and it is these carbon atoms that are the key to generating energy (ATP) in the mitochondria.

It doesn't matter what kind of fatty acid is involved when it gets *burned for energy*. It matters quite a lot if it is not burned but used for structure or is floating around for a while. Here is a key point: While the fats you eat go through a complex digestion process, the output that gets released into your bloodstream to be burned or stored also consists almost entirely of triglycerides. Importantly, *it contains exactly the same mix of saturated and unsaturated fats as what you ate in the first place*. That is, if you eat unsaturated fat, you get unsaturated fat in your blood, and later your body.

Most of the fat we eat contains a mixture of different fatty acids. Olive oil, for example, contains mono-, poly- and saturated fats, but the mono- and poly-unsaturated predominate. Seventy-five percent of avocado's fat is unsaturated, which makes it a terrific source of good fat. Butter or lard, on the other hand, is made up mainly of saturated fats.

Saturated and trans fats have straight carbon chains that hang down (closely packed) like straight hair. Mono- and poly-unsaturated FFAs are kinky and they are *much less tightly packed together*. As a result, they are also softer and more "fluid." Tightly packed, saturated fats are much *stiffer* and less *permeable* than unsaturated fats. This makes all the difference when you realize that fat makes up the walls of all cells, including muscle cells. For example, muscle cells receive a stunning number of messages from the brain that dictate just which one contracts or relaxes at what point, which dictates all movement, coordination, and balance. Those signals are essential to our basic ability to function. Those signals can get through the muscle cell membrane (or any other cells) more readily when it is made up of unsaturated fats.

What the muscles use for fuel is the FFA, which is part of the triglycerides inside these little fat globules. How to get at them? Most of our cells, including muscle cells, fat cells, and others, have enzymes on their surface (think of them as little "chompers" or "Pac-Men"), which bite off a chunk of the fat globule/triglyceride package and grab free fatty acids. That cell then burns them as fuel. When the muscles don't need any more fat for fuel, the other Pac-Men sitting on the surface of the fat cells bite them off and add the remaining triglycerides to existing fat cells, and that fat gets stored for future use.

Energy Storage

Here is an interesting chart that threw Chris into a tailspin when he first saw it. It shows where energy is stored in the body. It's shown under two different headings: carbohydrate storage (as free glucose or glycogen) and fats. This is the storage situation for a very fit-seeming,

Carbohydrates

Muscle glycogen ....2,025 kcals

Liver glycogen ....450 kcals

Blood glucose ....62 kcals

Fat

Subcutaneous fat ....73,320 kcals

Intra-muscular fat ....1,500 kcals

Adapted from *Physiology of Exercise and Sport*,
Wilmore and Costill, published by Human Kinetics

22-year-old man who weighs 143 pounds and has only 12 percent body fat (which is very low, especially for someone over 30).

First, notice how limited your storage of carbohydrate is. Now check out the "subcutaneous fat" number. Looks like a typo, doesn't it? That's what Chris thought. Especially when he read that that was enough energy to run twenty-eight marathons. Then he was horrified: He got to stewing about it and I got this urgent email at 4 o'clock in the morning: "Is this right?! How in the world is the body to get rid of all that fat? Especially when most middle-aged adults carry around about twice that amount of fat? All is lost."

Working with Chris has been an amusing process, let me tell you. Anyhow, the first "answer" is that the body does not have to "get rid of" all that fat. In fact if most of us had this "energy profile" we would be thrilled. A good chunk of this fat is permanent and that's just fine. Not all the fat in our body is destined for burning because it is structural. It is what we are *made of* when we are in good shape. It is there to insulate us from the cold, to sit on when surfaces are hard, to perform a lot of critical functions. Some fat is fine; it's indispensable, in fact. You need it to survive.

How little can we live with? Even for serious endurance athletes— long distance runners and cyclists—fat is going to constitute some 12–20 percent of their body mass. At 12 percent body fat, a woman usually stops menstruating—not a good sign. There goes reproduction, bone health, and so on. A man can go lower, but at about 6 percent— which is very lean indeed—men too have serious health problems. The point: Get over the notion that you're going to get along without fat in your diet or on your body. That too is not going to happen. At least I hope not, anyhow.

Protein

have a real penchant for protein. I spent years studying exercise physiology and muscle damage *before* spending another four years in a lab at Harvard Medical School, examining how a muscle grows and wastes away. You cannot do that without having a high regard for protein. It is what our muscles are made of. If your protein intake is inadequate, over time your body will "find it" in another place and cannibalize itself looking for more. And the first thing it does is to strip it from your muscles.

Beyond keeping your muscles intact, protein offers some big pluses: a strong sense of satiety, long digestion time, and it doesn't cause dangerous spikes of blood sugar. It also plays an important role in the body's signaling system. Finally, in a pinch, proteins can be broken down into amino acids in the body and these amino acids can be turned into glucose when our diets are carb-deficient.

So how much do you need? The fact is that most of us get plenty of protein simply by eating a balanced diet. Adding in extra in the form of shakes and pills or large portions of animal protein does no good. The excess is simply wasted because it's converted and stored as fat; the same is true for excess carbs and fat. Make your daily protein goal around 25 percent of caloric intake, which can come from lean meats, fish, beans, and legumes. Protein is also found in less thought-of food sources, including grains and cereals, and low-fat dairy. You will most certainly get the adequate quantity by following the eating guidelines in Chapter 9.

That's the lowdown on why it's so great to eat good food! Obviously there's more to it than what I've described here but the basics should be clear. Your carbs and fats serve as wonderful fuel sources, while proteins are used mainly as building blocks of cell structures. We have an amazing system at our disposal and the bottom line is we should take care of it by feeding it great fuel and exercising it for optimal operation.

CHAPTER SIX

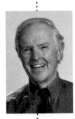

A Day in the Life:
Bash Bish Falls

Okay, here's the first of my "Day in the Life" chapters. They are a little goofy and random but they are designed to illustrate various messages in the book. And to give you a little break from the hard stuff.

I began my own journey exactly the way Jen and I urge you to begin yours: I made up my mind. And I meant it. How do you do that? I wish I knew, but I don't. I just did it, and there was a click. Off I went, and I never looked back. Okay, I looked back some, and fell off the wagon more than once. But mostly not. I began by giving the great flywheel of life a mighty spin. A line-in-the-sand exercise piece, to send myself a message and let myself know I had begun. I took a fifty-mile bike ride in the serious Berkshire Hills.

Hold it! you may sensibly say. I have put myself in the hands of a hundred-year-old lunatic who *starts out* with a fifty-mile bike ride on serious hills? What the hell is this all about?

Perfectly sensible reaction. But bear in mind that, unlike most of you, I already had a serious exercise habit, so this wasn't all *that* hard. The hard thing for me was the eating part. And dropping that fifteen pounds I'd been lugging around with such embarrassment for so long. For me exercise was easy—and eventually it will be for you. That's why this regimen works. In the end, exercise is easy. Exercise is the great driver of change.

So don't worry if my first-day exercise sounds nuts to you. It doesn't matter what you actually *do* on Day One, as long as it's serious for you. As long as you send yourself the message that you have begun . . . that you have made up your mind.

Look, let's start this a little differently, make it a little less scary. Take a look at a guy named Freddy Johnson. He was sixty pounds overweight, bone idle, depressed, and he hated everything, including his job, his ex-wife, and his dog. Well, not his dog, but everything else.

He also began by giving the great flywheel of life a mighty spin, but it did not involve a fifty-mile bike ride. He decided to walk to the office, a mile and a half away. He got halfway there, the first day, and hailed a cab. But here is the key piece: He really had made up his mind and he did the same thing the next day. And every day, six days a week, for the next two weeks. By week three, he did the whole thing—walked a mile and a half to his office. Excellent.

For the next year all he did was walk to—and then from—the office. Somewhere in there, he decided to cut down on eating crap, too. And booze. Cut back quite a bit on booze, like a lot of our "success story" people. Two years down the road he has lost sixty pounds, his energy is terrific, and his spirits are radically improved. His "numbers"—cholesterol, blood pressure, and the like—are much improved. He works out pretty hard, six days a week, and he looks terrific. The modest point: There are many paths to personal redemption. Start with an exercise piece that is serious for you. Because what we are really doing here is drawing a line in the sand of our lives: Before, we were one way—we were this man or that woman. Now we are another.

Back to my Day One. And—setting the format we'll follow throughout these "Day in the Life" chapters—we start and end with food. Exercise matters most, but exercise alone won't do it, as I well know.

What We Ate

Changing your relationship with food—not so easy. So it may be a good idea to do what I did and start with the easiest place to make significant changes, which is breakfast. The first, and most boring, thing to say about breakfast is that it matters a lot, just as you've always been told. Yawn. Your tank is basically empty, and you have to put stuff in it to get your body working right. Do not think for a second that skipping breakfast because you're not that hungry yet is a form of dieting. It works exactly the other way. Sooner or later, skipping breakfast makes you fat.

Breakfast is a great place to give up some of the worst stuff in your diet, *without* depriving yourself that much. Mercifully, there is stuff to eat at breakfast that is both terrific for you *and* tastes great. Like a lot of the meals we talk about, it is going to involve a little bit of cooking for yourself, not popping some crap in the microwave. You don't have to learn to "cook" a broad spectrum of elegant sauces and such, but cooking a *little* bit, which is stunningly easy, is an awfully good idea. It enlarges your menu options enormously and your chances of losing weight. So don't let your eyes glaze over when I mention that I cooked this or that. This is child-level cooking, and you can pick it up in the time it takes to read the words.

For example, this first morning I "cooked" myself some Quaker Oats (not the one-minute kind, which taste nasty; the Original, which take you a heartbreaking four minutes to cook. Eek!). [See box.]

There you go. You have had a great breakfast that will stand you in good stead until lunch. It

Quick Oatmeal

Put a half inch of water in a small pot, add a pinch of salt, and bring it to a boil. Then add a cup of oats and cook 'em, stirring some, for four or five minutes, until it looks edible and tastes okay. *Basic secret of all cooking:* Taste stuff. If it tastes raw and nasty, it's not done. If it tastes good, it is good. Now put the cereal in a bowl with an equal amount of blueberries (any berries will do) and skim milk. Eat. Oh, and make some coffee. Sit down with the paper, the kids, the dog, whatever you've got.

has a lot of nutrients, so your body is going to work this morning. It has fiber so it moves slowly through your body, which is curiously important. It's just about perfect. Nice going.

Once or twice a week, you can try eggs and a slice of dry whole wheat toast. I'm not nuts about eggs, but I make myself cook them, once or twice a week, for balance. If you are a coarse brute and don't know how to cook eggs, don't worry. It's a snap. See box; that's the *last* time we're telling you to look at the box. You're a *grown-up.*

That's the easy side of breakfast: eating stuff that's familiar and that you already like. Now the hard part: *not eating crap.* We have been trained since birth to think that breakfast means a Dead Food explosion. White flour–based bread. Or a croissant. Or a waffle. Or a bagel. Or a blueberry muffin. (The fact that it is *blue* or brown—or has some nuts or cranberries in it—does not mean it is good for you. It is still refined flour in there, and it is still a sugar bath. Extremely rotten for you.) Or some prepared instant bake horror that comes in a tube, perhaps with a separate container of *added goo*, as if the rolls weren't all white flour and sugar to begin with. The Pillsbury Doughboy and Betty Crocker—for whom I happily did a lot of legal work, years ago—are wonderful people, but they make Dead Food, the little rascals.

Same on most popular cereals. *Read the damn label*, not the lying headlines on the

Easy Eggs

Crack three eggs in a bowl and—with your bare hands, don't be shy—fish out one or two of the yolks and chuck 'em, so it's mostly egg whites. Add salt and a bit of water. Whip 'em up well with a fork or whisk till they're light and frothy. (Get yourself a whisk. And some decent pans. Men need toys; it is how they make commitments.) Melt a dab of butter, or use some spray like PAM, in a sauté pan, and cook 'em up, over low to medium heat, stirring constantly with a wooden spoon. Wood, so you don't wreck your new sauté pan. Add fresh pepper. (It is also okay, if you're a hell of a cook, to put in a bit of feta cheese. Or to cut up some chives or other green stuff. Stir in the green stuff as you stir the eggs so it cooks a little.) The whole business takes seven minutes.

front. Don't eat a cereal unless it says it is made from whole grain. If it doesn't say that expressly, it is made from refined flour, I promise. Also, don't eat it if the second or third item in the list of ingredients is sugar or some clever variant of sugar. Which means, don't eat most popular dry cereals, even if they have added some whole grains. Find the Good Stuff and add just a little of your own sugar, if you must; you'll put on much less than the manufacturers do.

In your new world of reading food labels, here's a good rule: The fewer ingredients (especially ones that you don't understand), the better. Here's a little scavenger hunt for you. See how many prepared or packaged foods you can find with exactly *one ingredient*. My list to date contains one such product: oat cereals, like Quaker Oats. Email me (see our website) if you find more.

Back to the Mighty Spin

We're doing a fifty-mile bike ride, up in the Berkshire Hills. Impossible for some, easy-peasy for others. This would not have been one bit serious for Jen, for example. She can walk fifty miles on her hands. Not my problem. *I* am my problem. And you, madam, you, sir, are *your* problem. Pick a start that is right for you.

One of the best pieces of advice I can give you is this: Exercise outdoors, in or on great gear as much as you can. Gyms are wonderful, a miracle of convenience in our lives. But if the weather is decent, go out the door. You get much better exercise (a real bike ride or a real hike calls for millions of micro-adjustments that recruit millions of muscles and signals to keep you balanced), and it's way more fun. You're far more likely to do stuff that's fun, over time. I am an expert on fun; I'd know.

Okay, I roll down my driveway and take a right up the hill into New York state, and then north on the never used Undermountain Road. Fairly flat and easy for the first ten miles. Some hills . . . my heart rate climbs a bit, but not bad. I'm going along at about 60–70 percent of my maximum heart rate.

Maximum heart rate? What the hell are you talking about? Well, one of *the* great measures of how hard you are working out, in aerobic workouts, is your heart rate. As you exercise more, your heart beats *harder*, which is to say more often. It does so to get more blood (and yummy food and oxygen) out to the little engines in the muscles that let you move. The dear old mitochondria, of which you have many millions. A core element of fitness—especially of aerobic fitness and the basic ability to *move*—is the ability to move *more* blood (and food and oxygen) to the muscles. Which is mostly a matter of making the pump, your heart, expel more blood each minute. So getting in shape, in significant part, is training your heart muscle to beat faster (without knocking you on your butt).

One of the weird new things you are going to want to know in life is your personal *maximum heart rate*, the most beats a minute you can do when you work out at your very hardest. You have an absolute maximum, and so does everyone else. Eventually, you'll want to figure out your own, unique max. In the meantime, you can use a formula to make a good, age-based guess. The best formula to figure out your max is to subtract 0.7 times your age from 208. Thus, if you are fifty, you subtract 35 (0.7 times 50) from 208 to get a max of 173. Wasn't that fun? The old formula—220 minus your age—is not as good. There are other, better ways, but forget about it till we get to the aerobics chapters.

Your maximum heart rate goes down as you age. It is on the "biological timeline," and you can't do much about it. Some, but not a lot. Part of the reason that there are no fifty-year-olds in the Tour de France is that their max heart rates drop. Their endurance goes down. Your endurance, too. You can put off 70 percent of aging till the end of life. But not all. Sorry.

But what you *can* do, regardless of age, is get the most out of your own heart at any age with training. You can train it to move more blood with fewer beats. You can train yourself to be able to work out for longer at higher levels. Thus I am a very fit puppy—for such an old dog—and I can go for a couple of hours with my heart thumping away at, say, 80 percent of my maximum heart rate. So I will probably be able to keep up with you, if we go biking, even though your max is a lot higher than mine. Working out at different levels is part of lifelong training. Some days you want to go "long and slow" with your heart rate mostly in the 60 percent of max level. Some days you want to hit it pretty hard—with hard "intervals," say—to take it up into the 80s and even the 90s. Serious aerobic fitness, you will learn later, is best achieved by alternating hard and soft days. One of the odd things that is going to happen to you if you get into all this is that you will start to have a sense of how hard your heart is beating. Matters a lot.

How do you know how hard your heart is beating? Most people rely on a subjective "sense" of it, called "Rating of Perceived Exertion" in the trade. Others, like me, wear a heart rate monitor, a gizmo that picks up the electric signal sent out every time your heart beats and registers it on a wristwatch. Easy-peasy. More details later on.

Okay, back to this stunningly beautiful road on a fine summer morning. The first twenty miles are an easy stretch. Not breathing really hard, no strain. I could carry on a conversation, as I pedal along, watching the cows and the morning mist rising in the fields. My heart rate is about 60 percent of my max, the first ten miles. Nice. There's a killer wind on my nose, but I don't mind . . . I am taking it easy on purpose.

An hour or so into it, I am sweating some, and I feel good. My heart rate is about 70–75 percent of my max, still pretty easy. I can bike to Canada at this clip. My legs are fine and my wind is always good. I stop, just for the heck of it, to get a cup of coffee and catch my breath at a modest place that says it is "Ted's Store." No one there at this hour but me and Ted.

We've never met before, but Ted is in his sixties and we have an oddly *limbic moment* . . . two old boys chatting, early in the morning, before anyone else is up. It is the old boys' curse waking up at dawn; nice to have someone to talk to. The word *limbic* is from the "Connect and Commit" chapter at the end of the book. Here's a tiny preview of an important subject we won't get to for a while.

We are mammals. With separate "limbic" or "mammalian" brains that do nothing but send and receive emotions. It was our great gift, us mammals, in the Darwinian crucible of survival, this ability to care about one another and therefore to work together. Emotions make that possible. We are designed to work together, in packs and herds and law firms. We get isolated at our peril, especially in the Third Act, when men in particular run a grave rise of getting isolated. Women, less so; that's probably why they live four years longer. Contact and connection are good; they send good signals. Isolation is bad; it sends bad signals. Makes you sick, actually. You'll want to remember that.

Ted's got nothing to do at this hour and, after a bit, darned if he doesn't tell me his whole life story. A bit of a surprise, but a treat, too. A free *limbic* dunking, early in the morning. I've got the time, and he's a good storyteller.

Turns out Ted was a cop around here, thirty years ago, and gave a ticket to the guy who owned the funky building we're in right now. The guy was weird—tried to persuade Ted to tear up the ticket and buy the building instead. Ted had no notion of buying this or any other building that morning, but the weird guy just kept it up. Went on and on. To make a long story short, Ted bought the building that very morning. Paid exactly one dollar that day and the balance of ten thousand dollars over ten years. And he's been here ever since, happy as a clam.

Ted moved in and started to fix the place up. A cute girl showed up one day, a personal trainer from Great Barrington. She and Ted start to talk (no surprise to me, may I say; Ted's a bit of a talker). She likes him and moves in. They fix up the store together. Marry. Live happily forever after.

Not quite. The pretty girl runs off with a client of hers, also from Great Barrington. Breaks Ted's heart. Briefly. Then darned if another pretty girl doesn't show up. They talk. She moves in. Yada, yada, yada. They fix the store up even more. All goes well. Till darned if *she* doesn't run off with another guy. Ted laughs at the story, bittersweet. I shake my head, sympathetic. "You better get going," Ted says, and I do. But I like him and I toss him one of my favorite lines in life as I climb back on my bike: "The market for love, Ted," I say casually as I clip into my pedals. "The market for love is *flawed*. You get stuff you don't deserve; and you don't get stuff you do deserve. It's what economists call a 'flawed market.'" On that odd note, I head off. Lord knows what Ted thinks of that bit of wisdom; he just nods pleasantly, and I am on my way. Up the brutal hill that climbs for miles beside the famous Bash Bish Falls. This is the planned crisis of the morning, Bash Bish Falls.

I am puffing almost at once; this is a tough, tough slog. But I am still thinking about Ted. And the market for love. I wonder why those women left him. Seemed like a good guy. A little chatty perhaps but pretty good. Well, the market for love, man. It's odd. And it makes all the difference. Curious.

The Bash Bish Falls road is beautiful but *way* steep. I have a triple or "granny" gear in front because I am old. But I almost never use it because I'm vain too, and I don't want people to see me (as if anyone would know or care). Today I use it all the whole way up. Glad to have it.

A mile up and my heart rate is in the 150s (according to my handy heart rate monitor), which means it is roughly 90 percent of my max. *This* is a serious climb and I am pushing hard. At the steepest pitch, I am in the granny gear *and* I am doing zigzags across the narrow road, which is like adding another lower gear. Talk about *interval training.* This is one long, brutal interval. The trick is not to go *so slowly* that the damned bike tips over. At one spot, there's a patch of gravel and the back wheel spins. That's steep. I finally get to a leveling-off place where I can look down at the falls. I stop. Check my heart rate, make sure I am not dying. I'm not. Not of a heart attack, anyway.

I hop back on the bike. I am full of beans now. Pulling like a train.

As I grind along, I remember another ride up this hill, with Harry and a heart doctor pal of his. I was up ahead a little and (Harry told me later) he was talking to the heart doc about mistaken attitudes toward aging in the medical community, especially among gerontologists (docs for old folks). "I wish every gerontologist in the country could bike up this hill with Chris. They'd get a new sense of how *very* good life can be." Do I like that story? Well, yes. Yes, I do.

Climbing *Up* the Waterfall

I liked the symbolism of this stretch: I am riding *up* the waterfall. In speeches—I give speeches *all* the time these days, on this revolution of ours—in speeches I talk often about "going over the waterfall." Meaning death. I am obsessed with death, I'm afraid. Want to put it off as long as possible. And then hit the waterfall at a hundred miles an hour, like Wile E. Coyote, flying off a cliff. I *love it* that on this special day, I am clawing my way *up a waterfall.* Into the tide of aging. Into the teeth of decay and rot. Into the teeth of death itself, by heaven. Not really, but sort of. Nice symbolic start for this regimen.

At the top, I swing right, along the ridge, to see a lovely old farm-house I used to own, in a different life, thirty-five years ago. It was a rickety place, back then in the mid-1970s, a wood cookstove in the kitchen, a small living room, and a warren of tiny bedrooms. An ice-house out back with a big wooden hot tub. It was the age of wooden hot tubs and a lot of other nice things. I put sliding barn doors on the corners of the icehouse so you could peel 'em back, look out at the fields in summer. Or at a snowstorm in winter. Pretty nice, being up to your neck in hot water, under a roof, looking out at the snow swirling around. Pretty good times up here.

The former owner had run the place as an inn for hunters. It was a Little Appalachia in the 1930s and 1940s. Babe Ruth stayed here regu-larly with his cronies in deer season. Mostly, he came to get away from his wife and act up. Drink, play cards. Maybe a woman or two, who knows. Toward the end of the week, the innkeeper, whose widow sold me the place, would go out and kill a deer for him—tie it to the fender of Babe's car. So his wife would know the trip was on the level. Which it was not.

Black Ice

One of the great pleasures of aging is that you see life in such depth. You're in the present, but also in the past about half the time. It's like a kid lying down on black ice in winter. Do you know about that? Probably not. It's something you only get up north. But for a kid from New England, it's *special*. What happens is that sometimes you get a hard freeze up our way when there is not a whisper of wind in the night. And the ice on the rivers and ponds freezes perfectly smooth and black and even. It happens only once or twice a winter, and it's won-derful. Wonderful for skating for slick black miles on the snow-lined river, through the cornfields and woods and past the occasional barn. But you can see through it, too, with amazing clarity. No air bubbles; that's why it's black. You can lie down on the ice and put your hands up to your face. And see the reeds and the grasses on the bottom. And, sometimes, a lost ball from last summer. Or a rusting cap gun or a cast-iron motorcycle that you liked a lot. Getting older is like that. You keep turning up in places where, if you want, you can lie down, like a kid on black ice. Put your hands up to your eyes, and see the toys you lost last summer. Or a lifetime ago.

I was a crazy man when I lived in this house, back in the 1970s, practicing law like mad, snatching the odd weekend up here. Married to this *wonderful* woman about thirty feet tall, just like Jen, and such a star. *Such a star.* How we loved each other. Had an awful lot of fun in that house. And in that life. Till I ran off like those girls down at Ted's Store. For no reason at all. The market for love, man. The market for love is flawed.

Which is a good thing sometimes. Catch a break you don't deserve, and hang on hard. Which is what I'm doing right now. Hanging on tight, by heaven, to a great marriage I don't begin to deserve. Not gonna go haring off this time . . . chasing after some different notion of myself. That's what so much of divorce is really all about. You're not sick of your spouse, you're sick of yourself, you silly bugger. You're divorcing yourself. Think that's gonna work? Not likely. You want change? Change yourself. There's a limbic message for you. I'm older. I'd know. Black ice.

Okay, twenty-five miles to go, a lot of it downhill. And then along the valley on the eastern side of this range. Even prettier than the western side. And that damned wind is at my back now. Easy lifting.

A last limbic moment on this special morning. You're probably getting sick of all this emotional stuff, but this one is nice. On the edge of my town, I stop to see a close friend, whom I buried a couple of years ago. Maybe my closest friend. He was a tough criminal defense lawyer with exquisite manners and meticulous morals. Good guy.

He used to do an odd thing. He'd come up to me when he hadn't seen me for a while. Give me a hug and say, "Missed ya, sweetheart. Love ya." And kiss me on the top of the head. Damnedest thing you ever saw.

He was Irish but no longer Catholic. So he's lying under a Celtic cross in the middle of our nice WASP graveyard. I bet it drives the dead neighbors crazy. I bike across the grass, silently tell him what I'm up to with Jen. Then I say what I always say: "Miss you, sweetheart. Love you." Blow him a kiss. Head home.

I get back to the big white Victorian on the hill where I am writing now: It was exactly fifty miles. I climb the hellish driveway

(10 percent grade), and get off. I adore this house, where Hilary is waiting, delighted and approving. Oh boy.

Two More Meals

Lunch was easy. I was *into* this stuff and I sure wasn't going to screw up *now*. Hilary and I dined handsomely on brown rice (leftovers from last night), a pile of perfect ripe tomatoes, and one chicken-based sausage. It is the tomato season, now, and it makes sense to eat tomatoes all the time until they are gone. Then, by the way, use canned ones, instead of those stones that come from Florida or Uruguay or someplace. If you get a good brand with no sugar, the canned ones can be surprisingly good. (Bottled may be even better.) And grilled spicy chicken sausage—not much fat, not many calories. Most stuff that is made out of one thing in hopes of making it taste like another thing (chicken sausages for pork sausages, turkey bacon for bacon) don't work worth a damn. But the best brands of chicken sausage are a miracle. Especially the spicy ones. Great meal.

For dinner we mostly go out, but not during this little crisis, if we can help it. So shrimp was the main course. Shrimp is one of the staples of the good diet in my view. Edible, good for you, and you can eat 'em till the cows come home and not gain weight. Fresh broccoli—another good staple of this life—with a teeny bit of butter (sorry). And a good green salad. Not exactly amazing but edible and pretty good for you—low calorie.

I am not the rule giver in this book; Jen is. But here are

Tasty Salad Dressing

Chop up a shallot, put it in a cup. Dump in a spoonful of mustard. Add a good squeeze of fresh lemon juice. And, of course, some good olive oil. But not much. Olive oil is a good fat, but it is fat. And it has lots and lots of calories. Use some for flavor but lighten up. (Two parts oil to one part vinegar is pretty tart, but I like it.) This dressing is very strong, and you only need a little bit to make the salad taste wonderful. Balsamic vinegar, if you like the taste, is another miracle of *strong taste*. You can get by with much less olive oil. Good.

two good rules for weight loss: (1) Eat at home as much as possible. (2) Learn to cook a little. I confess I've been cooking since I was ten, during World War II, so I'm odd for a guy, but it is *such* a help. Wonderful courting device, by the way, if you happen to be single. There is *nothing* more seductive than having someone lovingly cook you a decent meal and set it down before you. Glass of wine. Easy on the lights.

A word about salad. And spices. And salt, which is not as bad for you as you were told. In general, in my drive to change the way I eat, I do everything I can think of to crank up *taste* as I wind down the *fat and sugar* (which do taste wonderful to our sicko palates). This evening's salad dressing is a minor example.

We set the table in the big dining room for the two of us as if it were dinner for eight. Lit the candles, had water glasses and wine. A celebration. And drank one glass of pretty good red apiece (six ounces and no more). No dessert.

The wine is a close call, as I said before. Almost everyone who is serious about weight loss says you should stop drinking entirely. Which is probably right. But it is too depressing to me. Maybe we'll talk about it in the course of another meal. This one has dragged on long enough.

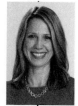

CHAPTER SEVEN

The Bad Stuff: What Happens When You Eat Junk

Y ou can eat almost anything once in a while and get away with it, especially if you're exercising on a regular basis. What you cannot do is eat Bad Stuff all the time, which is what too many of us do. It makes you sick, and ultimately it can kill you as it kills so many in this country. Before it gets that bad, a Bad Stuff diet makes you fat and saps your energy and enthusiasm for life. Not to mention it can wreak havoc on your looks.

Bad Stuff represents about 50 percent of the average American diet—and by that I mean fatty cuts of meat, especially red meat, fried foods, overly processed and refined grains (white bread and pasta), fast food, ice cream, butter, pizza oozing with cheese, heavy salad dressings, and many kinds of crackers and chips. Oh, and let's not forget the obvious—candy—from the beloved Twizzler to the infamous M&M's. Adults eat these, too. A whopping 35 percent of the total average daily calorie intake comes from added sugars and solid fats. Chris asked me to provide prioritized lists of Bad Stuff, which is difficult because there is so much of it readily available. However, here is a modest attempt at my "Short List of Rotten Food."

The Big Bad Five

#1: Fried Foods

The tiptop of the Mountain of Slop and Despair is very slippery, which is not surprising because it is made of grease *that comes out of a deep fryer*—French fries, onion rings, and most commercial chips, along with other foods that are coated with breading and plunged into a vat of boiling oil. Our appetite for this stuff is astonishing: There are places in the country (like the Iowa State Fair) where you can get a fried stick of butter, not to mention fried Twinkies. All of these items are loaded with artery-clogging fat, refined grains and starches, and are extremely calorie dense.

#2: Sweet Stuff

This list includes doughnuts, scones, cake, cookies, candy, muffins, and pastries of all kinds—and anything with a crust. What makes a great flaky crust? Crisco has got butter beat on that one according to many baking fanatic friends. Delicious and stone-cold bad for you because it contains, in part, trans and saturated fats, hydrogenated and partially hydrogenated soybean and palm oils. Of course, they are also high in refined sugars, including high fructose corn syrup (see the box on the facing page for my take on HFCS).

#3: Butter and Related Goop

Do what you can to avoid butter (which Chris adores). Ditto for all types of cream, sour cream, and mayo, including food made with these items, such as coleslaw, coated fruit salads, and potato salad. With deep, personal regret, I note that this group also includes my beloved ice cream. They are almost pure fat and/or sugar with a whopping number of calories. I confess that I cannot conceive of a life without ice cream (any more than Chris wants to live without butter), so I work like crazy to make it a special treat—even for my children. It is *not* easy.

#4: Processed and Cured Meats

Bologna, salami, sausages, hot dogs, and bacon are awfully hard for some people to give up, but it would be a great idea if they could. It may help if you see them the way I do: All these meatlike products come alarmingly close to being fat in a tube, or just fat altogether.

#5: Sweetened Drinks and Booze

The quickest way to get a blood sugar high and a subsequent low, *and* to take in a ton of useless calories, is to drink *soda and sweetened and artificially flavored juices and waters*. That goes for alcohol and foo-foo coffee drinks, too. These drinks contribute so many useless calories to our diets. Best to stay hydrated with no- or low-calorie beverages such as water, seltzer (my favorite), tea, and, yes, even coffee in moderation, without all the cream and sugar.

The Bottom Line on HFCS

'm sure it's not going to come as a surprise when I tell you that some researchers and nutrition writers blame high fructose corn syrup (HFCS) for the obesity epidemic. Well, maybe. Sure, there is an association between HFCS penetrating our food supply and the upswing of the obesity epidemic. It's also true that fructose is metabolized differently than glucose and that it may differentially affect fat storage. But HFCS can't be the only scapegoat; many factors are to blame. Before you demonize HFCS to the exclusion of all other sugars, let me point out that sucrose, or table sugar, is made up of an almost equal combination of fructose and glucose. And don't be fooled by "high" in HFCS, as it too is comprised of an almost equal combination of glucose and fructose.

Thus, both sugars likely influence your metabolism in very similar ways and one is by no means better than another. Sugar is sugar. The problem is simply the vast amount of products on the market that contain excess added sugars in any form. Avoid those foods and you'll surely be in a healthier place.

The trouble with a list like this is there are so many deserving candidates that are left out. One could reasonably say that the very peak of the Mountain should be crowned with an enormous fast-food place. Do not go to fast-food places, and don't give your kids a "treat" by taking them there. What you're really doing is training them at their most impressionable to see bad food as something special and wonderful. *That* is not good parenting. I actually freaked out about a year ago when our babysitter took my kids to Wendy's—yes, I admit, I might have overreacted. But do everything in your power to withstand the very real and seductive pressure from the advertisers who lure your children into wanting high-calorie garbage and the so-called free toys.

The Consequences of All Bad All the Time

Why is the Bad Stuff *so* bad? Obviously if you eat a little bit of these foods once in a blue moon, they won't kill you. However, every time you eat these things your body chemistry changes. Bad food does not dissolve or become something else. If you eat bacon, which has a high amount of saturated fat, the saturated fat gets digested and absorbed as saturated fat. The same with sugar—*you eat it, digest it, absorb it, and it circulates around as sugar. There is no magic. Solid fat and refined sugar* are absolutely dreadful for you, and they are not made any better or different in the digestion process. Your blood sugar or "glucose" goes up as result of eating sugar, and your blood fat or "lipids" content goes up from eating fat. It's not "normal" to saturate your bloodstream with sugar and fat. Your body goes a little nuts, and both the fat and sugar try desperately to find a place to go. The options are limited. Only so much sugar is needed to replace the glycogen stores in your muscle and liver, especially if you're idle and don't burn much. You need glycogen stores in your muscles for movement and a steady drip of glucose from your liver into your bloodstream to fuel your brain (your body is happiest when your blood sugar is between 80–100 mg/dL). What's left over has to go somewhere else. Similarly, you need only so much fat for the operation of your body and for fuel. Some is for cell structure and synthesis of other compounds. What happens to the excess sugar and fat?

All that homeless sugar and fat keep pumping through your body, and when levels get too high they cause damage but in different ways. Excess sugar initially gets converted to fat and stored in your fat cells. Much of it gets stored as adipose tissue including belly fat that comes with its own set of problems. When there is too much blood sugar, it starts coating everything in its path—from proteins to your DNA. Things that get coated with sugar do not work right. Even your red blood cells get a nice sticky coat of sugar.

Extra fat works a little differently. When you eat a lot of fat, it stays in your circulation longer. It promotes the synthesis of cholesterol, especially the bad cholesterol, the low-density lipoprotein (LDL). Your LDL rises and is more susceptible to attack by free radicals (molecules missing a critical electron, which search out and devour electrons from other molecules to make themselves stable). Once LDL is attacked, it becomes "oxidized" (damaged) and lays itself down along your artery walls. This is the critical first step on the road to heart disease. Moreover, when you overeat, and especially when you overeat fat, it is stored for future use. The potential storage is *huge* because fat cells are almost endlessly accommodating. A fat cell can swell to *fifty times its original size* to accommodate more fat. Then it can split in two and start the process again. We have the potential to hold an almost infinite amount of fat. It is a storage system that works much too well.

During the process of storing fat, it often accumulates around your middle. That development—more common with men than women before they hit menopause—may become your number-one health problem. Because belly fat, for some reason, is a great breeder of inflammation, and it's in an area right next to vital organs where it can do the most harm. You cannot see the inflammation, but you can see your belly. As a practical matter, you are looking at a depot of ill health.

Concept 1: "Runaway Fats," Sugar, and Insulin Resistance

This is a complicated topic that's worth learning about. Let's start with your body's stored fat, not fat in your bloodstream from recent eating, and how it causes things to go wrong. For most premenopausal women, it initially goes mainly to the lower half, to your butt and thighs. Not pretty but not too terrible for us. In men, it goes to the belly—the dreaded "beer belly" or gut. This fat is known to release high levels of inflammatory molecules that get into the bloodstream and readily target organs. And it is ideally located to do so because it surrounds all of your vital organs: your liver, kidney, pancreas, intestines, and so on. This stomach fat becomes much more common in women after menopause with the loss of estrogen. (Don't get me wrong—many women in this country have found a way to pack on excess fat everywhere well before menopause.) And sure enough, a women's risk of heart disease, which was so much less than a man's risk premenopause, shoots up. Once menopause hits, women's risk of heart disease is just as high as men's.

Not all stored fat is stored in the belly. But all stored fat is inflammatory, wherever it goes. And it goes everywhere—not only does it cushion your organs, it infiltrates them, like your liver and muscle. Fat cells grow like crazy if we overeat. As they get larger they release more inflammatory signals. When fat cells get really big, things get even worse. The oversized fat cells are attacked by an immune cell to basically do some home improvement—it wants to help rebuild the fat cells that you have "outgrown." In this rebuilding process, something scary happens: Some fat leaks back into your bloodstream. Runaway fats in the circulation have bad effects on muscle, and the liver, and pancreas, the major organs for fueling metabolism. In a healthy body, as you know, fats and sugars are taken up by the muscle for energy. Runaway fat in the bloodstream inhibits this process just as it inhibits basic metabolism. If the muscles for fuel can't take up fats and sugar, we can't move as easily. There is simply less energy available.

In the pancreas, circulating fats inhibit insulin secretion. You'll remember that insulin is indispensable for taking up sugar by the muscle cells. Obese individuals often have high blood sugar and need more insulin, but over time, less insulin is produced. They have less because the runaway fat in their bodies inhibits insulin production. This is one step in a very vicious circle.

Runaway fat hits the liver, too. In the liver, insulin typically inhibits glucose production, which is a good thing. Runaway fat inhibits insulin production, so more sugar is made, which you don't need. You are low on insulin and becoming insulin resistant, but your liver keeps on making glucose even when it is already high in your circulation because of the runaway fat!

Assume that the runaway fat has already inhibited the production of insulin in the pancreas. In the meantime, the fats have nowhere to go and spark more inflammation and other signals that further disrupt the normal pathways that would allow you to burn sugars and fats. At this point, cells that normally take up sugar become resistant to insulin and are slower to take up sugar or glucose. A person who has reached this stage is said to be "insulin resistant." The pancreas has worked its tail off trying to make more insulin to counteract the high blood sugar. It has been overrun and can't keep up.

The insulin-producing cells in the pancreas get worn down (partially through inflammatory mechanisms), self-destruct, and no longer produce insulin. At this point, you have become a person with type 2 diabetes. This is not a situation to take lightly. There is no such thing as a mild case of diabetes or having "slightly elevated" blood sugar— anything above normal has a negative effect on every cell in your body. Type 2 diabetes now accounts for 90–95 percent of all cases of diabetes: 26 million Americans have it, and 7 million of these don't even know it. A whopping 37 percent of adults are prediabetic. If you have diabetes, your life expectancy is about fifteen years less than people without diabetes. Moreover, it cripples you long before it kills you.

Here's a scenario to consider: Let's assume that you are either insulin-resistant or actually have type 2 diabetes. Then let's say that you chow down a gargantuan sugar-loaded muffin for breakfast that is extremely high in added sugars and solid fats. Your bloodstream is already high in circulating fats and sugar. Now you have added a lot more fat and sugar to the bloodstream, and you can't do anything with it. The muscle does not take it up because the runaway fats in your pancreas have destroyed the necessary insulin signal needed to take up glucose. Your blood glucose levels stay high for a longer period of time and your own blood becomes toxic: It has too much sugar in it and it wreaks havoc on any cell in its path. It causes large amounts of stress all over the place, not to mention more inflammation.

As for the glucose that does get taken up by the muscles, it is not used efficiently either, because the mitochondria are damaged from inflammation and are less efficient. The mitochondria actually change in shape, density, and function in such a way that they can't produce much usable energy. And when the mitochondria don't function well, they actually produce more stress signals. There is a virtual firestorm of inflammation and negative signals inside your body. Scientists call this "metabolic inflexibility." What it means, in sum, is that obese individuals can't handle sugar and carbohydrates anywhere near as well as they should. Eventually the sugar that cannot get taken up and used as a fuel goes back to the fat cells as yet more fat.

The extra glucose that stays in the bloodstream is not so wonderful either. That excess sugar in the blood has grave health consequences: renal (kidney) failure, blindness, amputations, and heightened risk of cardiovascular disease. Diabetes is the dominant cause of blindness and amputation in the United States. Too much glucose in the blood is like a slow-acting poison.

When glucose remains in the bloodstream too long, the sugar actually coats the red blood cell, a process called glycosylation. It makes the blood cell stiff and sticky. That interferes with blood circulation, causes damage to the artery walls and enables cholesterol to deposit there. Separate problem: If red blood cells are stiff, delivery of oxygen to working cells is compromised. It can take years for the damage to become apparent, but smaller, more fragile blood vessels such as those in the eyes, kidneys, and feet are most at risk, hence the risk of blindness and renal failure. As if all this was not bad enough, there is also the fact that bacteria thrive on glucose. You get sicker more often and stay sicker longer. Combine that with the loss of sensation due to glucose-related nerve damage, and you have a recipe for severe foot problems that could result in amputation. Eventually, even larger blood vessels can be affected, and even blocked, causing strokes and heart attacks.

Concept 2: Fats and Heart Disease

Decay into insulin resistance and diabetes is scary, but it is by no means the scariest thing out there for those who insist on eating like lunatics year after year. Cardiovascular disease kills us more than any other disease in this country, and it clearly begins with what you eat, as well as the exercise you're *not* getting. One and a half million Americans have a heart attack every year. It is a thunderclap when it happens. It strikes out of the blue or seems to. But that is anything but the case. More than 75 percent of American men have the beginnings of heart disease at age twenty! A woman's risk is equal to that of a man's after menopause. Autopsies of children have shown that the initial stages of heart disease can start as early as age five. The Great American Diet and the Great American Idleness in collaboration: What a terrifying duo.

You may want to know how this works, especially because there is a good chance it will become your personal story. You may want to have this in mind the next time someone tries to interest you in a saturated fat-centric Atkins-style diet or half a pizza, double cheese. Most Americans consume about 100–120 grams of fat per day, equal to a daily intake of 900–1,080 calories of fat, or close to half of our needed total caloric intake. When we eat fat, most of it is digested, absorbed as small components of fat (individual fatty acids) and repackaged into little fat globules that are released into the circulation. These globules transport fat around the body and can deposit fat where it is needed. Little Pac-Men, the "lipases," then work at different sites to chomp off pieces of fat when a tissue requires fat—whether this is to produce energy, make something that requires fat, or store fat. The remnants of the fat globules eventually end up at the liver.

That's not the end of the line. The liver is stimulated by these fat globules, that came from the food you ate, to produce cholesterol. This is an odd little process: The blood delivers the fat globules to the liver, which repackages them into another type of fat globule. The new fat globules are really high in cholesterol. How bad these are depends on whether they are high-density or low-density cholesterol (i.e., your HDL or LDL cholesterol). When your cholesterol is measured, it is typically analyzed as your total cholesterol, your HDL, and your LDL. This same screening usually also measures your triglycerides, the scientific name for fat. It is found in both the fat globules and cholesterol particles. All of these particles—your HDL, LDL, and triglycerides—have strong ties to heart health.

LDL is the bad cholesterol, responsible for depositing cholesterol throughout our body. But the real reason that it receives (and deserves) a bad rap is that it is also very susceptible to oxidation and damage, especially if it remains at high levels in your circulation. That oxidation process occurs in your arteries and creates plaque, which is the great precursor to heart disease.

HDL, in contrast, is known as the good cholesterol and works like a little vacuum, cleaning up the excess cholesterol in your body and sending it back to the liver to be recycled or excreted. When you go to the doctor for a cholesterol screen, you are getting a report on the state of the vacuum cleaner, the HDL, on the one hand, and the plaque builder, the LDL, on the other. You urgently want vacuum cleaners. You urgently do not want plaque makers. Eating fat and Dead Food creates more LDL. Eating Good Stuff and exercising creates more HDL.

That is a short telling of a long and intricate story, but the bottom line remains: Quit eating saturated fat and other Dead Food, and work out a lot. For those who want to know what really happens to cause heart disease, keep on trucking. It all begins with a little bit of damage, a little nick, chip, dent, or ding in the lining of the artery wall. The artery gets roughed up a bit from myriad things such as carcinogens and pollutants that you put into your body—like the ones you get from smoking or excess sugar and trans and saturated fats. The situation gets exacerbated by high blood pressure, which further wears away at the cells lining the artery walls.

The wear and tear is where you really run into problems. You continue to eat Bad Stuff, and this promotes the production of LDL. When LDL levels are elevated, it enters the walls of the arteries and becomes oxidized, or damaged. Damaged LDL, just like any other damage in your body, sends out inflammatory signals about the damage. A family of cytokines, which work much like hormones, leads these inflammatory signals. They promote the recruitment of white blood cells and other immune factors to collect at the damaged site. Immune cells respond to this damage by attacking (by the release of free radicals) and consuming the trapped LDL. These immune cells end up becoming engorged and become part of the arterial wall. This plaque releases even more inflammatory signals, which brings even more immune cells to the site and a vicious cycle ensues.

As more immune cells attack oxidized LDL particles, a yellow-ish fatty streak accumulates, with cellular debris and calcium also being deposited on the streak causing the arterial walls to harden. To make matters worse, diets high in refined sugar and bad fats promote inflammatory signals and immune cells to stay there. The deposition of fat over time is an extremely gradual process that can start as early as young childhood. This buildup of the fatty streaks marks the early stages of heart disease. It is bad from the get-go.

Over time, the fatty streaks calcify (harden) and a layer of connective tissue and smooth muscle is formed over the top of the fatty streak. As a result, the arteries narrow significantly and become gradually stiffer. Now your arteries are no longer able to expand and contract with normal daily blood pressure changes. Blood pressure rises in response to the stiffness, and the high blood pressure further exacerbates the damage within the arteries. The payoff (the heart attack) is not, as you might anticipate, that the walls of the arteries get so close that the blood cannot get through. Rather, at some point, a piece of unstable plaque breaks off and forms a clot. That *does* block the artery and prevents the blood flow to your heart. The heart must have a constant, steady supply of blood and nutrition or parts of it simply die. When blood flow is interrupted—by a clot—part of the heart muscle dies. It happens alarmingly fast. It takes only five minutes of blockage for that tissue to die. You lose part of your heart or, if the clot goes to your brain, part of your brain. End of story.

Inflammation: The Common Thread

Up to this point, we have hammered home the basic theme of how eating Bad Stuff makes you unhealthy, promotes a whole cascade of negative health effects, and of course makes you fat. The common thread running through these phenomena is that they breed inflammation, which is innately tied to biochemical pathways affected by our diet and our physical activity and, in turn, has a major effect on the progression of disease and how our body ages.

I hate to oversimplify, but it is appropriate here: Most of the time, inflammation really is the great Satan inside your body. And all the bad things—eating Bad Stuff, not eating Good Stuff, and being over-weight—create and promote inflammation. Think about it. (1) Excess sugar in your bloodstream promotes inflammation. (2) Excess fat in your circulation (triglycerides, LDL, and free fatty acids) promotes inflam-matory signals. And worst of all, in a way, (3) the fat stored in your fat cells, the fat cells themselves, release major inflammatory signals.

Why do we have an inflammatory response in the body? It is not always bad, as I say. It is actually a vital part of our immune system. We have special "immune cells," the white blood cells. The immune system is an intricate system designed to combat foreign pathogens like infections and other invaders. As it turns out, these immune cells release inflamma-tory signals that are important, and in this case good, for our health. For example, it helps to turn over damaged proteins like the ones in your mus-cle cells that get a bit banged up when you go a little overboard exercising or when you get a splinter in your finger. When it's an external wound, you may be sore, a little red, or even swollen and black and blue. In those instances, inflammation is good: White blood cells flood the site of injury and release free radicals to break down the damage and promote the repair of the tissue. There are minor side effects (soreness, fever, and/or swell-ing) that eventually dissipate, but the process is basically good. For your strained muscles, it is really good because it is a key step in the critical business of rebuilding your muscles stronger.

That's the good side of inflammation. However, chronic inflam-mation, the bad kind, works very differently. It is the version that leads to type 2 diabetes, heart disease, malfunctioning muscles, and mal-functioning metabolism—the works. It really is the root of almost all evil inside the body. It comes from eating slop, getting fat, and being idle. This may seem a little odd, but inflammatory signals are released from almost everywhere, beyond your white blood cells. They can be released from your muscle, bone, blood vessel walls, and even fat cells. And guess what? Excess adipose tissue, *being overweight, is the main contributor to most chronic inflammation.* Obesity is linked to almost every chronic disease and each is somehow associated with inflamma-tion: diabetes, heart disease, stroke, cancer, arthritis, and others.

Your fat tissue is not an inert substance. It is a living organ itself, and it lives to constantly generate and send out inflammatory mediators.

All fat tissue does this, and the fatter you are, the more inflammatory signals are released. The most active fat cells are those around your midsection, known as visceral fat. The bigger the belly you have, the more inflammation you have surging through your body.

Of the inflammatory signals released from fat tissue—including cytokines and hormones—some of the best researched include interleukin-6, tumor necrosis factor-α, leptin, and others. All of these can be released from fat cells and have an impact on other organs and tissues. They go to cells and promote or inhibit molecular mechanisms in the direction that often opposes health. The networks of signals that maintain health in a single cell are numerous, and most of these networks can be affected by inflammatory signals such as the cytokines that I mentioned, and likely hundreds of others, by something that you can't feel or see until it's too late (i.e., you have a heart attack or develop type 2 diabetes).

Some cardiac professionals see inflammation levels as a critical measure of susceptibility to heart attacks and stroke. Obesity is at the root of most disease-related inflammation, and yet not all fat people are sick. How come? Well, these processes are gradual; an inflammatory state promotes the quiet and gradual accumulation of decay. It takes a while, but it is going on right now. Remember that sewer around your middle. The fat in your midsection is lovingly enveloping all of your vital organs, the ones that let you survive: your liver, pancreas, intestines, and kidneys. It is a constant, powerful source of inflammatory signals, which are released in very close proximity to these vital organs.

Fat definitely hurts your vital organs. Autopsies of the obese clearly show the invasion of fat throughout these organs, especially the liver and heart. That is a given. And the situation is insidious because many of the negative inflammatory signals cannot be measured by your doctor, even in a lab—we have a few great markers, but they surely don't tell the whole story. The systems are amazingly complex, and we are still trying to decipher them. What we do know is that the signaling is going on, it is highly pernicious, and you should do everything you can to shut it down.

A healthy diet and physical activity are the two best ways to mitigate the proinflammatory signals—period! Which is good news when you think about it. Getting out of this appalling and vicious cycle is actually under your control. Not easy, but doable—and it's up to you. Exercise and nutrition work through very similar ways to help reduce inflammation. If we do both we are far more likely to cut down inflammation and the chaos it brings.

On the nutrition side, understand that consuming a pint of blueberries a day doesn't mean that you are quenching every free radical produced, especially if everything else you're eating is junk. Our diets have to be varied and balanced with several types of antioxidants from many different good foods (see the good foods list in Chapter 9). Plus, it is not the case that if we eat these items over the course of a few days or weeks, we will all of a sudden be "inflammation free." It doesn't work that way. It is more likely that all the signaling pathways within our bodies will start to work just a bit better so that we start turning the tide of negative metabolic signals. It is not just eating more of the Good Stuff; it is also eating so much less saturated and trans fats, which do such horrendous damage. It is a whole-diet approach—and exercise—that is going to work and not a temporary anti-inflammatory diet that lasts for a few weeks.

Exercise works in many similar ways to diet. It naturally increases our good cholesterol, the HDL that scavenges cholesterol and also has anti-inflammatory properties. Furthermore, exercise helps moderate immune functioning and balances the cytokine responses to stress. It inherently promotes anti-inflammatory cytokines and suppresses the inflammatory ones. Our immune system is primed and works better, and it is less likely to spiral out of control. Exercise also stimulates growth to our muscles and moderates insulin and blood sugar uptake, further diminishing inflammation in our bodies, which we talk about in greater detail later. Bottom line: Eating well and exercising hard will do a tremendous amount to fight inflammation. And that is a fight worth winning.

Diets and Other Fads

t's not just eating crappy food that can do you in. There are so many hucksters selling all sorts of crazy diet fads that also do damage to your system without resulting in the desired weight loss and fitness over the long term. First off, most fad diets are highly calorie restrictive and end up depriving you of vital food groups. That's why "no-carb" and "no-fat" diets don't work and are foolish for your health. Obviously, extreme all-ice-cream or all-grapefruit diets are also not balanced and therefore are not a good idea either.

Severe calorie restriction, the hallmark of most diet crazes, also puts you into starvation mode—you become more efficient at using every calorie which can slow down your metabolism. Weight loss becomes frustratingly difficult. When you are not eating enough it's also tough to fuel a regular exercise program. Let's face it: These kinds of diets are near impossible to sustain over the long haul, and then you find yourself right back where you started from, and sometimes with more weight piled on than when you started the darn thing. Diets that require you to buy and eat bars and shakes or frozen entrées can be filled with additives you don't need and are certainly not rich in whole, fresh foods. And they cost more than fresh food.

If you have understood all we've said about the role of balance in a sound diet, you don't need to know much more than that. But there are a few recent crazes you might have heard about that I do want to address.

Gluten-Free Diets

As I write this, on the cover of nearly every magazine in the grocery store checkout line is a celebrity claiming to have lost an unrealistic amount of weight with the latest and greatest fad, the gluten-free diet. In fact, even some athletes are going gluten free based on the advice of their trainers. Beyond that, the food manufacturers have caught on to the craze (always a bad sign). How many cereal boxes, cake mixes, and other processed foods in your grocery store do you now see that are labeled "gluten-free"?

The gluten-free diet is a valid, effective way of life for a very specific medical condition called celiac disease, an autoimmune disorder that affects digestion in the small intestine and is present in less than 1 percent of the population. Gluten is a protein found in wheat, barley, and rye, which these individuals cannot digest properly, leading to a whole host of symptoms. For those individuals, following a gluten-free diet is a way of life, not a "diet." Their symptoms disappear, and the illness caused by gluten can be reversed. But for those who follow the gluten-free diet for weight loss purposes, it's really nothing other than a rebranded low-carbohydrate diet due to the avoidance of wheat-based products. Not a good idea.

Here is the thing: If a gluten-free diet caused individuals to cut out refined carbohydrates and replace them with other whole grains, fruits, and vegetables, that would be great. But that doesn't always happen. Besides, whole wheat is not inherently bad for most people and has several health benefits: Loads of B vitamins (to boost metabolism) and fiber are prime among them. Unless equally fiber-rich whole grains such as brown rice, oats, or quinoa replace whole wheat, it is going to be very difficult to get adequate fiber, particularly soluble fiber (which is the type, by the way, that can help you lower your cholesterol).

There is nothing intrinsically healthier about a gluten-free diet, particularly if you end up replacing regular pretzels, cookies, and brownies with gluten-free processed alternatives. In fact, it could be worse for you. Watch out for all the other garbage on the market touted as gluten-free. Manufacturers of these products replace gluten with extra fat and/or sugar to maintain taste. Additionally, most gluten-free products are not enriched or fortified with micronutrients like B vitamins and iron, so you are losing out on vital nutrients. If you do have to go gluten-free for real health reasons, prioritizing gluten-free whole grains, fruits, and vegetables is key. If you don't have to follow a gluten-free diet, well then, prioritizing whole grains, fruits, and vegetables is still key. If you think you have a gluten problem, see your doctor and have some tests run. If you don't have a gluten problem, skip gluten-free.

High-Protein Diets

Very low-carb, protein-centered diets are still popular in the diet world. High-protein diets promise quick weight loss, which is mainly due to an elimination of another (inherently low-calorie) food group and water loss that results (you retain less water with high-protein intakes)—both of which are short-term fixes. As soon as you start incorporating other food groups, you may find the weight comes right back on again.

The other important idea to remember is that high-protein diets often require you to eat a lot of animal protein and red meat, which contains saturated fat, and I have already described how saturated fat is terrible for your health. A third important concept is that high-protein diets are basically repackaged low-carb diets, and low-carb diets don't fare well with an exercise regimen—you need healthy carbs to fuel movement! And low-carb is usually coupled with low fiber—not great for your health. You're likely eating adequate protein as it is. Bottom line: High-protein diets are not balanced and deprive you of the nutrients other whole foods provide. Besides, it's a boring way to eat. How long could you possibly stick with such a plan?

Cleanses

The idea that a detox can purge certain (unnamed) toxins that have invaded your body through a near starvation diet for a few days or even longer, lightened with a magical combination of juices and herbs, defies logic. You do some penance, scourge yourself with magical elements, and drive the evils out of your body. It is an appealing notion, so you can see why it has been around for a long time (the ancient Egyptians were doing it). It's also complete nonsense. There is no evidence that cleanses do you a bit of good. And—to those with some understanding of how the body works—it is hard to imagine how they could.

We have cleansing machinery in our bodies, especially the kidney and liver. How exactly do cleanses supplement the operation of those frontline systems? They don't. If your kidney or liver did break down, you would have a very serious problem, and I would need to see strong evidence that a detox cleanse would help in this or any other scenario.

By the way, what are the toxins that a cleanse claims to clean out? I know quite a bit about what can go wrong in the body, and I am on familiar terms with many of the evil forces that can raise hell with our health. None of them sound like the "toxins" that practitioners of the cleanse are talking about. What are these new toxins? And why don't the kidney and the liver pick them up? Very odd.

If you want to do a real "kick start" or a "detox," it is simple. Cut the real toxins you feast on: fast food, alcohol, too much caffeine, artificial sweeteners, cakes and cookies, trans fats, and heavily marbled steaks. Then simply go heavy on the fruits and vegetables and exercise and sweat like a lunatic. By the way, good old fiber consumption will increase the health of the bacteria and microflora in your large intestine. Nature's scrub brush, fiber, will definitely clean out your system.

Final Thoughts

The Great American Diet contains an astonishing amount of Bad Stuff. Here are a couple of details to put it in perspective: We consume over 22 teaspoons of *added* sugar per day and 5 tablespoons of solid fat per day. See what that looks like: Scoop out 22 teaspoons of sugar and 5 tablespoons of Crisco into a bowl. On the Great American Diet, half of your daily calories come from this bowl. It is the great breeder of fat and inflammation inside your body. Eating like this is insane. As are silly, unhealthy, unsustainable quick-fix diets that never work. Come on down off the Mountain, stop with the fads, and eat more veggies instead of doing a cleanse.

CHAPTER EIGHT

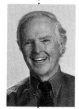

A Day in the Life:
A New Relationship
with Vegetables

ontrary to what everyone advises, and contrary to my own advice to you, I dove into Jen's regimen at the deep end and changed everything at once. Gave up all refined flour and sugar, all processed food, most meat, and most solid fat. All fried food (sob!). Ate a ton of veg and lots of whole grains, mostly brown rice, which I love. Cut my portions by about a third (depending on how virtuous the meal was; no need to cut back on broccoli). Cut booze to one whopping six-ounce glass of wine a night (sometimes two). All while exercising a little harder than usual. And writing down what I did. I got sick of writing stuff down, soon enough, but it was a help in the beginning, and I still do it some. Some people do it forever.

One important tip: Whether you go nuts like me or get into it more gradually, *have a fixed plan* about what you do and don't eat. And how much. Write it down. What you do not want is to be making fresh decisions, at every mealtime. You want to know in advance that you have given up all fried food, say, or all refined flour and sugar. Know that you are going to cut your habitual restaurant portions by a third, or whatever. Set out your own rules, and be tough about them.

A Quick Row on Twin Lakes

Exercise today is an early morning row on Twin Lakes, up in the Berkshire Hills. It's a perfect day for it, about sixty, clear and no wind. Hilary rows some but not today; she's sound asleep. The dog gives me a look, puts her head back down. I am on my own here, which is fine. A secret pleasure, actually. One of the privileges of getting older is that you're up so damn early, you "own" the morning most days. And it's a treat to a certain temperament. I make coffee, quietly, and have a dish of blueberries. Head out, barefoot, across the wet lawn to the car. Feel good.

No one rows anymore. Jen and I do, but almost no one. Too bad. It may be the best sport for your health and fitness of all the sports I know. And a pleasure? Oh, boy! You do it in beautiful places, there is a lovely, gliding motion you don't get in any other sport, and it is a superb whole-body workout. In earlier times, everyone could row—there were no outboards—and races in rowboats were a workingman's sport. Because workingmen were the ones who did it most and were best at it. They rowed light cargo here and there, took passengers out to the ships in the harbor. And across the wide rivers in New York and Boston, before the big bridges went up. Pulling boats, like my beautiful Whitehall skiff with the wineglass stern, were water taxis down on Whitehall Street on the East River. Hence the name. Pretty handy, those East River watermen a hundred years ago. And a hundred years before that, too.

Want to hear a nice story? A collateral relative of mine, John Glover, and a group of fishermen from Marblehead, Massachusetts, my hometown, rowed Washington's army—nine thousand men!—across the East River late one August night, in 1775, under cover of fog and darkness. And quite simply saved the Revolution. Thirty thousand British soldiers were going to sew 'em up the next morning and put an end to the rebellion. Except that Washington—in one of the great escapes in all military history—silently pulled his men back from the lines, marched 'em down to the landing, where the Brooklyn Bridge is today, and stole them away. He sat on his big horse, all night and into the morning, directing the evacuation. Glover and his men rowed back and forth, in the ferocious tide, the boats loaded to the gunnels with men and guns and, eventually, horses. Until every man-jack of them—and every horse and every cannon—got clean away. Washington, a handy sailor himself, was one of the last to board. When the British woke up in the morning, the trapped Americans were gone. The British simply could not believe it.

After that, in tough times (crossing the ice-choked Delaware on Christmas Eve, and other places) Washington would shout, "Where are my Marbleheaders?!" Handy men, by heaven. Just what you want for a revolution.

When gentlemen took up the sport, in the late 1800s and early 1900s, workingmen rowers were seen as a problem. There were actual rules to keep working stiffs out of the regattas. Grace Kelly's father, Jack, was a hell of an oarsman, but he was barred from the Diamond Sculls in England because he had once been a bricklayer. And of course he was Irish; that wasn't so great. Can't have "muckers," as they used to call them, in a gent's race. His son won the Diamond Sculls decades later, teaching the British another much needed lesson.

By the 1920s, single sculls didn't look much like a rowboat. The boats, made of the thinnest wood veneer, were twenty-six feet long, less than a foot wide, and weighed only thirty pounds. You could poke your finger through the bottom. Or your foot. They had outriggers to hold the nine-foot-long oars, which are the key to balancing everything. The boats look pretty much the same today, except they are made of fiberglass. Still a pretty delicate business. You skim along the surface, with those huge oars carefully balanced, like a waterbug.

Rowing, to an extraordinary extent, is a whole-body sport. It looks as if it were all arms and back, but it's not. Seventy percent of the power in your stroke comes from your legs, from that sliding seat. That's true of so many sports: The strength comes mostly from the legs, then gets carried up through your core to the arms and hands. Tennis is like that. Golf. Baseball. The legs and the core make all the difference. If the core is not stable and strong, the power coming up from your legs will dribble away. All strength-training exercise should be *core* exercise, if you can manage it. And you can, as you'll read later on.

The lake is only about a mile and a half long and narrow. No powerboats, no houses to speak of. A perfect rowing lake because, most days, it is out of the wind, tucked away in the vale of the hills. I head west, just paddling to start to warm up. And I let the curved oars skim the water on the "recovery," which stabilizes the boat wonderfully. The first ten minutes, it's like that—just paddling along, waking up the muscles—calling that signaling system back to work. And then the stroke gets a little longer. I reach a little farther toward the stern to the "catch," bending back deeper at the end of the stroke.

And then the stroke becomes somewhat more serious. When you get into it a bit, you hit the catch pretty hard and *pull* fast. *In-out* as hard as you can. And then slow and smooth on the recovery. As you get more serious, the oars are off the water on the recovery. Takes a while to be able to do that, to get your balance to that point. But it's faster. The boat has to be perfectly balanced at this point, and so do you. Hands, butt, shoulders, and arms—your whole body just so. But in passionate motion, too. It's complicated. You work like crazy on every stroke. And then you glide. Pull with all your might. And then glide. Silently and with perfect ease. The cranes, standing in the deep grasses to the side, look on approvingly. Nice sport. Nice day. I give it an hour and head back to the boathouse, put the boat away. Wipe it down. I feel sensational. I wish you all rowed, you would love it *so* much.

A New Relationship with Vegetables

L unch is sort of interesting. It occurs to me that—if this regimen of Jen's is going to work—I am going to have to see vegetables in a different light. Which begins today.

Asparagus is in season. I like it well enough, and I have laid in a bunch of it. Hilary is home; she is a much better cook, but I do most of the cooking for some reason. Because it's fun, probably, and I'm greedy. I am experimenting today. Lunch is going to be asparagus and whole wheat bread. Period. And it is going to be terrific.

Then—*quick*, while it's hot—to the table with Hilary. She brings water. Sparkling water with a splash of cranberry juice, in my case, as a substitute for the diet sodas with which I happily poisoned my body for decades. When I am a real grown-up, I will just drink water out of the tap, but that day is sadly far away.

Asparagus Lunch

take a deep sauté pan and fill it with about ¾ inch of water, add salt, and turn on the gas. Take two bundles of asparagus and break them off, pretty far up the stalk. Asparagus in season does not cost a lot and if you are going to change your eating habits, you might as well spoil yourself as much as possible. Cook the asparagus "on," not "in" water, as some wise man has said. You don't leach out quite so many of the nutrients and taste that way. And only cook them for a few minutes. You want them so they are firm to your teeth but not stringy or chewy. How do you get them just right? You taste-test them all the time. If you are going to cook—and it makes *so* much sense to do so—and if you are going to cook vegetables in particular, getting them cooked *just right* matters a lot. I put two thick pieces of terrific multi-grain bread in the toaster (about 150 calories a slice but nutrient dense and full of fiber). When the asparagus is perfect, I squeeze some lemon juice on it and add a tiny pat of butter. (Yes, children, a tiny pat of butter. So I won't be tempted to tip the whole thing into the garbage and go get a burger.)

And here is the nice thing: This simple meal is superb. If you sat down to a heaping plate of hamburgers, fries, and asparagus, you would mostly miss out on the delicate taste and pleasure of the asparagus. The other coarse stuff would drown it out. But today, that's all there is. And it's a treat.

Back to this simple veg lunch: I predict that you (like me) will develop a real sneaker for meals like this and that you will realize that you have just made yourself an elegant little meal that a cool chef in Provence would not sneer at. You didn't just "eat your vege-tables"; you made a meal of them. Try it again tomorrow with carrots or green beans or beets. Or—God help us—Brussels sprouts. Hey, I know that the chances of our getting all the way to Brussels sprouts are not great, but who knows? I am a coarse brute and look how far I've come.

Dinner: What to Do with
a Kid's Birthday Party

Supper presents an interesting challenge. We are having a pretty big birthday party for a kid who is turning seven. There will be about twenty people, half kids, half grown-ups. The mother—our dear pal and a houseguest—will bake the cake. I do supper. What to cook that will suit the kids, the grown-ups, and me? And honor Jen's Rules?

My answer was brilliant, up to a point: a vegetable, shrimp, and spicy (low-calorie, chicken-based) sausage sauce over a very modest amount of pasta. The great and all-but-invisible trick was the making of the sauce, with tons of crispy fresh vegetables, cut up small and cooked only to the point of soft crunch. In a sea of fresh-cooked tomatoes and a little canned pasta sauce. I have been making a variation of this dish forever. It's great for large mixed crowds (the littlest ones seem to eat just the pasta). And—strictly as a matter of taste and texture—I have added more and more vegetables every year. People go nuts about it. It reads like comfort food, but it is actually pretty healthy. The only difference now is that I am cutting back sharply on the amount of pasta served until it is almost an all-sauce meal. And the sauce is almost all vegetables and shrimp. People don't notice that they are eating something that is great for them.

The sauce is going to be amazing. And it is almost all veg and some low-calorie shrimp and chicken sausage. A sane portion—without any pasta, which you and I do not need—is basically a super-healthy diet dish. Yum. And no one knows. It looks like a *feast*. Not bad. Kids and the other grown-ups can have the usual ration of half pasta and half sauce or worse. But you, you clever devil, can just eat the sauce and be a great girl, great guy. Without a whisper of sacrifice or guilt.

The night is a great success. More people show up than expected. It's one of those perfect nights, in early summer. Our 1859 Victorian has never looked cozier. There are a dozen kids with croquet mallets, Frisbees, and baseballs, chasing around and around the house and down the hill toward the water, until dark. We fill our guests with modest rosé wine, which is just the wine for a night like this. The main hors

Pasta with Vegetables, Shrimp, and Chicken Sausage

For ten people, say (and you can double the amounts and have leftovers for weeks), cut up two or three big Vidalia onions into roughly ¼-inch pieces. (Here's how you dice an onion. Fast. First, sharpen the damn knife—makes all the difference. Then skin the onion, cut off the top and bottom, and set it on end. Then slice down, almost but not quite all the way through the onion. One set of slices down one way, another at right angles to those. Now—carefully holding it together with one hand—set it on its side and slice across the cuts. Not your fingers, you dope, the onion. Result: instant onion in ¼-inch bits. The bottom piece is a mess; chuck it.) Cut up two green or yellow or red peppers, same size. The same with a few heads [sic] of celery. Finally, open a jar of Kalamata olives, pit 'em, and cut them up, too. Put this vegetable mélange—which should account for more than half the mass of the sauce when you are done—into a huge frying pan, with a little olive oil and water and cook for fifteen minutes. Remember that you want the vegetables to be a little *crisp* when it's all done. Do not turn it into one of those all-day stews your Italian grandmother was so fond of. Add a couple of cans of chopped (not pureed) tomatoes. Or—in season—a ton of fresh sliced tomatoes (canned are surprisingly good, but nothing's ever as good as fresh). Then maybe a couple of jars of commercial sauce, if you like. Be sure to get a good one, which does not have *any sugar*. (Added sugar is the curse of cheap Italian sauce. Added sugar is the curse of *everything!*)

Separately, sauté the shrimp (larger ones are better; I get big two-pound bags of frozen ones, sixteen to twenty count if I can find them) in a different pan, with maybe some Asian spices, to confuse your Italian grandmother. Slice half a dozen sausages up in ⅓-inch thick slices and brown them separately. Throw the whole mess into a giant pot with the sauce, put on a lid and simmer over the lowest flame for a while so they can all get to know each other while you boil the pasta water, make drinks, be the great guy at the door.

---

d'oeuvre is fresh-made popcorn with no butter. (I have been making popcorn since 1944, like my father and grandfather before me, and it is apt to be tasty. I miss the butter like crazy.)

There's good cheese and some crackers for the others, but not for you and me. Drinks are out on the porch, under the big trees, where we can watch the kids churning around on the lawn. The fireflies are just beginning to show up. The pasta—and a dynamite salad Hilary made, with strong flavors of balsamic vinegar, mustard, and shallots, and not much olive oil—is dished up early and eaten inside. Great Italian bread and butter, but do I have a morsel of that? Of course not. I am on the program. I am Jen's guy.

There *are* two problems, however. Booze, first of all. It is so hard to be host and make drinks for everyone without joining in. Mostly people drink the rosé, not so hard to resist. But, in this part of the world, it is also cosmo season. Are you familiar with the cosmo? I hope not. The great thing about the cosmo is its innocent pink color and the fact that it is served in an ethereal martini glass. It looks as if it could not possibly hurt you.

The less great thing about the cosmo is that it is mostly made of vodka and it most assuredly *can* hurt you. I make a lot of cosmos (the trick is plenty of fresh-squeezed limes, not too much Cointreau, and just enough cranberry) and have a little flair for it. And sometimes I will take a little sip, to make sure that a given batch is okay. Tonight I have several sips. Not awful. About a dozen of 'em.

Second problem: This is a kid's birthday party and his mother made a birthday cake. A beauty, with a deep vanilla frosting. The smell has been in the house all day. I have been a near saint all night, but when the time finally comes to put the candles to the cake and sing "Happy Birthday," I am not quite drooling, but close. I am not nuts about dessert, but I adore birthday cake. Especially this very kind. I do not know what you would have done, but I do the only honorable thing under the circumstances: I go up to my study, find my old service revolver, and blow my brains out.

No, I don't. I have a *modest* piece of cake. Wash it down with rosé.

Interesting thing. I weigh myself with dread, the next morning, assuming I have gained a pound and blown off a day of virtue. Not a bit of it. I get clean away with the whole thing: *lost* a pound on the day. Oh, boy! That lovely row, man. And the amazing, no-sacrifice sauce. Yum.

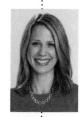

CHAPTER NINE

The Thinner This Year Eating Plan

You see, Chris can survive a birthday party, drinks, and cake—and so can you. Once you know what to eat and how much of it to put on your plate, you can really just stick to this plan for the rest of your life, allowing room for life's little celebrations.

The good news is that you'll find an *ocean* of great food out there to eat *after* you quit eating the bad stuff. With the tools here helping you make the right choices, and with practice and patience, our way of eating will become second nature—you'll do it without thinking that much about it. I don't like the word *diet* because it implies a temporary fix. What we're suggesting isn't something you do for a couple of weeks before you revert back to the "convenience" or prepackaged foods that were the centerpiece of your diet before. This plan is for keeps. The two weeks' worth of meal plans at the end of the chapter get you started and in the rhythm of the plan, so when you're on your own you'll know how to select food to create your own delicious meals.

The varied nature of the plan—and variety is the spice of life—makes the point that there are no single *perfect foods*. You hear about magic foods—kale or blueberries or pomegranate juice—but taken on their own, they don't provide everything you need. Sure, there are plenty of superfoods, nutrient-dense produce, grains, and fish that are high in certain essential vitamins, minerals, and antioxidants. But you have to eat a wide variety of whole foods to really benefit from what they have to offer nutritionally. As you'll learn in Chapter 11, nutrients work best in combinations.

As Chris said, you may have to learn to cook or brush up your skills in the kitchen. I don't advocate fancy chef techniques, which is why there are no difficult recipes in the book. (Heck, if you *want* to become a master behind the stove, I'm all for it.) Good quality, fresh food needs very little manipulation to taste good. Basic skills like boiling water, chopping, steaming, sautéing, grilling, and roasting are all that's needed. Cooking is as easy as following directions—treat yourself to a basic book of healthy recipes and try them. The Internet is also a rich source of ideas. Dive in.

A huge number of us could afford to lose some weight. Those with bellies simply have to. Setting a goal and being serious about weight loss is essential. For some of you, an interim goal will be as far ahead as you can think. But I hope that many of you will choose to go all the way to your ideal, permanent weight. Get below a BMI of 25. That is the most crucial target. But an even better goal is to get back to what was probably your best you, what you weighed when you were twenty-two. Get back to your best *you—when you actually looked and felt great.* Maybe you will want to lose in stages, but I hope you always have the big goal in mind. Meanwhile, Chris has some suggestions for less ambitious goals. Pick a goal; that's the main thing. Then make up your mind to meet it.

Here are the *Thinner This Year* eating plan basics.

Eat Significantly Fewer Calories

One of the simple reasons we are fatter today than we were thirty years ago is that we eat about 20 percent more than our parents probably did, often without realizing it. Take a look at the calorie consumption chart on page 99. It provides a guideline on how much you should eat to *maintain* the recommended healthy weight depending on your age, gender, and activity level. It's not perfect, believe me, but it does give you some reasonable context. Find where you fall because the range tells you a bit about why you're overweight.

The calorie guide is also in sync with the eating guidelines presented here, which are designed for an active person. That means you don't really have to do calorie counting as much as you just have to be fully present and notice how much good food you are doling onto your plate. In our consistently overbooked daily lives—often fully packed with time spent sitting and not moving behind a computer or phone, or in front of a TV, even a steering wheel—we EAT. Mindless eating has a clear link to weight gain and has to stop. You know how easily you can finish off a bag of chips or cookies without realizing it. Plan meals, don't multitask while eating, and enjoy your food by paying attention to it.

Now what is interesting about this plan is its unfairness. As you get older, you can't eat as much as you did when you were younger, no matter what. Thankfully, the difference is a relatively small one. And there's more good news: Notice the bump you get for being moderately active or active, as opposed to sedentary. The spread for men is a whopping six hundred calories a day; for women, four hundred. Over time, as your metabolism improves, you might even do better than that. Here's how the numbers on the chart shake out in real life. If you want to stop gaining weight—the one or two pounds a year you put on after age twenty-five that is the American norm today—you have to cut back roughly 20 percent from what you've probably been eating. For a moderately active man in his fifties or sixties, it might mean eating 2,200 calories a day to maintain weight, and for the same age woman it might mean sticking closer to 1,800 calories per day. Depending on what you're eating now, that probably means knocking off between three hundred and five hundred calories to reach those daily maintenance numbers.

One size does not fit all, however. You have to experiment with how much you need to cut and how much you need to exercise, perhaps with professional help. For those who need to lose weight beyond what would normally have been gained since college days, say from fifteen up to twenty-five pounds, you probably have to cut back a full third, at least for a while until you hit your goal weight. That adds up to knocking off a bit more, about five hundred to seven hundred calories per day because you've likely been eating more than the person who has just been adding a pound or two a year.

Admittedly, losing weight is hard work, but keeping it off is much more challenging and much more important. Large national studies including the National Weight Control Registry have demonstrated that most successful weight losers—meaning the ones who both lose weight and keep it off—have cut calories by the five hundred to seven hundred calories a day we recommend. That seems to be the sweet spot for long-term permanent weight loss, *if*, that is, you pair it with a 300–500 calorie-burn-a-day exercise habit to produce *real and substantial* weight loss within a reasonable time. One pound a week—week in and week out—is a healthy miracle. The real goal is to *lose this weight forever.*

Those of you who are seriously overweight, more than thirty pounds, may have to cut back even more aggressively. If you are such a man and typically consume around 3,000 calories or more per day, and are inactive, cut 1,000 calories from your diet to get to 2,000, start exercising, and the scale will go down. If you're a fifty-something woman in a similar position, slash about the same 1,000 calories a day (from 2,600 to 1,800 to 1,600) along with a regular exercise program. It seems aggressive, but it's doable if you make smart food choices. A combined calorie reduction of 1,000 calories a day is a glorious 6,000 calories a week. That will lose you almost *two pounds a week,* which is acceptable for someone who is very overweight (or obese). Once you hit your goal, you can return to maintenance eating—2,200 for men, 1,800 for women.

Success at cutting calories is in great part a matter of choosing foods with a lot of water and fiber content and therefore more "volume"—exactly what produce has going for it. These foods make you feel fuller longer than Dead Foods that don't have much fiber or water like high-sugar donuts and starchy fries. Even if you ate the same volume of foods from the food list I offer later in this chapter as you had been consuming when you were dining on the Mountain, you would still be eating many fewer calories than before. That's one of the beauties of this plan. Take note of the low caloric density of most nutrient-rich foods. The foods that are best for you generally have the fewest calories. It is a deep win-win situation.

**Recommended Daily Calorie Consumption
by Gender and Physical Activity Level**

Age	Males			Females		
	Sedentary	Moderately Active	Active	Sedentary	Moderately Active	Active
41–45	2,200	2,600	2,800	1,800	2,000	2,200
46–50	2,200	2,400	2,800	1,800	2,000	2,200
51–55	2,200	2,400	2,800	1,600	1,800	2,200
56–60	2,200	2,400	2,600	1,600	1,800	2,200
61–65	2,000	2,200	2,400	1,600	1,800	2,000

Adapted from 2010 Dietary Guidelines for Americans/Institute of Medicine

It's also a matter of portion control. Portions have gotten ridiculous—at restaurants and at home. Take bagels, for example. About twenty years ago, the average bagel was three inches in diameter and about 140 calories. That's fairly reasonable. Today the average bagel shop or grocery store offering is about five or six inches in diameter and about 350 calories. Food inflation is everywhere. You see it in pizza parlor slices, movie house popcorn, chicken Caesar salads, bottles of soda, and even coffee. We have to reframe our idea of what a portion is. You might be surprised at first when you actually see the quantities I suggest—they will likely seem much smaller than you're used to. You have to adjust both your eyes *and* your brain. Once you do that, the need to fuss over calories is eliminated.

Eat out less often. When you do, shoo the breadbasket away *before* the server places it on the table. Choose the same kinds of whole foods as you would at home—start with a green salad with balsamic vinegar instead of a creamy dressing, and then order a piece of grilled salmon with lentils or brown rice. Studies have shown that if you start a meal with a salad or a clear soup, you eat less. Skip dessert. When the main course comes, push at least a third of the food—and in most restaurants, a half—to the side of the plate. Then take it home for tomorrow's dinner. Another handy tip to control portions is to check out the restaurant's menu online before you leave the house, and choose your food beforehand so you won't be tempted by specials and extras when you get there.

Eliminate Dead Food

We've said this before and, believe me, we'll say it again: More than half of our diet is composed of Dead Food. The crowning glory (or should I say gory) of the Mountain of Slop and Despair is the astonishing amount of food that is cheap, calorie dense, addictive, and almost nutrient-free. It comes in three sometimes overlapping categories: filler, processed foods, and fast foods.

Filler includes refined grains such as white or refined wheat flour, white rice, white pasta, and corn products. It includes almost all bread, bagels, chips, crackers, croissants, pancakes, breakfast cereals, muffins, cakes, cookies, snack foods, and pasta. I call this huge category "filler" because that's what it is for most of us: It fills up our plates and us—with calories, not a heck of a lot of nutrition. Filler foods are not inherently poisonous (a cup of white pasta will not kill you), but eating a diet heavily based on these items, as many people do, is no good over the long haul.

The *processed food* category is huge, comprising some 80 percent of the food in the middle of your supermarket except for the spice, dried and canned bean, and pasta aisles (and a few cereals are winners, too—look for oatmeal or whole-grain, fiber-rich, no-sugar brands). Center aisles are filled with packaged goods, from chips and cookies to dry baking mixes to frozen dinners. Frozen entrees, with a few organic exceptions, are of particular concern. Not only are many of them unhealthy (not to mention not very tasty or satisfying), they are completely overpackaged—as bad for the environment as the food is bad for your body.

Fast food: It is possible to eat vaguely healthful foods at fast-food places, but only if you stay clear of French fries, soft drinks, milk shakes, deep-dish pizzas, burritos loaded with sour cream and cheese, triple-decker burgers, griddle cakes, and anything else that can be put in a fry-o-lator or slathered up with mayo or cream sauce.

Keep Your System Going with Steady Fuel

Do not skip meals! Eat regular meals and focus on high-fiber, nutrient-dense foods—whole grains, vegetables, legumes, and lean protein. You will be hungry less often and feel better and more focused throughout your day. Eat these lower glycemic index foods and meals to avoid the dreaded sugar highs and lows. You will find these foods on our master food list later in this chapter. Many Dead Foods—like sodas and refined flour products like white bread and pastries—have a high glycemic index and will punch up your blood sugar temporarily, followed by a more extreme sugar low, the terrible "sugar spikes." One reliable way to avoid sugar spikes is to eat a decent breakfast. When people skip breakfast, they tend to eat more calories throughout the rest of the day. Studies have shown that people who eat breakfast are better able to maintain a healthy body weight versus those who skip it. Breakfast is not only key, it is an easily controllable meal. See Chris's Chapter 6 and the meal plan here for suggestions.

Make Vegetables and Fruit Account for 50 Percent by Volume of Your Diet

Replace Dead Food with vegetables and fruit. For some of you, that is going to be a huge change and a challenge to achieve. Think about it this way: One category of food makes you gain weight and is terrible for you; the other makes you thin and is great for you. That ought to be a no-brainer, but it is not.

As I said earlier, I am neither a vegan nor vegetarian, but if I were going to look at any one dietary component to get the best snapshot of someone's health, it would be vegetable and fruit intake. Vegetables and fruit are big on volume and nutrient-dense and, in general, also wonderfully light on calories. The upshot: You can eat your fill, especially of veggies, with little concern about expending your energy budget. Experiment—try at least one new veggie a week. Check out the local farmers' market in season and ask questions—you'll learn more about produce than you ever dreamed. In other words, if you can make the switch from Dead Food to vegetables and fruit into an adventure, eating fewer calories will more or less take care of itself.

Make the Other 50 Percent Count

So where does the other 50 percent fall? About 20 percent of your diet should come in the form of whole, not processed, grains. There is a world of whole grains to choose from, so you never have to fear getting sick of brown rice. Think amaranth, barley, buckwheat, bulgur, brown rice, farro, millet, and quinoa—and those are just a few examples of what's out there. Read Chris on farro, a major new pleasure in his life.

Another 20 percent should come in the form of lean protein, including legumes and tofu, fish, and some poultry. Cut way back on red meat, no more than once a week or, better yet, once every other week. If you must have red meat, switch to 90 percent lean or, better, chemical-free grass-fed beef. Eliminate processed and cured meats like bologna, bacon, salami, hot dogs, and anything that has been squeezed into a casing like sausage. Although Chris can't resist a dog here and there, I'm not a fan. Most of these items are loaded with saturated fat and calories. Try leaner choices such as turkey, chicken, and some cuts of lamb and pork. In general, eat much smaller portions of all meats—treat it as a side dish to accompany your vegetables, not as the centerpiece of the plate.

The remaining 10 percent is rounded out with low-fat dairy like fortified skim milk and nonfat plain yogurt, and healthy fats. Fat, one of the basic building blocks for your body, makes foods more palatable and more satiating. Pleasure and satisfaction surely count. But fat is also calorie dense (twice as "bad" as carbs). Translation? You absolutely do need fat in your diet but not 35 percent of your dietary intake. As I said earlier, aim for 25 percent, with most of it coming from unsaturated and plant-based sources.

You should—you *must*—eat healthy fats from fish and oils. Some fats are absolutely essential, such as omega-3s and omega-6s. Most of us get enough omega-6s from many of the oils that we consume, but we don't get quite as much omega-3 fats, which is why I am asking you to make it a goal to eat fish at least once or twice a week. Fish such as salmon, sardines, mackerel, and even whitefish are ideal and yummy choices. As for fats—definitely opt for oil over butter, and when using oil, avoid the tropical oils and go for vegetable and nut oils such as olive, soybean, canola, flaxseed, avocado, grapeseed, and walnut.

Sugar should be used sparingly. Unfortunately, it has a way of sneaking into the food supply—it's in everything from ketchup to sugar-sweetened beverages to hamburger rolls to flavored yogurt and often times in the form of high fructose corn syrup. Whole foods like fruit, which contain natural sugar, are fine. Added sugar, however, greatly increases our calorie burden and may be one of the most important contributors to silent weight gain over time. To avoid it, read labels of packaged or processed items because it's jammed into almost all these foods. If you need sugar, and humans do have a natural sweet tooth, control it by adding it yourself like in your coffee or to plain yogurt. It will likely be far less than what food manufacturers routinely put in. Honey, agave, maple syrup, and raw cane sugar are good natural choices, used in moderation.

Let's not forget about herbs and spices—get carried away with them! They add flavor and nutrition with minimal or zero calories. Fresh garlic, parsley, basil, and thyme add perky flavor to foods and are packed with nutrients. Spices like turmeric and cumin are also micro-nutritional powerhouses that can help a simply grilled chicken and turkey breast become that much more exciting. Once again, become a food experimenter like Chris if your idea of seasoning is limited to salt and pepper.

Don't Drink Your Calories

Most people don't realize how many calories beverages contribute to their daily intake. People may forgo the afternoon Snickers, but they are less likely to give up their morning full-fat latte even though it has the same number of calories. Many of us could easily consume 800 calories per day on beverages alone: the morning latte (250 calories), the lunchtime soda (150 calories), your late-day energy drink after the gym (300 calories), and the glass of wine with dinner (150 calories).

Here is the real kicker. Research has shown that calories consumed via beverages are not registered as well by our internal feeding systems. For instance, if we guzzle that morning latte, we are less likely to be "full" compared to eating a bowl of cereal, even though both items have the same number of calories. The drink *does not register*.

Whether your beverage of choice is a Coke, a martini, fruit juice, or a so-called health drink, know that they're full of the extra calories that help pack on the pounds. Colas and other carbonated soft drinks, sports drinks, and mocha-whatevers have zero nutrition and a lot of calories—all of it in the instantly digestible, sugar-spike–causing form of sugar. Even with fruit juice, which does contain nutrients, you are much better off eating the fruit, not drinking the juice. The fiber slows down digestion, which is critical to giving you the sensation of fullness. Diet sodas aren't the answer either because they mimic sweetness, which may prompt a craving for the real thing. Besides, they're loaded with chemicals you can and should live very nicely without.

As for alcohol, not only is it calorie dense (7 kcal/gram, almost as high as fat), it has no satiety factor. For those who can manage it, it is okay to drink with moderation—say, two glasses of red wine a night for men; one glass for women. Drinking at those levels actually has been

Before You Begin: A Clean Slate

Consider purging the junk from your pantry and fridge—this may be tough for some of you. I understand it might be difficult to toss out what seems like perfectly good food. However, it's much more wasteful to fill your body with cookies and cake mix, peanut butter pretzels, crackers, super salty canned soups (some with more than 40 percent of the RDA of sodium *per serving!*), candy, and other items that fall into the Dead Food category. Once you eliminate the bad stuff, you won't be tempted to eat it—and there will be plenty of room for the good food that's going to make you thinner this year.

shown to have some health benefits. Wine or beer should be reserved for savored enjoyment, not as thirst quenchers. There is another reason to cut down on your alcohol consumption: It blows away your resolve. Which is why I'm going to give you this challenge: To kick-start your weight loss and to lose weight, don't drink alcohol at all. After that, if you can control it, have a glass of wine at night every once in a while. If you don't drink now, don't start.

Feeling truly thirsty? Try water, coffee with skim milk, seltzer with lime, tea with lemon and a wee bit of honey—you get the picture.

A Long List of Great Things to Eat

ere's a list of really good food that will become one of your most important tools in terms of changing the way you eat and making the right, balanced choices. Although you can't eat "all you want" off this or any list, these foods pack a wonderful nutrient punch. They're very, very good for you. You still have to eat less, but these foods aren't calorie dense, which makes choosing among them far less stressful than selecting from "low-fat" or "low-calorie" items in the packaged food aisles. You still have to exercise like crazy because it keeps your machinery in shape.

When thinking about using this list, keep in mind the proportions of foods I talked about earlier. Any given meal should be made up of 50 percent produce by volume, 20 percent from grains, 20 percent from protein, and 10 percent coming from dairy and/or some healthy fat. This is a guideline. Some meals might be heavier on produce (a large veggie salad for lunch perhaps), whereas others might be packed with more protein (egg white omelet for breakfast), but at the end of the day—literally—you want to end up with the basic proportions recommended. Also note that the calorie counts given for each food are for 100 grams and not necessarily the serving size indicated, so you might have to do a bit of math. Check out the Quantity Counts sidebar for information about quantities—again this is a tool to help you reorient yourself to new normal portion sizes. These guidelines are also in sync with both the caloric recommendations and the meal suggestions in this chapter. And remember: You still have to exercise!

Quantity Counts

Here's an at-a-glance general guide to how much you should be eating in each category of food. It's been such a long time for many of us since we've actually seen a normal portion size, our understanding of what a serving means is completely out of whack. Familiarizing yourself with what the right portions look like makes it so much easier to get your head around the eating plan—and eliminates the need to count calories.

LEAN PROTEIN
Men: 4–6 ounces per serving; 2 servings a day

Women: 4–5 ounces per serving; 2 servings a day

VEGGIES
Men: 1 cup per serving; 3 servings per day of nonstarchy veggies, 1 serving of starchy veggies per day (peas, lima beans, corn)

Women: 1 cup per serving; 2½–3 servings a day of nonstarchy veggies, 1 serving of starchy veggies per day (peas, lima beans, corn)

FRUIT
Men: 1 cup or 1 piece of hand fruit (apple, pear, peach); 2 servings a day.

Women: 1 cup or 1 piece of hand fruit (apple, pear, peach); 1½ servings a day.

WHOLE GRAINS
Men: 1 slice of whole-grain bread, 1 cup of ready-to-eat cereal, or ½ cup cooked rice or other grain, cooked pasta, or cooked cereal; 3 servings a day.

Women: 1 slice of whole-grain bread, 1 cup of ready-to-eat cereal, or ½ cup cooked rice or other grain, cooked pasta, or cooked cereal; 3 servings a day.

DAIRY (OPTIONAL)
Men: 1 cup of low- or nonfat milk, yogurt, or soymilk, 1½ ounces of natural cheese; 1–2 servings a day.

Women: 1 cup of low- or nonfat milk, yogurt, or soymilk, 1½ ounces of natural cheese; 1–2 servings a day.

FATS
Men: 2 tablespoons per day of healthy oil or fat, which can include nut butters and nuts, and avocado.

Women: 1½ tablespoons per day of healthy oil or fat, which can include nut butters and avocado.

Vegetables and Fruit

(50% of intake)

Vegetables	Nutrients	Caloric Density	Serving Size
Artichoke	Fiber, Antioxidants	53 cal/100 g	1 medium cooked (120 g)
Arugula	Vitamins A & K	25 cal/100 g	½ cup raw (10 g)
Asparagus	Inulin (prebiotic), Vitamin K	22 cal/100 g	½ cup cooked (90 g)
Beets	Antioxidant, Carotenoids, Folate	44 cal/100 g	½ cup cooked (85 g)
Broccoli	Fiber, Vitamins C & K, Carotenoids, Phytochemicals	35 cal/100 g	½ cup cooked (78 g)
Brussels Sprouts	Fiber, Vitamins C & K, Carotenoids, Phytochemicals	36 cal/100 g	½ cup cooked (78 g)
Carrots	Beta-carotene, Vitamin K, Fiber	41 cal/100 g	1 cup raw (128 g)
Cauliflower	Potassium, Riboflavin, Vitamins B_6 & C	25 cal/100 g	1 cup raw (100 g)
Corn	Carotenoids, Fiber, Folate, Niacin	131 cal/100 g	1 cup cooked (141 g)
Garlic	Selenium, Sulfur compounds	149 cal/100 g	1 tsp raw (2.8 g)
Green Beans	Carotenoids, Vitamins C & K	35 cal/100 g	1 cup cooked (125 g)
Kale	Vitamins A, C & K, Calcium, Antioxidants	28 cal/100 g	1 cup cooked (130 g)
Mushrooms	B vitamins, Selenium, Zinc	28 cal/100 g	1 cup cooked (156 g)
Onion	Selenium, Sulfur compounds	40 cal/100 g	1 cup raw (160 g)
Red Cabbage	Fiber, Antioxidants, Carotenoids	29 cal/100 g	½ cup cooked (75 g)
Red, Yellow, Orange Bell Peppers	Beta-carotene, Vitamin C, Soluble Fiber	31 cal/100 g	1 medium raw (119 g)
Sea Vegetables	Fiber, Iodine, Vitamin K, Iron, Calcium, Antioxidants	43 cal/100 g	⅛ cup raw (10 g)

Spinach	Carotenoids, Calcium, Nonheme Iron, Vitamins A, C & K	23 cal/100 g	1 cup raw (30 g)
Summer squash	Magnesium, Potassium, Vitamins A, B_6 & C	16 cal/100 g	1 cup chopped (124 g)
Sweet Potato	Beta-carotene, Vitamin C	92 cal/100 g	1 medium cooked (114 g)
Swiss Chard	Antioxidants, Vitamins A, C & K	19 cal/100 g	1 cup cooked (175 g)
Tomatoes	Lycopene, Vitamin C	18 cal/100 g	1 cup raw (180 g)
Winter Squash	Beta-carotene, Carotenoids, Vitamin C, Fiber	37 cal/100 g	1 cup cooked (205 g)

Fruits	Nutrients	Caloric Density	Serving Size
Apples	Fiber, Antioxidants (polyphenols)	52 cal/100 g	1 medium (182 g)
Avocado	Carotenoids, Monounsaturated Fat, Vitamin E	160 cal/100 g	1 medium (201 g)
Banana	Potassium, Fiber	89 cal/100 g	1 medium (118 g)
Blackberries	Fiber, Potassium, Antioxidants	43 cal/100 g	1 cup (144 g)
Blueberries	Vitamin C, Fiber, Antioxidants	57 cal/100 g	1 cup (148 g)
Cantaloupe	Vitamin C, Beta-carotene, Fiber	34 cal/100 g	1 cup diced (156 g)
Cranberries	Antioxidant Phytonutrients, Vitamin C	46 cal/100 g	1 cup (100 g)
Figs	Calcium, Potassium	107 cal/100 g	1 cup dried (259 g)
Grapes	Antioxidant (Resveratrol), Manganese, Vitamin K	69 cal/100 g	1 cup (151 g)
Guava	Vitamin C, Lycopene	68 cal/100 g	1 medium (55 g)
Kiwi	Vitamin C, Fiber	61 cal/100 g	1 fruit (2" dia) (69 g)
Lemons/Limes	Vitamin C	29 cal/100 g	1 fruit (58 g)
Mango	Vitamins A, B_6, C	65 cal/100 g	1 fruit (207 g)

Oranges	Vitamin C, Potassium	49 cal/100 g	1 fruit (140 g)
Peach	Niacin, Potassium, Vitamins A & C	39 cal/100 g	1 medium fruit (100 g)
Pink Grapefruit	Lycopene, Vitamin C	42 cal/100 g	½ fruit (4" dia) (123 g)
Plums	Vitamin C, Antioxidants	46 cal/100 g	1 fruit (2" dia)
Pomegranate	Potassium, Phosphorus, Antioxidants	83 cal/100 g	1 fruit (4" dia) (282 g)
Prunes	Vitamin A, Fiber, Potassium	107 cal/100 g	1 cup (248 g)
Raspberries	Fiber, Potassium, Antioxidants	52 cal/100 g	1 cup (123 g)
Strawberries	Vitamin C, Fiber, Potassium, Antioxidants	32 cal/100 g	1 cup (144 g)
Watermelon	Beta-carotene, Vitamin C, Potassium	30 cal/100 g	1 cup (152 g)

Whole Grains
(20% of intake)

Whole Grains	Nutrients	Caloric Density	Serving Size
Barley	Fiber, Beta-glucans	123 cal/100 g	1 cup (157 g)
Brown Rice	Fiber, Selenium, B Vitamins, Gluten-free, Magnesium Manganese, Antioxidants	112 cal/100 g	1 cup (195 g)
Buckwheat	Fiber, Antioxidants	92 cal/100 g	1 cup (168 g)
Farro	Fiber, Protein, Magnesium	373 cal/100 g	½ cup cooked (54 g)
Oatmeal	Fiber (Beta-glucans)	71 cal/100 g	1 cup (234 g)
Quinoa	Protein, Fiber, Magnesium	120 cal/100 g	1 cup (185 g)
Spelt	Fiber, Niacin	127 cal/100 g	1 cup (194 g)
Whole-Grain Bread	Fiber (Beta-glucans)	247 cal/100 g	1 slice (28 g)
Whole-Grain Cereals	Fiber (Beta-glucans)	367 cal/100 g	1 cup (Cheerios) (28 g)
Whole-Wheat Pasta	Fiber, Selenium, B Vitamins, Magnesium, Manganese, Antioxidants	124 cal/100 g	1 cup (140 g)

Fish, Animal, and Vegetable Protein
(20% of intake)

Seafood	Nutrients	Caloric Density	Serving Size
Salmon	Protein, Omega-3 Fatty Acids	231 cal/100 g	3 oz (85 g)
Sardines	Vitamin D, Vitamin B_{12}, Omega-3 Fatty Acids, Protein	208 cal/100 g	1 can in oil (3.75 oz)
Shellfish (Shrimp, Scallops, Lobster)	Protein, Omega-3 Fatty Acids, Vitamin B_{12}	119 cal/100 g	3 oz (85 g)
Tuna	Protein, Omega-3 Fatty Acids	130 cal/100 g	3 oz (85 g)
White Fish (Cod, Halibut, Haddock)	Protein, Omega-3 Fatty Acids, Vitamin B_{12}, Niacin	111 cal/100 g	3 oz (85 g)

Animal Protein	Nutrients	Caloric Density	Serving Size
Buffalo	Protein, Vitamin B_{12}, Iron	113 cal/100 g	3 oz (85 g)
Chicken (Skinless, White Meat)	Protein, Niacin, Zinc, Selenium	148 cal/100 g	½ breast (98 g)
Grass-fed Beef (Sirloin, Tenderloin, Steak)	Protein, Vitamin B_{12}, Selenium, Zinc, Iron, Phosphorus	219 cal/100 g	3 oz (85 g)
Lamb	Protein, Vitamin B_{12}	192 cal/100 g	3 oz (85 g)
Turkey (Skinless, White Meat)	Protein, Niacin, Zinc, Selenium	135 cal/100 g	3 oz (85 g)
Venison	Protein, Vitamin B_{12}, Iron	149 cal/100 g	3 oz (85 g)

Vegetable Protein	Nutrients	Caloric Density	Serving Size
Black Beans	Fiber, Protein, Folate	132 cal/100 g	1 cup (172 g)
Garbanzo Beans	Fiber, Protein, Folate	138 cal/100 g	1 cup (158 g)
Kidney Beans	Fiber, Protein, Folate	82 cal/100 g	1 cup (256 g)
Lentils	Protein, Iron, Fiber	114 cal/100 g	1 cup (198 g)

Pinto Beans	Insoluble Fiber, Protein, Folate	114 cal/100 g	1 cup (277 g)
Soybeans	Protein, Iron, Fiber, Phytoestrogens	122 cal/100 g	1 cup (155 g)
Tofu	Protein, Iron, Phytoestrogens	145 cal/100 g	½ cup (126 g)

Eggs & Low-Fat Dairy	Nutrients	Caloric Density	Serving Size
1% Cottage Cheese	Protein, Calcium, Vitamin D	72 cal/100 g	1 cup (226 g)
Eggs	Protein, Choline	144 cal/100 g	1 large (50 g)
Feta Cheese	Calcium, Protein, Riboflavin, Vitamin B$_{12}$	263 cal/100 g	1 ounce (28 g)
Yogurt (low-fat, plain)	Protein, Calcium, Vitamin D, Probiotics (depending on brand)	63 cal/100 g	1 cup (245 g)

Nuts, Seeds, and Oils
(consume in moderation)

Nuts, Seeds, & Oils	Nutrients	Caloric Density	Serving Size
Almonds	Monounsaturated Fat, Vitamin E, Manganese	575 cal/100 g	1 oz (28.5 g)
Cashews	Magnesium, Copper Monounsaturated Fat	553 cal/100 g	1 oz (28.5 g)
Flaxseeds	Omega-3 Fatty Acids, Fiber, Manganese	534 cal/100 g	1 tbsp (10 g)
Oil (Olive, Canola, Grapeseed)	Monounsaturated Fat, Polyphenols	884 cal/100 g	1 tbsp (13.5 g)
Peanuts	Monounsaturated Fat, Niacin, Folate, Protein	567 cal/100 g	1 oz (28.5 g)
Pistachios	Thiamin, Vitamin B$_6$	557 cal/100 g	1 oz (28.3 g)
Pumpkin Seeds	Magnesium, Fiber	559 cal/100 g	1 oz (28.5 g)
Walnuts	Omega-3 Fatty Acids, Phenols	654 cal/100 g	1 oz (28.5 g)

Beverages
(those with calories, consume with moderation)

Beverages	Nutrients	Caloric Density	Serving Size
Water	Water	0 cal/100 g	8 fl oz
Black Tea	Antioxidants	0 cal/100 g	8 fl oz
Green Tea	Antioxidants	0 cal/100 g	8 fl oz
1% or Fat-Free Milk	Protein, Calcium, Vitamin D	42 cal/100 g	1 cup (244 g)
Fortified Soy Milk (plain)	Protein, Calcium, Vitamin D, Phytoestrogens	41 cal/100 g	1 cup (242 g)
Cranberry Juice	Antioxidants	54 cal/100 g	1 cup (253 g)
Pomegranate Juice	Antioxidants	54 cal/100 g	1 cup (249 g)
Red Wine (in moderation)	Antioxidants	83 cal/100 g	5 fl oz (147 g)
Grape Juice	Antioxidants	60 cal/100 g	1 cup (253 g)

Spices
(use at will!)

Spices	Nutrients
Basil	Antioxidants, Vitamin K
Chili Powder	Capsaicin
Cinnamon	Antioxidants, Manganese
Cloves	Antioxidants
Dill	Antioxidants (Flavonoids)
Ginger	Gingerols
Mint	Perillyl alcohol
Parsley	Antioxidants (Flavonoids), Vitamin K
Rosemary	Antioxidants (Flavonoids)
Sage	Antioxidants (Flavonoids)
Thyme	Antioxidants (Flavonoids)
Tumeric	Curcumin

Two Weeks and Fourteen Good Meals

To get you started, I've outlined fourteen days of breakfast, lunch, and dinners, along with several snack suggestions. These meals have some variation in quantity; men and very active people can eat a bit more. If you follow what's outlined here to the letter, you will be eating a fairly aggressive calorie-reduced plan. In that case, think of it as a kickstart to your weight loss effort. Once you have reached your goal weight, you can eat a bit more food to maintain the weight. That may mean adding another two hundred calories to your daily intake, which means an extra ounce of fish, a bigger salad, an extra half cup of grains or beans, and maybe an extra piece of fruit per day.

The key to changing the way you eat and maintaining those changes is to find what works for you. This is highly personal, and you have to craft your own solutions, almost every time. You won't be able to sustain any changes you make unless you feel satisfied and enjoy the food you are eating. If you don't like the nutty flavor of quinoa, replace it with whatever whole grain you like best. You don't like fish, fine; you are missing out, but include whatever lean protein you want in its place including tofu or beans. Each meal plan also includes two snacks—one at mid-morning and one in the afternoon. Therefore, the plan was also written to give you an idea of how your new meals based on whole foods should look.

Fats to Avoid

Butter
Milk fat
Beef fat (tallow, suet)
Chicken fat
Pork fat (lard)
Stick margarine
Shortening
Partially hydrogenated oil

DAY 1 MENU

Breakfast

1 cup oatmeal made with water, ½ cup blueberries; medium (7-inch) banana; coffee with ½ cup nonfat milk

Lunch

Arugula salad: 3 cups arugula, ½ cup chopped tomato, 2 tablespoons shredded Parmesan, 1 tablespoon olive oil, ¼ lemon squeezed, 3 ounces rotisserie chicken breast; 1 4-inch whole wheat pita with 2 tablespoons hummus; 8-ounce glass unsweetened iced tea

Dinner

4–6 ounces salmon baked with 1 cup cooked baby spinach and ½ cup tomato sauce; ½ cup steamed broccoli with 1 teaspoon olive oil; ¾ cup quinoa with mushrooms and onion; 12-ounce glass sparkling water or seltzer with lemon wedge

DAY 2 MENU

Breakfast

One 6-ounce low-fat vanilla Greek yogurt; ½ cup sliced strawberries; 1 piece dry whole-wheat toast with 1 teaspoon trans-fat–free olive oil–based spread; coffee with ½ cup nonfat milk

Lunch

2 cups barley soup with mushrooms and kale; 12 ounces unsweetened iced tea

Dinner

4–6-ounces 99 percent lean all-white-meat turkey burger (no bun) with 1 slice low-fat Swiss cheese; 1 cup steamed green beans with 1 teaspoon olive oil; 1 cup whole-wheat couscous; 1½ cups mixed green salad with 2 ounces low-fat balsamic vinaigrette; 12 ounce glass sparkling water or seltzer with lemon wedge

DAY 3: VEGETARIAN MENU

Breakfast

Mixed berry smoothie: 1 6-ounce low-fat vanilla Greek yogurt, 1 cup sliced strawberries, ½ cup blueberries, one 7-inch banana, ½ cup nonfat milk

Lunch

Chef's salad: 3 cups mixed greens, 1 cup cherry tomatoes, ½ cup chopped carrots, ¼ sliced avocado, 2 tablespoons shredded Parmesan, ½ cup garbanzo beans; 1 tablespoon olive oil

Dinner

Vegetable stir-fry: 1 cup broccoli, 1 cup sliced white mushrooms, and ½ cup edamame sautéed with 1 tablespoon olive oil and 3 tablespoons soy sauce; 1 cup steamed brown rice; 12 ounces water or seltzer with lemon

---

DAY 4 MENU

Breakfast

Half a grapefruit with cinnamon broiled for 1 minute; egg white omelet (3 eggs) filled with a handful of chopped fresh baby spinach; 1 slice whole-grain toast with 1 teaspoon olive oil spread; coffee with ½ cup nonfat milk, or black tea

Lunch

Pita pizza: Top a 4-inch whole-wheat pita with ¼ cup plain hummus, 3–4 thin slices of tomato, and 3–4 thin slices of zucchini. Bake at 350°F for 6–7 minutes and top with 2–3 basil leaves sliced into thin ribbons; ambrosia salad of one small banana sliced and combined with ½ cup mandarin orange slices (drained and rinsed if from a can) and 1 teaspoon coconut flakes; 12 ounces unsweetened iced tea or seltzer with lime

Dinner

4–6-ounces baked herbed wild Alaskan salmon; ¾ cup cooked green lentils combined with ¼ cup diced carrots and ¼ cup chopped mushrooms; 6–8 asparagus spears roasted with 1 teaspoon olive oil, lemon juice, salt and pepper; water or seltzer with lime

---

DAY 5 MENU

Breakfast

Apple cinnamon oatmeal: 1 cup of quick-cooking oatmeal cooked
with ¼ cup unsweetened apple juice, ¾ cup water, ¼ teaspoon
cinnamon, ¼ cup dried cranberries in a saucepan. Bring to a
simmer; then cover and cook 3 minutes. Let stand 3 minutes
before serving; small navel orange; coffee with ½ cup nonfat
milk, or black tea

Lunch

Tuna and avocado tomato salad: Toss 5 ounces chunk light tuna
with ½ small avocado, cubed, ⅛ teaspoon pepper, ½ tablespoon
freshly chopped dill, 1 tablespoon feta cheese crumbled, and juice
of half a lemon. Scoop out a medium-sized tomato to create a shell
and stuff with tuna mixture and top with feta; 1 cup of red and
green grapes; cup of green tea

Dinner

Tricolor salad: For two servings, microwave 1 cup fresh green
beans, ends trimmed and beans cut in half, for 2 minutes on high.
Drain and rinse 1 15-ounce can black beans. Defrost ½ cup corn or
use kernels from one small ear. Toss beans and corn together
in a bowl with 1 teaspoon Italian seasoning, ¼ cup chopped fresh
cilantro, 2 tablespoons fresh lemon juice, and 1 tablespoon olive
oil, ¼ teaspoon salt, freshly cracked pepper to taste; serve over a
bed of undressed mixed greens; 1 cup your choice mixed berry fruit
salad (blueberries, blackberries, raspberries, strawberries); cup of
green tea

DAY 6 MENU

Breakfast

Banana-citrus parfait: Slice one small banana and layer it with
slices of a small navel orange and top with ¼ cup low-fat granola,
2 tablespoons low-fat plain yogurt, and 1 tablespoon slivered
almonds; coffee with ½ cup nonfat milk, or black tea

Lunch

Pasta primavera: Bring ¼ cup water or vegetable broth to a boil in large skillet. Add 2 cups fresh baby spinach, ½ small zucchini julienne, ¼ cup julienne carrots, and 3 mushrooms sliced. Cook over medium-high heat until tender, about 5 minutes. Stir in 2 tablespoons dried Italian seasoning, ⅔ cup crushed tomatoes, and ¼ cup chickpeas. Simmer until heated through. Meanwhile prepare 3 ounces whole-wheat pasta. Serve pasta and sauce together; 12 ounces unsweetened iced tea

Dinner

Asian-inspired chicken slaw salad: Shred 4–6 ounces broiled or poached skinless, boneless chicken breast into a bowl. Toss with ½ red pepper seeded and sliced thinly, ½ cup shredded carrots, 1 cup shredded Napa cabbage, 1 tablespoon chopped cashews, and ¼ cup mandarin oranges drained and rinsed. Drizzle with 1 tablespoon low-sodium tamari or soy sauce, 1 tablespoon rice wine vinegar, and ½ tablespoon toasted sesame seed oil; toss to coat and serve immediately atop ½ cup steamed brown rice; cup of black tea

DAY 7 MENU

Breakfast

1 cup yellow grits (or farina) with water, drizzled with 1 teaspoon real maple syrup and 1 tablespoon raisins; ½ pink grapefruit; coffee with ½ cup nonfat milk

Lunch

Curried sweet potato: Bake a medium sweet potato and top with ¼ cup plain Greek-style non- or low-fat yogurt with ½ teaspoon curry powder and 2 drops hot sauce. Garnish with squeeze of fresh lime juice; 12 ounces unsweetened iced tea or water

Dinner

4–6 ounces of cod or other white fish broiled with 1 teaspoon olive oil, juice of half a lemon, 1 teaspoon capers, 1 tablespoon freshly chopped dill, freshly cracked pepper; ½ cup quinoa seasoned with ¼ cup freshly chopped parsley; 1 cup steamed broccoli; seltzer with lime

---

DAY 8 MENU

Breakfast
1 slice whole-grain toast with 1 tablespoon sugar-free peanut or almond butter; 1 cup blueberries; coffee with ½ cup nonfat milk

Lunch
The big salad #1: Toss 3 cups mixed baby greens with ¼ cup shredded carrots, ¼ cup diced celery, ¼ cup chopped raw broccoli, 1 tablespoon dried cranberries, 1 ounce crumbled feta, 1 tablespoon chopped nuts of any kind; ½ tablespoon olive oil; 2 tablespoons balsamic vinegar; 12 ounces unsweetened iced tea or seltzer water with lime

Dinner
4–6 ounces turkey cutlet grilled with 1 teaspoon olive oil, sea salt, and freshly ground pepper served with rainbow veggie rice salad: ½ cup brown rice tossed with ¼ cup freshly chopped parsley, 1 cup steamed diced carrots, and 1 cup steamed and halved snap beans; cup of green tea

---

DAY 9 MENU

Breakfast
Orange berry smoothie: 6 ounces low-fat plain Greek yogurt, 1 cup sliced strawberries, ½ cup blueberries, 7-inch banana, ½ cup orange juice: Whir in a blender.

Lunch
Mango turkey pita: 4–6 ounces sliced or diced turkey, 2 large romaine leaves chopped, ½ cup diced mango, tossed with ¼ cup plain low- or nonfat yogurt and ¼ teaspoon curry powder to fill a small whole-wheat pita; 1 small navel orange; cup of green tea

Dinner
4–6 ounces grass-fed sirloin steak grilled and served on a bed of 2–3 cups chopped Swiss chard, steamed with lemon, and 1 small baked sweet potato garnished with 1 tablespoon low-fat Greek-style yogurt; 1 3-ounce glass of red wine (optional)

DAY 10 MENU

Breakfast
Half of a pink grapefruit; 1 cup oatmeal made with water garnished with 1 tablespoon dried cranberries and 1 tablespoon chopped walnuts, ¼ teaspoon cinnamon; coffee with cup nonfat milk

Lunch
Spinach salad: 3 cups baby spinach leaves, 1 large hard-boiled egg chopped, 1 ounce feta cheese crumbled, 1½ tablespoons balsamic vinegar whisked with 1 tablespoon plain hummus; 12 ounces unsweetened iced tea

Dinner
4–6 ounces grilled chicken breast served with pepper medley: Sauté 2 cups of red, orange, yellow, and green peppers with 1 small onion in 1 tablespoon olive oil served over ½ cup yellow grits made with water or low-sodium veggie broth; seltzer with lime

DAY 11 MENU

Breakfast
Citrus Sundae: Combine sections of a small navel orange and ½ pink grapefruit and top with ¼ cup low-fat Greek-style vanilla yogurt and 1 tablespoon slivered almonds; coffee with ½ cup nonfat milk

Lunch
Waldorf lettuce wraps: Fill two large romaine leaves with 4–6 ounces boneless skinless chicken cubed, tossed with ¼ cup low-fat plain yogurt, 1 tablespoon raisins, ½ cup apple diced, 1 tablespoon chopped walnuts; 12 ounces unsweetened iced tea

Dinner

4–6 ounces Alaskan wild-caught salmon poached in a sauté pan with ½ cup veggie broth and ½ cup good dry white wine (the alcohol cooks off), 2 tablespoons fresh dill leaves, 3–4 whole peppercorns uncovered for about 10–12 minutes; serve with 1½ cups roasted halved Brussels sprouts (toss with 1 teaspoon olive oil and roast at 425°F for about 10 minutes) and ½ cup brown rice or bulgur wheat

---

Tip: *Think ahead when cooking grains—make a few days' worth of portions. Cooked grains can be stored in the refrigerator for up to one week.*

DAY 12 MENU

Breakfast

Fruity crepe: Egg white omelet (3 eggs) stuffed with ¼ cup blueberries, ¼ cup sliced strawberries, topped with ¼ teaspoon cinnamon; 1 slice whole-grain toast with 1 teaspoon all-fruit apple butter; coffee with ½ cup nonfat milk

Lunch

Curried shrimp primavera: 4–6 ounces of shrimp tossed with ½ cup steamed chopped broccoli, ½ cup shredded carrots, ½ cup red or orange peppers julienned, 5–6 red seedless grapes, halved, ¼ cup low-fat plain yogurt with ½ teaspoon curry powder; serve chilled; 12 ounces unsweetened iced tea

Dinner

Beans and greens: To make two servings, combine 1½ cups of canned pink or red beans drained and rinsed well, ½ cup low-sodium veggie broth, ½ small onion diced, ¼ teaspoon chopped garlic, and ⅛ teaspoon nutmeg in a deep saucepan. Place 4 cups chopped kale or collard leaves on top of beans and bring to a boil. Cover, reduce heat to low, and simmer slowly until kale or collard is tender, about 15 minutes. Remove from heat and fold in

½ teaspoon olive oil and sea salt, freshly ground black pepper, and Tabasco sauce to taste. Finish with a cup of green tea and a piece of fruit.

Tip: *Rinsing canned beans under cold water for a minute removes 40 percent of the sodium.*

DAY 13 MENU (VEGETARIAN DAY)

Breakfast
Southwest tofu scramble: Sauté ½ small onion diced in 1 teaspoon olive oil until just soft, add 6 ounces light firm or extra-firm tofu crumbled and ½ cup veggie salsa and cook for 2–3 minutes until heated through; add freshly ground pepper to taste

Lunch
Big ol' bowl of chunky veggie soup: Simmer 1½ cups of your favorite veggies (green beans, carrots, peppers, onions, Swiss chard, etc.) diced in 3 cups low-sodium veggie broth with ½ cup chickpeas until heated through and veggies are al dente; medium piece of seasonal fruit; 12 ounces unsweetened iced tea or seltzer with lime

Dinner
Cauliflower-millet mash with tomato sauce (this tastes *better* than mashed potatoes!): For 2 main course servings bring ½ cup millet and 2 cups cauliflower florets to a boil in 3 cups low-sodium chicken broth for about 12 minutes until millet looks fluffy. Remove from heat and let stand 12–15 minutes; then mash until fluffy. Top with ½ cup sugar-free tomato sauce.

Tip: *Easy tomato sauce: Simmer one 28-ounce can crushed tomatoes with 1 tablespoon Italian seasoning, and 1 tablespoon capers in brine until heated through. Will keep refrigerated for one week in a tightly sealed container.*

DAY 14 MENU

Breakfast
Secret smoothie frost: One 7-inch banana cut into chunks, 1 cup frozen or fresh blueberries, 1 handful baby spinach leaves (you won't taste them, promise!), ½ cup cranberry or pomegranate juice, 3–4 ice cubes. Whirl in a blender until smooth.

Lunch
The big salad #2: Toss 3 cups chopped romaine and baby spinach leaves with ¼ cup shredded carrots, ¼ cup shredded zucchini, ½ cup lightly steamed and cooled green beans, 2 dried apricots chopped finely, 1 ounce crumbled feta, 1 tablespoon pistachio nuts chopped, ½ tablespoon olive oil, 2 tablespoons balsamic vinegar, 12 ounces unsweetened iced tea or seltzer water with lime

Dinner
Tropical cod: Top 4- to 6-ounce codfish with 1 teaspoon canola oil, 1 teaspoon flaked coconut, and ½ teaspoon ground almonds; bake for 15 minutes at 350°F or until flaky. Serve with black bean mango salsa: ½ cup black beans tossed with ¼ cup corn kernels, ¼ cup mango diced, dressed with 1 tablespoon red wine vinegar and ½ tablespoon olive oil, sea salt, and pepper to taste; 12 ounces unsweetened iced tea

Smart Snacks

S elect a couple of these snacks as part of your daily plan—one at mid-morning and one at mid-afternoon. Healthy snacks help keep your blood sugar on an even keel, and they stave off hunger so you don't pig out at mealtime—or fall off the wagon completely and eat a cinnamon bun on your way through the train station. Remember too that you can always grab a piece of fruit or a handful of baby carrots as a quick healthy snack.

- 1 100-calorie bag of microwave popcorn
- 3-inch-diameter apple; low-fat mozzarella cheese stick
- 1 cup baby carrots; 3 tablespoons hummus
- 1 7-inch banana; 1 tablespoon all-natural peanut butter
- 1 raw bell pepper sliced; 1 tablespoon low-fat ranch dressing
- 1 medium pear and 1 8-ounce carton of skim milk
- 23 raw almonds
- ¼ cup black beans combined with 1 tablespoon salsa, 1 tablespoon cottage cheese, and ⅓ cup diced avocado; serve with 4 celery stalks
- 1 "large" hard-boiled egg (not more than once a week)
- 1 cup unshelled edamame
- ½ cup pumpkin seeds in shell
- 20 frozen red or green grapes
- 1 vanilla-almond shake: Blend ½ cup skim milk with ½ cup frozen yogurt and 1 drop almond extract
- 1 cup unsweetened applesauce

CHAPTER TEN

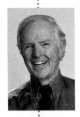

What Do You Say We Drop a Couple of Pounds?

en has given you the deep orchestral themes of the book: eating less, eating right, and exercising more. That is the gravamen (as lawyers like to say), or *center of gravity*, of the book. Then the question arises: How the devil do you actually do it? Jen's diet is your guide to what to eat, but there are still some things to think about. Do you jump in all at once? Do you begin gradually? Do you get a trainer or a friend? Where do you start?

This modest chapter is designed to give you a little practical help with questions like those. Some of this is what they call "small ball" in baseball: you know, stealing bases, running out every ground ball, bunting the runner along. Stuff like that. Small ball wins a surprising number of ball games. Helps here, too. In the end, losing weight—even quite a lot of weight—is mostly a matter of small changes over time. A matter of not taking in a hundred calories here and burning an extra hundred calories there. In a funny way, weight loss is always—as the Duke of Wellington said of his victory at Waterloo—"a close-run thing." Victory may be in the details.

The Conceptual Framework: Small Changes Over Time

One way to get a sense of just how "close-run" this whole business is may be to look at the conceptual framework once again. The way weight goes on throws light on the way it is going to *come off.* And the great message is *small changes over time.* Look at the conceptual framework, and then look at a hypothetical. You'll see what I mean.

The iron rule of weight gain and loss reads like this, *in its entirety*: Eat more calories than you burn and you will gain weight. Burn more calories than you eat and you will lose weight. That's it. Anything else is smoke and mirrors. There are *always* new books and articles saying this rule is not correct, but they are wrong. There are variations and surprises and some tricks, which Jen will tell you about, but the rule is the rule, and there's no way around it.

How come? That's interesting. We are internal combustion machines, with a deeply ingrained *fuel-saving mechanism.* We take on fuel to burn in the engines of our bodies (mostly the billions of mitochondria, as you now know, out in the muscles), but we have a mechanism to *save what we don't use.* As fat. Too bad, you could say. Too bad that we *save* the extra as fat and don't just chuck what's left over at the end of the day. But we were designed for the Darwinian crucible of survival where almost every species and almost every individual died from starvation, not for a world with a McDonald's on every corner. In the crucible, every scrap of energy was too precious to be wasted. Our bodies evolved to save it as fat. It was a miraculous adaptation when you think about it—perfect for the crucible when there was never enough to eat. And lousy for now when there's too much.

How We Got Fat

Now think about this hypothetical. Let's assume that you were in good shape and at your ideal weight, the number Jen talked about, when you were twenty-two (or even thirty). Let's say you weighed

170, if you're a guy; 120 if you're a girl. Doesn't matter. Assume your weight in your twenties had been stable for a while *because you burned every calorie you ate*: roughly 2,500 calories a day for men; 2,000 calories or so for women. You did not gain or lose. Congratulations.

Now assume a tiny, tiny change. You began to eat *ten calories a day more* than you burned. You are out of balance, to the tune of ten lousy calories a day. Much less than a tenth of 1 percent. Big deal.

But watch. That minuscule change will add a pound in one year. It takes an extra 3,500 calories to add a pound of fat. Eat an extra ten calories a day for 365 days, and you're there, just as sure as God made little chocolate-covered raisins. Keep it up for ten years: You gain ten pounds. Twenty-five years: You gain twenty-five pounds. Hey, congratulations! *You're fat!* You did not change your diet *at all* or at least not in a way that anyone would notice. And you're twenty-five pounds overweight. *Yikes!* You can get the same huge change if your metabolism slowed down by 10 calories a day, which it surely did, for most of you, as you got older and less active.

Here's the lesson again: *Tiny changes, over time, make a huge difference. Gradual, steady change—plus time—is the key.* And it works in both directions: for weight gain and for weight loss.

To reverse that gain, you have to make modest changes in the other direction. Not 10 calories a day because you don't have twenty-five years to do it. But something relatively modest. A *serious* change of the kind we're talking about would look like this: Do 300 calories or more a day of exercise. That is fairly easy. That's like forty-five minutes to an hour of exercise. There are good reasons to work out harder and burn closer to 400 calories a day. But even an easy workout can burn 300 to 350 calories a day. Now suppose that, in addition, you drop 300 calories of intake a day. Again, that is not tough at all. That's a couple of soft drinks (or a hard one). That's shifting ever so slightly out of Dead Food and into the Good Stuff. But—taken together over just six days—that's 600 calories a day and 3,600 calories a week. Enough to take off a pound a week. Do that for six months as we suggest and *bingo*: You've lost twenty-five pounds and changed your life. Not quite small ball, on a day-by-day basis, but damn near. And look what you just did for yourself. Nice going.

Know Yourself: Set Rational Goals

As easy as we say that is, it's not. It's hard to hold steady for six months. It's sort of hard to develop an exercise habit and it's *really* hard to quit eating the addictive slop of a lifetime. There is also the fact that the body seems to have mysterious set points and plateaus of resistance at various levels which, for some people more than others, make it hard to follow the simple path we set out. Our suggestion—of twenty-five pounds in six months—may be too much for you. So set another goal, one that's realistic for you. Setting a realistic goal is of the essence.

The only reason to set goals is to *motivate* yourself and keep track. If you set an unrealistic goal—one that makes you want to quit tomorrow—it is not a good goal. We think tough goals are great, just the thing a lot of us need. But if they break your resolve, they're useless. One obvious thing to do—and this is Jen's idea—is to give yourself up to a year to lose that twenty-five pounds instead of six months. I worry that you'll lose interest if you give yourself that much time, but she thinks not. Especially if you're good about keeping a log or journal. Anyhow, there's one easy alternative. Lose as much as twenty-five pounds in a year, and you have still done a hell of a job. Do it our way and it will last forever.

The 7 Percent Solution

Another one that is going to make sense for many is what I call the 7 percent solution. It is a solution that is designed to recognize— a little bit—the brute fact that so many of us put on some weight as we age and have a hell of a time reversing it. This goal "makes peace" with a gain of up to 7 percent, from the time you turned twenty-two, say. Not ideal but maybe realistic, in a useful way. Here's what you do. Figure out your ideal weight (either by going back to what you weighed at twenty-two or going to your BMI of 23–25). Then take 7 percent of that number and add it to your ideal weight. That's your goal. Or at least your initial or interim goal. Do the numbers for you; they may look sane and appealing. They may be a great motivator to make real change without going completely crazy.

Or—especially if you are seriously overweight—think about drop-ping 10 percent of your body weight. That's a huge achievement. A lot less than our twenty-five pounds for most, but an honorable goal and a good motivator. Do the numbers. See if it's right for you, especially as an interim goal.

Caveat

If you are setting a goal that takes you down to a level *above* your ideal weight, watch out for two things. If the goal still puts you at a BMI of 30 or higher—keeps you obese, that is—it has to be an interim goal *at best*. Still being obese (but less so) may be the best you can do for a while, but being obese is still so god-awful that it would be nuts to settle for that for life. Shoot for that in the first six months or year or whatever. And then keep on going. Fight like a steer until you get yourself below a BMI of 30. So important. A BMI of 25 or less would be a lot better.

Now What?

Okay, now you know how it's done—in small increments. And you have a sane and achievable goal; what do you actually do? Do you jump in at the deep end? That is, do you try to give up *all* Dead Food on day one and cut way back on meat and quit drinking and all the other stuff? While jumping into a lunatic exercise program?

Probably not. Frankly, that's what I did and I more or less got away with it. But dietitians and weight loss experts say that's mostly dumb and won't work. Fundamental change of lifestyle habits is hard, hard, hard. Take it a step or two at a time. Except for one thing. Exercise.

Jen and I are of one mind on this one: Start working out six days a week from the get-go, and never stop. I know you're getting sick of hearing this, but it is *so* key. You do not have to work out hard at the outset. Indeed, if you have not exercised for a while (or ever), you should get into it very gradually indeed. But it still makes a world of sense to start the six-days-a-week habit in the beginning, even if you don't do that much on a given day. Do some damn thing every day. It doesn't have to be a heavy workout, but *change into exercise clothes—* that's the minimum—and *do something, six days a week.* Even if the early workouts are puny, you are sending yourself a message every day, which is mysterious but deeply important. That's what makes our system work. No exercise, no success.

Eating: Gradual Changes in the Early Weeks

C hanging the way you *eat*, however, you should probably do a step at a time. It may make sense to go ahead in two-week increments, during each of which you give up one of the rotten foods you love or the family of rotten foods. And hit the most dangerous—to you—first.

Do you know what your worst eating enemies are? You probably do, but just in case, keep a *meticulous food diary* for a few days where you write down everything (this is not the same as the much simpler permanent log we'll talk about later). Write down absolutely everything that goes into your mouth, without fear or favor. Then sit down at the end of a few days and take a look at what you've written. Then look over Jen's meal plan and the Bad Stuff chapters. The answer—the list of enemies—will jump out at you. Write down your own "List of Enemies" and rank them in terms of awfulness. Then pick them off, one at a time, starting at the top. Quit them cold.

For example, see if you're a serious soft drink and fruit juice and sport drink user. Sugary soft drinks are the number-one source of calories in our diet, worse than cake, cookies, and pizza. Worse than anything. So if you're still drinking that stuff (including sugary sports drinks and lots of regular orange juice), make them enemy number one and *quit.* You'll save a ton of calories. (And by the way, *do* get your kids off the stuff. And heaven help us, their schools! Get that stuff *out of their schools!*) Or maybe your little weakness is booze, enormously popular in big fat piggy circles. Or fried food (French fries, calamari, clams, breaded this and that); fried foods are certainly the great Satan for some of you. Or go straight to the top of the Mountain and take on

SoFAs, solid fats and added sugar in prepared foods. Just stop eating almost all the stuff in the center of the supermarket. Great idea. Or ice cream (sorry, Jen). Or, desserts generally. Or—perhaps best of all, if you're into them—all fast foods. If you have a bad fast-food habit, there is no more obvious or deadly an enemy; put that at the top of your list. Or refined flour and sugar in all their dreadful guises. (That happens to be my number-one enemy. I *so* love white bread of all kinds. And butter.)

Sink the Carriers!

A t the outset of World War II, the Japanese made a sneak attack—a preemptive strike—on Pearl Harbor. Putting treachery and rottenness to one side, it wasn't a bad idea from their point of view: Destroy our Pacific Fleet on Day One and go on from there to win the war. Except for one thing. The American carriers got away. They were not at Pearl Harbor that Sunday morning. Six months later, at Midway, the carriers that had slipped away from Pearl destroyed the Japanese fleet. And basically won the war in the Pacific.

Here's the message: When you pick the *first* food or *worst* food to attack in the first two weeks, be sure to pick your most serious enemy. *Sink the carriers?* Do that, and the rest will be doable.

The Bad Carbs Fallacy

Y ears ago, there was a mighty war on eating fat in this country. Reasonable enough, except that it was coupled with the dreadful advice to take up the slack by eating more carbohydrates. It was a disaster. You have to eat plenty of carbs, as you know, but there are good and bad carbs. What happened in the anti-fat wars is that huge numbers of people cut back on fat. And dug in on rotten carbs. Carbs in any form were hot, fats were not. Not a good idea. Swapping out Dead Food works only if you swap *in* Good Food.

Otherwise, don't bother.

Stupid Eating Tricks

When you go out to eat—and are confronted by those monstrous restaurant portions—take your knife or fork and divide your portions in half. Literally push half to one side of your plate. Eat what's left. Chuck the rest. Or take it home for tomorrow's lunch. Or give it to the dog. Whatever. Do not worry about making the server or the chef feel good. Worry about you.

Quit the Clean Plate Club!

The worst and most sinister organization in the country is not the Ku Klux Klan or the American Nazi Party. It is the Clean Plate Club. And your own precious mother is the driving force behind your chapter. I don't know a hell of a lot about your mother, obviously. But she does have one flaw. She is a crazed member and promoter of the dreadful Clean Plate Club. It's going to be hard to make this change, but try it: Everything you leave on your plate is a little victory. See it that way.

Keep a Log

This is different from that meticulous three-day food diary. This is permanent, if you can bear it. It makes a ton of sense to keep at least a summary diary of what you ate and what exercise you did or didn't do every day. Write a couple of lines, every morning. Sailors who keep a good log do not get lost at sea.

Have a Circle of Friends

This is a genius idea . . . maybe the best in the book. Put together a small circle of friends to do this with you. People from your church, the job, the neighborhood. Share your plans and performance. Tell one another *everything*. Help one another out. This is *structure*. This is magic. It's the mammal's gift: Use it.

Eat on Purpose; *Decide* Every Time

The great temptation is to zone out when we eat . . . let our powerful, reptilian brains take over and let 'er rip. Don't do it. Try this instead. At every stinking meal, stop and *think*: What am I doing here? How much am I going to eat? And what? *Decide* every time. It's like saying grace at the beginning of the meal, only you're praying you can eat like a human being for once, not like a slimy crocodile.

Make Up Your Mind

L et me end this odd chapter on a particularly odd note. A friend and I have been studying the surprising number of emails and Facebook comments we get from successful readers of *Younger Next Year* books. People who have really gotten in shape, lost a ton of weight, and so on. We call them the "You changed my life" letters because virtually everyone had some variation of the line, "Hey, man, thanks for writing those books. You changed my life."

But here's a curious thing about them. A surprising number of them contained this casual aside: "Once I made up my mind, it was easy." The writers didn't make a point of it, but those words came up often and usually in those very words: Once I made up my mind, it was easy. As if making up your mind was some separate magical thing. The sheer numbers were impressive. But the idea really had resonance for me because I had had exactly the same experience. I had been fooling around with that fifteen pounds forever. But at last—with the writing of this book—I took a deep breath and really made up my mind. Then it was easy. Huh! What's that all about? I have no idea. But I am struck by it, enough so to mention it here.

All right, there you go: a few tips and one bit of magic, to go with Jen's science. Go for it.

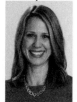

CHAPTER ELEVEN

Nutrients: They Make the Body *Work*

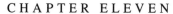

here are places around the world, tragically, where people really are starving in "the old-fashioned way" because there are simply not enough calories to eat. In this country, we have plenty, but we are starving, too. Starving for nutrients. Did you see the movie *Super Size Me* about the guy who ate exclusively at McDonald's for thirty days? He started out a very healthy guy, but by the end of four weeks, he was very sick indeed. He gained weight and his blood pressure and cholesterol levels went through the roof. Few if any of us eat as extremely as that, but just the same, Dead Food wears down your system until it comes to a grinding halt, often prematurely. The combination— too many calories and not enough nutrients—makes us sluggish, fatigued, fat, and eventually sick.

Nutrition is a fast-paced science, and we still don't know quite enough about it to give up completely on eating a broad range of foods. Consider that we've been omnivores for a very long time; it's an evolutionary strategy that has helped us advance in many positive ways. A balanced diet of good food also supplies *essential nutrients*, which means some thirty vitamins and minerals. These nutrients are critical for allowing your body to function properly; they are called *essential* because they *are*. If you don't consume each of them, things start to go terribly wrong, sometimes in funny places: You could go blind, your skin gets scaly, your nails become brittle, and your hair falls out, to name a few unpleasant outcomes. I have to admit that when I was a teenager in high school I'd eat a minimal breakfast and save my lunch money by skipping that meal, and my hair *did* start falling out! Eat right, however, and you will look better, live longer, better, and more effectively because the machine will work the way it was designed to work, efficiently and powerfully. Nutrition is one of the great keys to the good life.

The good news—the *great* news—is that your body is astonishingly resilient and responsive to change, especially when it comes to your diet. Start eating rationally and embark on a solid exercise program and you can make profound changes in the quality of your life in a matter of weeks. Your cholesterol and blood sugar levels can plummet to healthy levels, and that's just the beginning. The longer you do those good things, the better off you will be. So think it over hard and make a serious decision. Be serious with yourself or don't bother; it won't work. And if you are up for a major decision and a major undertaking, make it soon, and begin. The Third Act can be remarkable.

Vitamins and minerals are not energy sources, but they perform thousands of unique functions within the body. They are not separate comestibles; you cannot sit down to eat a plate full of vitamin K and riboflavin, no matter how much you need them. You can get them only by eating nutrient-rich *foods,* especially fruits, vegetables, whole grains, and legumes.

You can't really get them from pills, either, a topic I discuss at length later on. Supplement makers have tapped into the notion that we need nutrients and sell billions of dollars worth of vitamin E, selenium, B complex, or whatever. But frankly—and there will be howls about this from those with a huge financial or emotional stake in the industry—supplements mostly don't work. We love the idea that we can take a fistful of pills and all will be well. With a couple of important exceptions, you simply have to eat good *food* to get effective nutrients. You can take a vitamin C pill and you will get some vitamin C. But vitamin C in an orange is much more powerful and much more effective. Just how much more we don't know, but we do know enough to know that food is far better and more effective than pills, almost every time.

The Myth of Perfect Foods

Here is another important point: Different *good* foods have different *good* nutrients, and you need them all. That's what nature's bounty is all about. Spinach and kale—stars on everyone's lists of super-foods—are loaded with vitamin C, vitamin K, beta-carotene, calcium, lutein, and other antioxidants; spinach is also high in iron and folate and flavonoids that are potent antioxidants. Broccoli is a great source of vitamin C, vitamin K, and fiber, but it's not so hot for the B vitamins and protein. Edamame, or fresh soybeans, offer high fiber and protein. Oatmeal—Chris's and my breakfast standard, especially served with berries—is high in soluble fiber, B vitamins, and iron. Quinoa, which is one of my favorites, is actually a plant and unique among plants (beyond soy) in that it is a complete protein with all nine essential amino acids and is high in iron, phosphorus, and magnesium. Black beans are loaded with fiber, magnesium, and folate and are a good source of healthy carbs and protein.

Skim milk (for dairy consumers) is a great source of calcium, vitamin D, the B vitamins, and protein, and—if you are as concerned with saturated fats as you should be—you'll be relieved to know that it has only trace amounts and not even enough to end up on the food label. Lentils are high in fiber, folate, iron, manganese, and phosphorus and, like black beans, a great source of healthy carbs and protein. Blueberries—another perennial star on lists of superfoods—are high in antioxidants like vitamin C, vitamin K, fiber, and many other things. More protein: Egg whites have zero fat or cholesterol. Egg yolks are high in vitamins B_{12} and A, and they are also a complete protein. Eating eggs once or twice a week, especially if you go with egg whites only some of the time, is a good idea. Kiwi, that weird furry little fruit, is worth getting to know. It has twice the vitamin C of an orange and all the potassium of a banana. Walnuts pack an omega-3 punch! Not a "perfect" food but awfully good—and satisfyingly crunchy, too.

All these foods are great, which is why most of them made it to our good food list on page 107. We want you to eat them. It's well worth going out of your way to eat a lot of them. Yet taken individually they don't have everything you need, which is why it's so important to eat a rainbow of produce and add in protein and whole grains. It's the only way you can be sure, without doing crazy calculations every day, that you're getting the right combination of nutrients. Besides, eating a variety of foods is much more fun than limiting yourself to narrow choices. Think of this plan as a wild adventure—your chance to try lots of new things, as Chris has been doing.

Nutrients and Metabolism

Among the most important things that nutrients do inside your body is enable metabolism to work. They make the process of burning carbs and fat happen. They are key components in hundreds of reactions within the metabolic systems. For example, think of the role of *whole grains* in aerobic metabolism, the burning of carbs or fat with oxygen, our most used metabolic path. Aerobic metabolism relies heavily on nutrients in whole grains to work. Whole grains are chock-full of B vitamins—thiamin, niacin, and riboflavin—all of which are essential microcomponents of enzymes in your metabolic pathways. No details on this one, but trust me: If you are low on whole grains, you will almost certainly be low on most B vitamins. And if you are low on B vitamins, your metabolism will slow down and *you* will slow down.

Nutrients as "Structure"

In addition to being *enablers* or catalysts, nutrients also help to *form structures*. For example, magnesium, phosphorus, and calcium become essential parts of your bones. And I don't mean they help a little; they are *essential to the framework*. No magnesium, phosphorus, and calcium and your bones become weak, they get thinner, they collapse. It's as simple as that.

These are not isolated instances, by a long shot. They are typical of thousands of critical reactions and processes in which nutrients are essential. Think about this: For almost *every substance in our body*, there is an essential nutrient that is needed to make it work right. If we don't have enough of any one of them, a critical piece is missing, and things *don't work*. Worse than "don't work," they fall apart.

What Key Nutrients Do

To bring the nutrients story home, I thought it might make sense to go into real depth on a handful of them. Then keep in mind that this is just a small part of the story, and there are forty more that we have not touched. The point? Nutrients matter much, much more than most of us can begin to comprehend. Eat a wide variety of wholesome fresh food and you will get the right mix of nutrients.

Iron

Iron is one of the most abundant metals on earth and a critically essential element in your body. You only can get it from nutritious food. If you don't, you pay a price. Iron deficiency is the number-one micronutrient deficiency in the world. It affects as much as 80 percent of the world's population. Iron is important because it is a critical element in hemoglobin. Hemoglobin is the stuff in red blood cells that carries oxygen from your lungs to your heart and working muscles. Oxygen is the "fire" of your life, in the mitochondria. Remember, oxygen is needed to burn fats and the majority of carbohydrates. Iron, therefore, is a key part of your metabolism and your ability to produce energy. No iron, no hemoglobin. No hemoglobin, no fires in the mitochondria and no movement. And even beyond the hemoglobin, iron is part of important enzymes within your mitochondria that allow ATP to be formed after the combustion of carbs and protein. You can perhaps imagine how critically tied iron is to staving off fatigue, keeping you alert, and promoting exercise performance. Iron brings the oxygen to help burn fuel and also catalyzes the final steps in making those carbs and proteins turn into energy the body can use.

Beyond carrying oxygen to our tissues and promoting energy metabolism, iron plays several other major roles. Iron is required for the enzyme that synthesizes estrogen. It helps to metabolize drugs and alcohol, substances that your body needs to quickly detoxify; iron is the drinker's friend. It is involved in the synthesis of brain neurotransmitters such as serotonin, dopamine, and epinephrine (adrenaline). Here you can see the link between iron deficiency and depression. In kids, it is of particular concern because it is critical in cognitive development, failures that may not be reversible. The immune system also relies on iron for immune cells that fight infection. If iron stores are low, the ability to fight off infection plummets.

To get iron, you have to eat iron-rich foods. The obvious ones, which you probably know about, are meat, poultry, and seafood. Red meat is a particularly good source of hemoglobin. In meat, the iron is bound to "heme" in the hemoglobin, and the heme structure allows for increased absorption and bioavailability of iron once it is consumed.

You can also get iron from plant sources. To the annoyance of vegetarians (and to me), iron is found in a different form in plants, where there is no heme, so it is much less bioavailable. The best plant sources of iron include lentils, beans, leafy vegetables such as spinach, tofu, chickpeas, quinoa, fortified bread, and fortified cereals. You should eat a variety of plants to get the iron that you need if you are on an all plant-based diet.

Iron is important, but the requirements are not difficult to achieve. The iron requirement for women drops to 8 mg/day after menopause (no iron losses from menstruation)—the same requirement needed by men. Iron is a heavy metal and in high doses increases oxidative stress and inflammation, which you'll read about later in this chapter. Bad business. Luckily our bodies are equipped with an elaborate system to moderate our absorption of iron, but if you must take iron supplements (which is generally unnecessary), a physician should monitor your intake. Most adults who are eating a balanced diet get enough iron.

Calcium

Calcium's number-one role is to provide structure. Ninety-nine percent of the calcium we take in goes to the makeup of bones and teeth. It supports their hardness and is an integral part of their architecture. Without ample calcium, our bones and teeth get soft and—with age—porous, fragile, and brittle. That is, we become more prone to osteoporosis.

Maintaining bone strength is terribly important and not totally easy. By the age of thirty we have reached our peak bone mass. After that, your bones will never be as big or as strong again. Depending on how much you exercise, especially strength train (discussed in the exercise section), you lose bone mass steadily every year. It is particularly serious for women after menopause, but for men, too. Osteoporosis leads to more than 1.5 million fractures each year in this country, and their consequences can be grave. After age sixty, there is a 50 percent chance that a woman who falls and breaks her hip—a very common injury—will never walk unaided again.

Calcium is also key to muscle contraction, cell signaling, and the transmission of signals from your brain to the rest of your body. Furthermore, calcium is used to help blood vessels move blood throughout the body and to help release hormones and enzymes that affect almost every function in the body. With muscles, the actual contraction is initiated when calcium binds directly to tiny muscle filaments to enable a cycle that generates force. This happens thousands of times per second. No calcium, no muscle contractions. You should know that it is so critical, that your body cannibalizes itself if you do not eat enough—that is, it takes calcium out of your bones and teeth to use everywhere else it is needed. You do not want that to happen. Strength training is an excellent defense against this decay, although consuming enough calcium in your diet along with strength training is even better.

The great food sources of calcium are dairy products. You can get it from plant sources as well including tofu, fortified orange juice, broccoli, kale, collard greens, almonds, quinoa, and beans. But it is still hard to get enough without some dairy. Trouble is, of course, many dairy products are high in saturated fat and cholesterol except for nonfat products. Diets high in cheese, whole milk, and ice cream have an impact on blood lipids, namely your LDL, or "bad cholesterol," and triglycerides. This puts people at added risk for heart disease and other ailments. They are also calorically dense; as Chris says, they make you fat. That's why I am not against low-fat dairy products like skim milk and low-fat yogurt. In one eight-ounce glass of skim milk or a six-ounce cup of yogurt, you get 300 mg of calcium. Cheese is even better: In just two ounces of Swiss cheese, you get 530 mg! Think of a little feta on your salad—lots of taste without much fat.

You'll eat many calcium-rich foods if you follow our eating plan. That means including plenty of alternative sources of calcium on your plate. However, if you want to eliminate dairy completely, you will likely need a calcium supplement of some sort, especially if you are over the age of fifty or sixty. This is another exception to my no supplements rule, which you'll read more about later in this chapter, but a necessary one.

Antioxidants and Free Radicals

I want to talk about the great war that goes on inside your body—the war that we have touched upon with inflammation and disease—the war between free radicals and antioxidants. Because one side in that war, the antioxidants, is trying to save your life, and antioxidants can be recruited only by eating Good Stuff, whereas free radicals mostly destroy and are produced in response to eating Bad Stuff.

A free radical is a molecule that is missing a critical "piece" (an electron, to be precise), and its great purpose in life is to find and devour an electron from another molecule to make itself stable again. Good for the free radical, and extremely bad for the victim molecule and for your body in general. In a desperate effort to make itself whole, a free radical tears lots of other things apart. When it grabs a vulnerable piece from, say, a cell membrane or part of your DNA, they get seriously damaged. Cells quit working. Signals don't work. Pathways are inhibited and don't produce energy.

A favorite target of free radicals is your mitochondria. When they are damaged, we don't metabolize foods for energy as well. In general this process—of free radicals wandering around and biting off chunks of other cells—is called *oxidative stress*. Free radicals and oxidative stress have been implicated in everything from aging and cognitive decline to cancer, diabetes, and cardiovascular disease. Free radicals are produced during inflammation. Oxidative stress is bad. Free radicals do not directly cause cancer and heart disease and adult-onset diabetes. But they are an essential part of the process. Big time. They are your sworn enemy.

So where do these devils come from? All over. They can be produced in response to environmental pollution in the air that we breathe and via ultraviolet (UV) exposure. Mostly they come from our own most basic functions, a by-product of breathing. When we take in oxygen, pass it into the blood, and burn it with carbohydrates and fat in aerobic metabolism, an unavoidable by-product of the process is free radicals. Of all the millions of molecules of oxygen that we inhale and consume in the metabolic process, about 4–8 percent of them end up as free radicals. We are constantly producing them.

Now that I have just ranted about how awful free radicals are, let me clarify that life is complicated and not all free radicals are bad. They also have a positive role in the operation of the immune system, for example. Small numbers of free radicals fight off foreign invaders and clear debris. Large numbers cause oxidative stress, which is why we are so nuts about antioxidants. Antioxidants eat free radicals and balance "stress" and inflammation. And thus they fight cancer, heart disease, adult-onset diabetes, and Lord knows what else.

A diet high in antioxidants provides your first line of defense against free radicals because the antioxidant donates what is missing and the free radical is no longer radical. What remains of the antioxidant that donated a piece of itself is simply recycled in many cases.

Antioxidants are found in foods in natural combinations and often in conjunction with other antioxidants that work together. You can't buy them in a bottle or get enough of them from a single source. Different antioxidant foods offer different benefits depending on which antioxidants they contain. Vitamin E is a fat-soluble vitamin and found in nuts and oils (that makes sense because these are sources of healthy fats) and is a potent antioxidant in the membrane of your cells. Vitamin C, in contrast, is a water-soluble vitamin and found in high concentrations in fruits such as oranges, cantaloupe, and strawberries. Vitamin C works best on the inside of your cells—in the aqueous environment. Beta-carotene and other carotenoids are also antioxidants and help to form vitamin A.

Carrots and kale are great sources of beta-carotene. Spinach is high in another carotenoid called lutein. Don't skimp on carotenoids because they are beneficial in combating damage to your eyes and brain. The point: You must have a variety of foods that are high in different types of antioxidants to have it all work. Think green tea, which is high in catechins; flavonoids are found in berries, coffee, and chocolate; tomatoes are high in lycopene; and red wine is high in resveratrol—the list goes on and on, and more are constantly being discovered.

Supplements: A Few Good Ones and a Lot of Expensive Junk!

I f I really wanted to make some money in the nutrition business, I would not be writing this lifestyle book with Chris or endlessly writing grants to fund research projects. I would be making supplements. Seriously. According to the *Nutrition Business Journal*, the dietary supplement market was $28 billion in 2011. Half of the U.S. population takes some form of dietary supplement, and the percentage increases the older we get. It is a mega business in this country. Sure, a multivitamin has *some* merit, but there are millions, including some of my closest family members, who take all sorts of other things, and it drives me bonkers. Year after year, I continue to be stunned that Americans have not caught on to what I see as basically a scam.

By and large, supplements don't work. There are no magic bullet pills. With minor exceptions, supplements are a waste of money and time. I know that some of you will never be convinced. Many people cling to the perceived power of supplements as a matter of near-religious faith backed with stunning amounts of money. That's why I usually decline to discuss the subject because there's little use in arguing about matters of faith.

Every supplement picks its claim to fame, such as its ability to increase energy, enhance performance, lose weight or reduce body fat, relieve symptoms of fatigue and stress, and, of course, eliminate signs of aging—similar to a lot of face and body creams that women spend millions of dollars on, right? Most supplements are sold without traditional scientific evidence of the benefit that is touted, but who wouldn't want to believe that they work? The supplement manufacturers can say these things, just as long as they do not claim to *prevent a specific disease*. Just like those fancy lotions and body creams.

Here are some great examples: chromium, guar gum, green tea extract, and I don't even want to list some of the crazy names that they've come up with. They all sound cool and effective, and some actually use the biochemical names from which the manufacturers derive their purported functions. Supplement manufacturers cue off the use of real molecules to make their misleadingly broad claims. For example, "pyruvate" is a popular nutritional supplement said to achieve weight loss by burning fat while also stimulating energy for exercise performance. Of course this has to be so because pyruvate lies at the intersection of several key metabolic pathways. Genius. It sounds cool and it would be cool if it actually did all those things. We would be all set.

But it just does not work that way. What is forgotten is that each little molecule within our metabolic pathways is tied to several other molecules, so one in isolation does not exactly change things. Second, taking pyruvate may not be "limiting" because, among other reasons, we already have plenty of it and consuming more won't change a darn thing.

The trouble is you also don't know what you're buying. A supplement can consist of any "dietary ingredient" intended to "supplement" the diet ranging from essential vitamins and minerals to herbs and botanicals, to amino acids, enzymes, and metabolites. You can find all of these ingredients as extracts or concentrates in all sorts of mediums: tablets, capsules, soft gels, liquids, powders, bars, you name it. Your pharmacies, supermarkets, health food stores, and gyms are loaded with them—and they are often astronomically expensive.

The FDA does not consider supplements as "drugs" and therefore they are not regulated like a drug, even though many of us treat supplements like a drug—a cure for almost any ailment. Under the Dietary Supplement Health and Education Act (DSHEA) of 1994, the FDA in fact places dietary supplements under the general umbrella of foods the same way it categorizes an apple or a tomato. Think about it. The FDA

Read the Label

S tories of false labels and even contamination are alarmingly common in the dietary supplement world. United States Pharmacopeia (USP), a nonprofit public health organization, manages the Dietary Supplement Verification Program (DSVP) that conducts random off-the-shelf testing for integrity, purity, dissolution, and safe manufacturing. A USP certification does not mean that the product works, but at least the bottle contains what it says it contains. If you are going to take a supplement, look for this label. Better idea: Skip supplements and eat good food.

does not closely monitor what is placed in a supplement unless there is affirmative evidence that it is dangerous.

The fact that there is seldom any solid proof that a given supplement does what they say it will is bad enough. Far worse, in my mind, is the fact that, even today, many supplements do not have in them what they claim to have and may even contain hazardous substances. Here's a scary aside. It is entirely possible that some of those inexplicably popular protein powders that young people and athletes take have been contaminated with steroids. Actually, if some kids knew that a given protein powder contained steroids, they might take even more. Which is all the more reason this field should be regulated. And why you and your kids should mostly stay away from it until it is.

Doesn't it just make sense to stick with food? For example, not only does a tomato have high levels of vitamin C, it also has lots of fiber, beta-carotene, and lycopene. All act as potent antioxidants. There have been studies of tomato consumption and possible links to reduced risk of certain cancers and heart diseases. Populations that consume high amounts of tomatoes and tomato products have been found to have a lower risk of getting these diseases. No surprise then that some researchers went on to study the individual ingredients in tomatoes to determine which of them conveyed the health benefits to the consumer. Some studied lycopene, others studied beta-carotene, but as it turns out, none of them worked in isolation. That's the critical point: It took all of these nutrients in a natural combination found in the tomato to have the health benefit. It was not one ingredient alone or something synthesized in a lab. So when a supplement says "all-natural ingredients," I am not impressed. Tomato off the vine—that is "all natural."

Are there times when we should say "yes" to a supplement? *Sometimes.*

Supplements with Special Consideration

There are comparatively rare circumstances when it may make sense to take specific supplements. This is such a thorny area that it may be helpful if I try my hand at some rules on the subject. Here you go.

1. You do not need to consume any dietary supplements unless you are clinically deficient in a particular essential nutrient. That deficiency should be diagnosed and monitored by a qualified physician.

2. Consumption of individual nutrients at high doses puts you at risk for toxicity and can interfere with the absorption of other essential nutrients.

3. It's a low-risk habit, but don't bother to take multivitamins as an insurance policy. Far better to learn to eat better.

4. Nonessential nutrients and herbals are not necessary. The science on them is either nonexistent or extremely fuzzy, and the purity of the product is uncertain. They are unproven and risky.

There are nutrients that are *essential* to your health—that is, the *essential vitamins and minerals that you cannot live without.* And there are times when you may not get enough from food alone. Supplementation is warranted when you cannot consume essential nutrients in your diet on a regular basis or choose not to. For example, people (often the elderly) with low-calorie intakes may find it very difficult to eat enough of a variety of foods to cover their nutrient needs. Vegans who avoid all animal products may require more calcium, iron, zinc, vitamin D, and B$_{12}$ to prevent deficiencies. One of the reasons why I am not totally vegetarian is that I hate the thought of having to take a pill or a shot to round out my diet.

Pregnancy and lactation require more iron as well as folate. There may be other special situations: There are people who have milk allergies or are lactose intolerant; they often have to take extra calcium and vitamin D. The same is true for individuals who are concerned about osteoporosis. But they are the exception, not the rule. The rule is: Do not use supplements, except in the case of special needs. Let me talk for a minute about some of the most popular supplements and consider the pros and cons.

The Multivitamin

An astonishing one third of us in the United States take a multivitamin as an insurance policy. They are particularly popular among those who are conscientious about good diets and need them the least. They are also popular among people who know that they eat like crap, realize that their hair is falling out, their nails are brittle, and their skin is scaly but are too lazy to eat better. So they pop in a multivitamin. Both camps would do so much better to save the money, and spend it on good food or a personal trainer.

Take-home message: Multivitamins can serve a purpose for some and for the most part are safe. They can fill in gaps for those of us who don't consume many calories (for example, it is hard to get all necessary nutrients from food on less than 1,200 kcal/day) or those who can't eat particular food items or avoid certain food groups. In these cases, taking a multivitamin is preferable to taking individual supplements. Multivitamins typically provide doses of nutrients that are within reason—usually around 100 percent of the Daily Value as opposed to megadoses that you often see with individual nutrients. But if you are eating a well-balanced diet rich in fruits and vegetables, whole grains, and lean protein, save your money and hit the gym.

Protein Supplements

Almost the first thing you see when you walk into most gyms are big vats of protein supplements that promise to stimulate your muscles into a chronic state of bulk and flex. Walk on by. Do yourself a favor and have a turkey sandwich instead. I tell *all* my athletes, including my little brother who played Division I football at Oklahoma, the same thing: Eat protein-rich food, not protein supplements.

Protein supplements usually contain a lot of other garbage, and we have no idea what those additives do to you over the long haul. But the basic reason not to take protein supplements is that most of us simply don't need them. High intakes can also stress our kidneys and result in calcium excretion. In addition, if carbohydrate intake is low, this may result in an unhealthy metabolic state known as ketosis. In the United States, we generally get plenty of protein from what we eat. Protein is not only found in meat and fish but also in eggs, soy, legumes, beans, dairy products, and grains.

The one exception may be some older people. There are studies that show protein intake tends to decrease with age, which may warrant the use of a supplement. There has been an explosion of research examining the impact of supplementation with protein, specifically whey protein, on muscle mass in older adults. Whey protein is simply isolated protein from the liquid material that is a by-product of cheese production. Cow's milk, for instance, is made of 80 percent casein protein and 20 percent whey protein. These studies are usually done in conjunction with a strength-training program to build muscle and strength in older individuals at a time when they are losing a great deal of muscle mass due to sarcopenia.

Most of these studies do show a benefit to older people from consuming essential amino acids, namely branched chain amino acids, which are found in complete proteins, like whey or beef protein, either before and/or after a resistance training bout to help stimulate muscle protein synthesis—*on a molecular level.* How much this translates into improved muscle mass, function, and the ability to live a high-quality life is still a big area of investigation.

Take-home message: Most of us do not need any protein supplements at all. It's far better to eat a balanced and colorful diet. Do pay attention to eating a certain amount of animal products and fish, and if you don't consume meat, concentrate on a healthy intake of soy, beans, and nuts.

Omega-3s and Fish Oil

Fish and other seafood are great sources of the long chain omega-3 fatty acids, docosahexaenoic acid (DHA), and eicosapentaenoic acid (EPA), and consumption of fish one or two times per week has been directly linked to heart health and reduced risk of all-cause mortality. *Nice.* The omega-3s exert their powers via lowering blood pressure, triglycerides, and even inflammation. That is nothing to pooh-pooh for sure. There is also a strong association with brain health, especially in

Supplement Cheat Sheet

Calcium: The Recommended Daily Allowance (RDA) for women and men over age thirty is 1,000 mg/day; the RDA increases for women over fifty and men over seventy to 1,200 mg/day. It is not necessary to consume calcium from diet and supplements combined in amounts greater than these doses. Women and men over fifty should consider a calcium supplement of 500–1,000 mg/day if their dairy consumption is low. Caution: High intakes of calcium in men have been linked to prostate cancer risk, so don't overdo it. Note: Calcium is best absorbed if consumed 500 mg or less at a time.

Vitamin D: The new RDA for vitamin D has been set at 600 IU/day and 800 IU/day for those older than 70 years. Vitamin D is difficult to consume in foods, unless you eat fish and drink fortified milk. If the four main risk factors for deficiency (living at northern latitudes, older age, darker skin pigmentation, and being overweight/obese) pertain to you and/or your dietary intake is low, you should get screened by your doctor. If you think you may be insufficient, supplement with 1,000 IU/day.

Vitamin B_{12}: Many people older than fifty do not have enough hydrochloric acid in their stomach to absorb the vitamin B_{12} naturally present in food. The best sources of B_{12} then become fortified foods or supplements, where the B_{12} is bioavailable even to those with low hydrochloric acid. Animal foods are the only natural source of B_{12}. Vegetarians should consider supplementation. A multivitamin or B complex vitamin typically contains at least 100 percent of the RDA of 2.4 mcg/day. That'll do it.

developing fetuses. The verdict is still out on direct ties to cognitive function, depression, and dementia in adults. So fish are good. But how about pills said to contain the omega-3s from fish?

The short answer, again, is no. We should really be trying to *eat fish*, not taking pills. You do not get all the other benefits that fish has to offer from a pill. Fish is a great source of healthy calories, and it is certainly nutrient dense. In addition to being a source of omega-3s, fish is a great source of vitamin D, selenium, and protein. And eating fish as a protein source is more heart healthy than eating a hamburger.

What about the stories about cancer-causing polychlorinated biphenyls (PCBs) and methyl mercury in fish? It is a concern but here is the thing: Harvard School of Public Health professors Drs. Mozaffarian and Rimm did a comprehensive analysis of studies that looked at fish consumption and risk of cancer and heart disease. They found that if 100,000 people ate farmed salmon twice a week for seventy years, the extra PCB intake might cause about twenty-four extra deaths from cancer, but it would also prevent at least 7,000 deaths from heart disease. Eating fish is a reasonable risk. A separate analysis by the FDA, the Institute of Medicine (IOM), and the Environmental Protection Agency (EPA) found that current evidence is insufficient to recommend limitations on the amount of fish we eat in terms of mercury exposure. The best recommendation I can give is to eat different varieties of fish two or three times a week and stick to smaller breeds that have less mercury. When buying salmon try to find Alaskan wild-caught species, which have very low levels of mercury. Avoid swordfish, tilefish, and shark, especially if you are pregnant or likely to become so, because the risks are a little different.

You should also know that omega-3s (alpha linolenic acid) are found in walnuts, flaxseeds, green leafy vegetables, soybean, canola, and flaxseed oil. The omega-3s from plant sources are a little different from the omega-3s in fish, but both convey health benefits.

Take-home message: Taking fish oil supplements is unnecessary. Eat two 4- to 6-ounce servings of fish per week, and balance it by adding some walnuts or flaxseeds to your salad, and cook with canola, soybean, and flaxseed oils.

Vitamin D

Vitamin D has been hot in nutrition research lately. And—full disclosure—I am studying vitamin D, including vitamin D from *a supplement*, in a clinical trial funded by the federal government. Here's why. It happened to be the middle of winter when I was doing research on the fitness and heart health of urban schoolchildren from the Boston area and I stumbled across the fact that most of them were vitamin D deficient. These were *growing children* so the finding scared the dickens out me, and prompted me to study vitamin D on a larger scale. As it turns out, it seems like the rest of the population is not getting enough vitamin D either. What is going on here?

Interestingly, our greatest source of vitamin D is not from our diets but from the sun. Sun exposure for as little as ten to fifteen minutes provides about 80–100 percent of our daily vitamin D needs. In climates north of 42 degrees latitude like Boston and much of the Northeast, however, we synthesize absolutely no vitamin D from sun exposure from November through March. The angle of the sun is simply too low to convert the vitamin D precursor that is found in your skin to the active form. You could lie naked on the ski slopes in Vermont in January and you still wouldn't synthesize vitamin D. In addition, these days, we slather on the sunscreen and often stay inside way too much even if we live in warmer climates. Beyond that, darker and older skin are both less efficient at synthesizing vitamin D. And here is the kicker: Your fat tissue binds vitamin D and makes it unavailable. Basically, if you are obese, you are more likely to be vitamin D deficient. You may also have a problem if you don't eat fish or drink fortified milk, the best food sources of vitamin D.

The Balanced Diet of Good Food

There are so many more nutrients to discuss that I feel as if I am short-changing you by not talking at length about niacin, riboflavin, vitamin C, vitamin E, zinc, phosphorus, magnesium, part of the other forty-two to forty-seven essential nutrients, if you also include essential amino acids and a few essential trace elements. They function throughout the body and are involved in absolutely everything, including forming structures, metabolizing fuels, promoting immune function, creating and dissipating inflammation, and forming hormones. They are called essential because they all play key parts in virtually every body function.

Briefly, you should know that zinc is a component of insulin. Selenium is an essential component of an antioxidant, and zinc and copper are components of other antioxidant enzymes. Magnesium alone is involved in the order of three hundred enzymatic reactions. For example, it is needed to synthesize DNA, your genetic code, and is also involved with hundreds of reactions involving ATP, your energy currency. And as I did mention, it helps to build bone. There are probably a hundred Ph.D.s in this country alone whose whole life is the study of magnesium, and it's a good use of their time, too.

Ultimately, you will have to take it on faith: Without these nutrients, we simply don't work, and I hope I've done my job in convincing you that there's no perfect one food or group of foods. I return to my message that a varied diet made up mainly of real, unprocessed foods is not only the healthiest way to eat, it gives you a built-in guarantee that you have all the tools to function. They say there's safety in numbers, and that theory applies to food types—eat an assortment of produce, grains, and lean protein to protect your health.

CHAPTER TWELVE

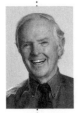

A Day in the Life: In the Land of Dreamy Dreams

This happened last summer, just a month into my struggle. Nice night. Bum result. Could happen to you. *Will* happen to you. Get ready.

Let's get at it this way. Assume for a moment that you were a little fool last night. You fell off the wagon. Not the worst guy in America, not the worst woman. But your mind wandered a little and, *bang*, you lowered your muzzle into the trough and turned into a little piggy for a while. Lowered your whole *body* into the trough, to tell the truth, and rolled over and over in it, absolutely delighted. Showed your bare bottom to the whole wagon train, as the song says (Do you remember "Sweet Betsy from Pike"?). You drank everything in sight, ate buckets and buckets of dreadful slop, and jeopardized all the wonderful work you've been doing. Today, you feel awful—paralyzed with guilt. What to do?

First, take a long shower, and wash the last of that slop out of your hair.

Second, get over it. This happens to everyone who embarks on profound change. That's not to say it isn't important; it is. But it isn't *fatal*. Unless you let it run away with you. The most weight you can gain in a day is, say, two pounds. In three days, you might gain four, if you were a real hound. And it is an "unstable" four pounds, too: easy on, easy off. If you act fast enough, it can be off as fast as it went on. It can be gone before your body can fall in love with it. So get back on the horse, no matter how wretched you feel. Gallop around. Get a little wind in your hair.

Third, bear in mind that the worst *potential* impact is psychological—no longer thinking of yourself as this wonderful new person. You think you betrayed yourself so *profoundly* last night that you'll never get the good feeling back. Well, yeah, you sure are an awful mutt. But the hell with it. The hell with guilt and weird psychological consequences. Just jump back on the damned old pony right now, and let's get out of here. Today, we're just losing a little weight, and that's mechanics. *C'mon!* Let's go.

Fourth, go back to basics: Give the great flywheel of life a mighty spin, just as you did when you began. Exercise is real. Do it and you can see that you mean it. Never mind the hair shirt and the scourge. Get back on the bike. This is one of the places where exercise really does its job. It is so *tangible*. Exercise is also the great mood lifter. It can pluck you out of the doldrums and get you on your way again. And incidentally, if you have the time to do a "long and slow" work-out, you may actually get to reverse some of the nonpsychological damage, the actual pounds gained. Or minimize it, anyway. But don't worry too much about that. And for sure, don't wait for the weekend when you'll have time to do the Long and Slow. Get back on the pony now *and* do the Long and Slow this weekend. Get back some of what you lost.

Fifth, recommit, more ferociously than before. If you can manage it, *double down*, as they say in gambling circles: Double your commitment to the program. And do the best you can to mean it. Do not assume you did not mean it the first time. You did. You just got a little buggered up, is all. Just slipped off into the Land of Dreamy Dreams. You don't know what that is? Sure, you do. It's just that the name is unfamiliar. I'll remind you, 'cause I have been there. Lately.

The Rapture of the Creep

had had a terrific week. Had worked out like crazy, had followed Jen's Rules all week. And had lost another *two pounds*, which is the outer limits of safe dieting. I am virtually *there*, where I want to be. I feel great. *Bulletproof*, in fact. I truly believed that I had learned the secret of life. I had learned *how to lose weight* and be strong. This feeling of smug euphoria, by the way, is not unusual among early-stage dieters. It is known as the Rapture of the Creep. And it is dangerous.

It took me when I was feeling particularly strong, even a little self-satisfied. See me, standing there last night—proud, erect, and serene—by the stove. I am cooking dinner for ten and I am preparing a great, sane meal. Salmon, beets, salad, brown rice. And a couple of yummy French baguettes for our guests. I do not eat white bread anymore, as you know. And if I did—which I do not, as I say—I would not put butter on it. I am not sure there is any butter in the house. In fact, such is the force of my resolve, I am not sure there is any in this part of the state. I no longer eat butter.

People arrive. I cook away, make drinks for them. Hilary meets and greets. She and I are loving hosts. and people like to come here. Oh, and the popcorn has just been popped. Good news. It is my signature hors d'oeuvre, and people have gotten used to digging their fists into the huge red bucket, which is used only for this purpose. It's good. Not good for you, but good. Without butter it is not even that bad for you, but I did put butter on it tonight. For the sake of my guests, not me. I am no longer that kind of chap.

On nights like this I sometimes make a special drink that I urge folks to try. Cosmos, for example. Or Manhattans—drinks you do not get every day. A little treat and a mood setter. I do not drink much myself these dieting days—when I am almost perfect—but that's no reason for them to suffer. Same as the popcorn. The drink I am pushing tonight is interesting. Do you know what sliders are? The little baby hamburgers that are appearing in bistros these days? They are adorable. You can eat one, or a hundred of them. Scarcely notice.

The drinks I was making were a little like that. Miniatures. Hilary found a bunch of martini glasses in the attic the other day, about a third the size of the modern ones. It pleased me to serve little bitty martinis in them, an amusing *homage* to the slider concept. Slider martinis, in fact. Try one: The whole thing is just a few sips.

They are a great hit. Everyone is trying them. They are going down like sake shots. It's going to be a good party. Shake, shake, shake. Pour, pour, pour. Let me top that up. Oh, thank you. Oh, these are lovely.

In the excitement of the moment—and because I was anxious to test their miniature proportions—I had one of the little fellows myself. One of my rules during the weight loss phase of my new life is no hard booze. But surely that did not apply to these little guys. Especially when I had been such a great chap all week. I whistle one down. It is perfect. Not a surprise; this is not my first rodeo. And the popcorn is good, too. Oops—without a thought, I am eating the forbidden popcorn. Didn't decide to, just did it. To go with the little martini maybe.

In the Land of Dreamy Dreams

A s surely as Harry Potter walked through the wall to get the train to Hogwarts, I downed that teeny little martini and slipped into the Land of Dreamy Dreams. Where we are all wonderful creatures. And we do not have to think. Or decide to do this or that. We are there, and we do what we do. Like a man in bed with a pretty girl with his duds off, we are no longer thinking things through.

I say it was the slider martinis, but there were several things all at once. Somewhere in there I forgot the sacred "no buttered popcorn" rule. Somewhere in there I forgot the "no hard booze" rule. Somewhere in there, I forgot about watching and weighing every single bite I put in my mouser. Somewhere in there, I slipped away from the Land of High Resolve and Long-Term Goals, and into the Land of Dreamy Dreams. A lovely place where you do *whatever you like, you adorable creature.* Because you have been such a little star these two weeks past. And can quickly unwind any little mistakes you make because you know the secret of life. Didn't you bike twenty-five miles this morning? Aren't you *entitled* to a little treat? I did not ask those questions, but they were in the air. *Hubris* was in the air.

Then, without a moment's thought or a whisper of reproach, I sat down at the table. Picked up the long hot baguette nearest me. And ate it. The whole damn thing. With butter. And more sliders. Best thing I ever put in my mouth.

Do you remember in the *Odyssey* where Odysseus and his lads come to Circe's island and drink this amazing nectar that she has on offer? It is the best thing any of them have ever tasted. And the only drawback is that it turns men into swine. Literally. The fun crop on Circe's island is opium. The cash crop is pigs. Pigs who used to be men. In America, the fun crops are bread and fries and snacks—buttered popcorn, say. And the cash crop is pigs. The cash crop is us.

Doubling Down

So, it's the next day. What to do? Well, it's the litany of things I said at the head of this chapter. I got out of bed, wracked with shame. Had a long shower and dressed for the day. In my usual tasteful superman suit (Lycra biking shorts and shirt, gym shoes) I go out to our little gym, in the barn in the backyard. And work out, hard, for an hour. Then—because I am so ashamed of myself and because I do not have a day job—I change the gym shoes for biking cleats and bike for an hour. Then I come home, have a rational breakfast (blueberries and Greek yogurt). Congratulate myself. And resume living.

There you go, kids. Can't fall off the wagon once a week and survive, but you can get away with it a couple of times. I would know.

Two More Meals

So what does one eat for lunch and dinner after a blowout like that? If you can manage it, just more Good Stuff. There is a risk that you will be ferociously hungry the next day, a variation of the sugar spikes Jen mentioned. If you can comfort yourself with apples and other Good Stuff for snacks, instead of the more traditional day-after meal of greasy cheeseburgers and fries, it will be a blessing. Sometimes the worst excesses come the day after the blowout. Try to duck that bullet. It helps to snack on apples and such, to drive those old hungers away.

For lunch, I pandered a little to the yearning for hair of the dog by having scrambled eggs and fresh sliced tomatoes. And two slices of whole-wheat bread, dry.

Dinner was not exactly riotous. Chicken breasts in lemon butter (mostly lemon). Fresh carrots and more whole-wheat bread. Dry, by heaven. And one sturdy glass of wine. Went to bed semi-early. And only mildly shamefaced. Did not wake up at 3 a.m., the way I had the night before.

Is there any moral in all this, apart from what we've talked about? I'm not sure. The obvious one, I suppose, is that recovery from sloth and self-abuse is possible.

More important, if more elusive: In a new life of small ball, where tiny swings to one side or the other count a lot, you really do have to pay fairly close attention all the time. The price of losing significant weight after fifty is eternal vigilance, or close to it. Once you get where you want to go, I believe it makes sense to "plan"—or at least leave room—for the occasional night like that. Life has got to be fun, after all. And the occasional blowout is fun. Especially if you happen to survive it.

Last observation: Do you remember when I first looked on the slider martini and concluded that my own rule against hard liquor did not apply in the case of such a small and innocuous drink? Well, here's another rule of near universal application:

Whenever you conclude, for whatever excellent and compelling reason, that a given rule does not apply in a particular case, it does.

CHAPTER THIRTEEN

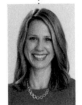

Exercise:
The Magic Bullet

A s Chris discovered, exercise is truly a magic bullet and for two very important reasons. First, exercise changes your fundamental physiology—your ability to work well—and second, with those changes, exercise enhances your ability to lose weight. Why? Because it changes your infrastructure, your machinery, and your metabolism. If these networks are optimized through avid exercise, you simply function better. The more you burn, the stronger you become and the more you are likely to burn even more calories with subsequent workouts. It becomes a vicious cycle—a *beautiful one*! The whole complex business is a remorseless and effective burner of calories. And will make you *thinner this year and for a lifetime.*

When you find out how and why exercise is so helpful to maintaining health and healthy body weight, you just can't help feeling motivated. Chris likes to separate the concept of exercise for health and exercise for fitness, for emphasis and organization, which is fine. But for me, they are simply too interconnected to break apart.

The moment you start exercising you get fitter and healthier, no questioning that. Sure, you see a tall sinewy twenty-year-old swimmer in a Speedo and you say, "Wow, now that guy is *fit.*" That may be true, but the slightly doughy-looking woman next door who power-walks her dog every night for an hour may be very fit compared to what she was three years ago when she didn't have a dog and couldn't even think of walking longer than ten minutes at a time. The swimmer may be at his peak and will never get fitter than he is now, and the woman still has plenty of room for fitness gain, but they both are reaping health benefits, just on a different scale. There is a *fitness continuum.*

What happens to both of these individuals as they increase their exercise and their fitness? What will happen to you? So many good things, on both fronts. Your muscles get stronger and your heart pumps blood more efficiently and your aerobic capacity increases—but there are a lot of other things that *work* better and enable you to avoid dreadful diseases. Adding in a nutritious diet further compounds the positive effects of getting your body moving. Much of this is explored in Chapter 18 on muscle, but it is so important to get it in the mix here.

Exercise Changes Your Fundamental Physiology for a Much Better You

Your muscles, blood vessels, hormones, signals, and receptors are all deeply and positively affected by exercise. Even though I have studied the mechanisms of several of these changes, the whole orchestration of events is still quite mysterious and magical, even to me. But one thing is clear: You will be hard-pressed to find a system where exercise is detrimental. Almost every week, I read or hear about a study that finds a new positive relationship between physical activity and good health. Exercise has a favorable impact on many deadly conditions, whether they're genetic or linked to lifestyle: coronary heart disease, hypertension, lipid disorders, type 2 diabetes, colon and breast cancer, depression, osteoporosis, frailty, sleep problems, Alzheimer's disease and other cognitive problems, and obesity. Exercise is used in cardiac rehab with stunning results. Rheumatoid arthritis patients' symptoms are relieved, and these individuals get much stronger. Those who exercise during pregnancy have quicker births, recovery, and less weight gain. I know that last one, firsthand. I am a very serious exerciser, and my two kids wanted out *fast*. I didn't even have time to think about an epidural.

Structurally, major changes occur with exercise. Your heart gets stronger and the left ventricle gets larger; it has an increased capacity for filling and for pumping out larger volumes of oxygen-saturated blood per beat (the "stroke volume"). You will see your resting heart rate decrease because of this change and your heart rate at a given workload will decrease with increasing fitness. Your blood volume increases and your red blood cell number also increases. The network of capillaries that bring the oxygen-rich blood to every single muscle fiber in your body multiplies. The ability of your muscles to extract the oxygen from the capillaries is also increased. Each muscle fiber has more capillaries surrounding it, which enhances the supply of nutrients and oxygen to muscle fibers and facilitates the removal of by-products of metabolism and waste.

Your muscles themselves undergo dramatic changes depending on the type of training you engage in. With resistance training, the individual muscle fibers increase in size within a particular muscle group (like your quadriceps, for example) and with greater size, they are able to produce more force. The ability to activate contraction in that muscle also increases because the nerve is better able to signal the muscle to contract. The "connections" between nerves and muscles change and you are better able to recruit muscle that you never knew you had.

With these changes, energy utilization is enhanced. Your muscles store more ready reserves of glycogen and triglycerides, and the enzymes needed to burn them as fuel multiply and are more active. Even the lipases, the Pac-Men, that pull fat from the bloodstream down into the muscle increase and are more active—they are primed to tap into those fat stores and burn them a lot sooner during movement, holding off on the breakdown of the precious muscle glycogen. And because the breakdown of fat requires oxygen, myoglobin content also increases, which offers a limited supply of oxygen right within your muscle. Energy is more readily available to you when you want to move!

Outside the muscle, a multitude of biochemical, hormonal, and enzymatic changes occur as well. Those "lipases," or Pac-Men also exist around your stored tummy fat and are more active in breaking it down and releasing it into the circulation for use as fuel in your muscles. With exercise, they actually develop a preference for using the visceral fat, the dangerous fat around your middle! That one change is huge for your health. The hormonal environment to promote this fat loss also changes: Growth hormone increases, which assists with fat metabolism; your insulin sensitivity is also enhanced. When you eat sugar from any type of food, your muscles are much better able to scoop up the glucose from your circulation, keeping it from damaging other molecules and causing higher insulin release. Less insulin is used, and therefore the equilibrium between high blood sugar and a high insulin response is kept in place. What is even cooler is how muscle contraction alone actually assists with the translocation of the little glucose receptors to the surface of the muscle cell (Chris' little buttercups again).

Exercise increases your good cholesterol, your HDL; the "vacuum cleaner," if you remember, scavenges cholesterol from your arteries and helps to rid it from your body. HDL is also known to have anti-inflammatory properties. Triglycerides and LDL, your bad cholesterol,

The Set-Point Theory

The set-point theory of body weight control says that we have a highly individual internal control system based on our genes, hormones, and our physiology that helps dictate how much fat we carry. It's a kind of thermostat for body fat. The theory goes that whereas some individuals have a high setting (efficient at storing fat), others have a low setting (not as efficient at storing fat). If I have a high set-point, my body might fight to stay between 155 and 165 pounds. If I have a low setting, it might try to stick around 125–135 pounds. Experts speculate that high set-point dieters in particular often hit a stubborn plateau or put weight back on after initially losing it because trying to overpower the internal fat thermostat is hard to do with dietary changes alone. Exercise is the one strategy that shows promise in lowering high set-point individuals and helping them reach new set-points and maintain goal weights.

also typically see a drop. Physical activity also promotes the production and activity of your body's naturally occurring antioxidants, antioxidant enzymes, which help quench free radicals and further promote an anti-inflammatory state. Your body becomes more resilient to damage during this process. Immune function is enhanced with regular moderate-intensity physical activity—your immune cells that naturally fight off infection and foreign invaders are more numerous and active. You will get sick less often, a major bonus.

Exercise Is Key for Weight Loss— and a Thinner, Healthier You

Let's think a bit about how all of these physiological changes will confer a metabolic advantage that will also promote weight loss. Weight loss alone gives you a physiological advantage, but weight loss with exercise packs a much more powerful punch.

Exercise is hard. For some of us it has become unusually unnatural. But physical activity *is* natural. It is also the key to losing weight and maintaining a healthy body weight. Exercise is our powerful ally in combating weight gain and promoting weight loss. And it is an impressive list, from the sheer calorie burn, to changes in metabolism and physiology, to the afterburn. *It fundamentally changes you.*

You Build Muscle

Exercise leaves a prolonged imprint on your whole metabolic profile, starting with how it changes the muscle machinery. Here's the fundamental fact I introduced in Chapter 3: *Muscle is more metabolically active at rest than fat.* Each pound of muscle burns approximately 6 calories per day per pound, whereas fat burns about 2 calories per day per pound. If you increase your muscle mass, your resting metabolism will likewise increase. The differential in calorie burn between fat and muscle tissues is not mind-blowing, but the extra calories of burn add up to something significant over time. Serious resistance training— done with intensity and progressive weight increases—is a terrific way to build healthy muscle. Start slowly, but go for it. Study the strength training chapters with care and follow them as best you can. Our advice about working out *hard* is eventually going to do amazing things for you when it comes not just to weight loss and muscle development, but sarcopenia and inflammation, too. Sound good? It is.

You Improve Muscle Metabolism

Here is what really happens when you exercise and build muscle. You build a lot of other things, too, including the infrastructure and muscle machinery, meaning the muscle fibers have more molecules working efficiently as well. If you are entering the business of building things, you need energy. Clearly exercise is a powerful stimulus to your skeletal muscle. The more it is worked, the more force it generates and the stronger it becomes. Neural networks are enhanced, and you're better able to stimulate muscle fibers that you never knew existed. The capillaries that extend from your arteries to supply blood, oxygen, and fuel (sugar and fat) expand their network around the active muscle fibers—they grow, too. They actually dump the needed oxygen and fuel quicker to the hungry muscles, further increasing the efficiency of fuel delivery and utilization.

Once these capillaries have effectively delivered oxygen and fuel to the muscle, dramatic things also happen inside the muscle. When energy needs are high in the muscle, mitochondria increase in size and multiply. Because we are better able to burn fuel, we are able to exercise at higher intensities and for longer, in turn, increasing calorie burn. When energy use is low, as it is when we don't exercise regularly, mitochondria become inactive or are destroyed. Enzymes slow down and so do we.

You Burn More Fat

Stored fat is your great enemy BUT exercise burns stored fat. Here's the story: With the growth of new muscle from exercise, more oxygen and nutrients are delivered to the growing mitochondria. Our general metabolic profile shifts. The proteins/enzymes that are needed to burn fat increase in number and activity, a process called lipolysis. (Chris has been dropping that word into his conversations at cocktail parties for weeks now. He claims to clear entire rooms with a sentence or two.) In sedentary individuals, the body defaults to burning carbohydrates because it takes much longer and it's harder to figure out how to use your fat for energy. Fit people catch a major break.

Here's a kicker: Idle people who diet and lose weight take a curious and deeply unfair beating. With calorie restriction and weight loss, fat burn for idle people typically goes down. The metabolism of the deconditioned dieter actually slows down and the ability to burn fat *decreases.* Here is the great news for the dieter who also exercises: Studies show that those who both diet and exercise do not have this problem. Achieve a moderate calorie reduction (less than seven hundred calories per day) and exercise, and you will show no diminution of the ability to burn fat. Research has not yet taken the next step, but I am confident that the ability to burn fat, while dieting, goes up for the seriously fit and active dieter. Win-win for our side. As Chris would say, "and richly deserved!"

Finally, this wonderful and fundamental difference in "fat burn" goes on for a while. Exercise seems to remodel the metabolic pathways that determine how the body stores and utilizes food. It goes like this: *Exercisers burn more fat after their meals, whereas non-exercisers burn more carbs. Nonexercisers let more fat in meals be put away as "stored fat," whereas exercisers burn more of it.* It's a *very* powerful reason to exercise hard when you're trying to drop that poisonous gut of yours.

The Afterburn

Here's something else to keep in mind: Not only do you burn calories *during* exercise (and more calories at rest because of the growth of your metabolic infrastructure), but there is also substantial evidence showing that *an additional calorie burn on top of your usual metabolic rate persists for the 24 hours or so after an intense exercise bout.* It's hard to pinpoint just how long this effect lasts; people vary. Those who exercise a bit longer and harder get a bigger postexercise calorie burn.

The fit get fitter. "Virtue rewarded at last!" Chris says. I'll buy that.

Here's an example. After forty-five minutes of intense cycling, Chris is likely to have increased metabolism for another fourteen hours or so, *even when he is sleeping*. There have been some interesting studies of this phenomenon done in metabolic chambers (don't ask). The excess calories burned following vigorous exercise in young men were found to be almost 200 calories extra and in us older folks, perhaps it is a wee bit less, say 150–175 calories. This halo effect is delicious to contemplate. If you add up those extra halo calories burned over the course of a week, assuming daily exercise, it is a very big deal. Chris writes beguilingly about the joys of bicycling around his Berkshire Hills. Add this little halo business, and he *really* has something to feel great about. Exercise is the gift that keeps on giving, *all the time*.

Your Insulin Is Under Control

Here's another great boon from serious exercise. Let's revisit our good old friend and foe, insulin. Insulin has been pointedly blamed for weight gain, central adiposity (the open sewer around our middles), and obesity. It is a little odd to blame insulin, frankly. What they are really talking about is the fact that when you eat a ton of carbohydrates—and especially the refined ones with the high glycemic index—they increase your blood glucose like crazy, which leads to a sharp insulin surge. If you have a sugar spike, then you'll surely have an insulin spike soon after. That's how it is supposed to work. There are terrible things about insulin spikes, but the villain is the Dead Food you ate, not the insulin.

The difficulty is that insulin's fundamental job is to store energy, whether fat or sugar. With insulin, muscle and fat cells take up fat and sugar. We want sugar going to the muscles. Fat going to fat cells is just what we *don't* want. But the real difficulty with this slanted telling of the insulin story by so-called diet experts is that it is so utterly and importantly incomplete. It blatantly ignores how exercise fits into the mix because so many diet people—of whatever level of seriousness— just don't get it about exercise.

With just one bout of exercise we increase our "sensitivity" to insulin. That is a term of art in nutrition. What it means is that your body needs less insulin to suck up sugar into your muscles. You will have less of an insulin surge in response to elevated blood sugar. Insulin, in effect, works more efficiently, and you need less of it to get the job done. That is subtle but important because less insulin floating around in your blood means less storage of excess glucose as fat. That's less storage of fat, period.

One other predictable outcome of a sugar spike, followed by an insulin spike, is that it leads to a *hunger spike.* The insulin spike (in response to a flood of fast-digesting carbs) wipes out *too much* sugar in the blood. The body cries out for more (even though you just ate some), and you are ravenously hungry. I know this is getting complicated, but the bottom line reads like this: The more you exercise, the less need for insulin. With less of an insulin spike there is less of a sugar drop; therefore you won't experience hunger spikes.

And what is even more beautiful is that the effect of exercise lasts. *Following an exercise bout, the good impact on insulin lasts for up to three days!* That's why you want continuing bouts of exercise throughout the week to prolong these good effects. Throw in some vigorous activity, and the burn gets even better. Weekend warriors—those who work out only a couple of days a week—cheat themselves of these benefits.

So here is the take-home message: Eat better, and you will be better able to exercise. Exercise more and you will get more healthy and fit. With increased fitness, organ systems, hormones, enzymes, and your resulting health are optimized. You will gain strength and lose the most dangerous fat. We have said again and again that exercise is the flywheel of the good life. Now you know the details. And the slogan is not just a slogan. It is profoundly and importantly true.

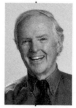

CHAPTER FOURTEEN

A Day in the Life: Intervals, "Periodization," and Kedges

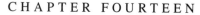

ife is long, thank God, but that pleasing fact has some implications for all this training we are talking about. And for the notion
that you are going to be doing this stuff, six days a week, for the
rest of your life. Does anybody think that you can really, really do that
without going nuts? And quitting? Well, yes we do. But you have to
take some steps. Most training regimens—including ours—talk often
in terms of your getting stronger, faster, having greater and greater endurance, as if that were going to go on that way forever. But that is not
going to happen. Certainly it is not going to happen in the Third Act,
that's for sure. Serious trainers of serious athletes recognize there have
to be peaks and valleys in even a full-time athlete's training life. They
train their people to build for this or that great race in the summer or
fall. Then taper off and do something different for a spell. Then swing
back into spring training or whatever it is. They call this *periodization.*

If you are a master athlete and going into actual competitions, like
Jen, you can do that, too. But most of us are not. For us there has to be
something different. For us—as luck would have it—there are kedges,
which as some of you know, are serious physical events—one to three a

year, depending. A ski trip to Stowe or Aspen, say. My Ride the Rockies bike trek or any good bike trips. Running a half marathon, whatever.

The notion is to set yourself a task or a goal. Something that will be fun but a serious challenge, too. Something that you will have to train for. But—because it will be such a kick when you actually do it—something deeply motivational, too. You train and you build up your strength, your endurance. You peak out on the great event. And then you taper off, go on a maintenance basis for a while. In maintenance mode, in the Third Act, you're just trying to hold your own. At my tender age, much of the year I am in maintenance mode. I'm a good kid about doing something every day for an hour or more. But I am not exactly trying to get stronger, faster, fitter, forever. I'm trying not to go to hell. In maintenance mode, I am not increasing the weight load or the speed when I do strength training. And I am mostly not doing intervals. But when I set a new kedge, a new goal for myself, I am apt to do all those things. And they will be tailored to the event, whether it's a major ski trip or a single scull race or a big bike ride.

When you periodize—or set kedges—what you are doing is avoiding getting stale. Or losing interest in the whole damn thing. You are dramatizing your physical life a little. And it is a blessing and a joy. The central pleasures in my year—year after year—are apt to be the kedges. Some are better than others, but they all work miraculously well. The subject of this Day in the Life chapter is interval training, and the fact is that I am doing a lot of interval training these days as I work on this chapter. The reason is that, once again, I am going to go on Ride the Rockies, a hellish six-day bike trip (only three days for me this year, thank heaven), of up to a hundred miles a day, over the highest mountain passes in the country. I have done a bunch of these, and they never disappoint. This year is going to be tough because I have been working so hard on other things and I have been in maintenance mode far too late into the season. Now I am playing catch-up. And catching up for an aerobic event like this is—most important—doing intervals.

Actually, we are going to canter through three very different interval days, in different locations, to give you a sense of some possible variations. It's hard to get a sense of how intervals work, just from reading Riggs's excellent programs. So here are some living examples.

The plan for the first one is simplicity itself. I am going to do the first (and easiest) of Riggs's intervals, set out in Chapter 17. But it will still be plenty tough. Intervals are hard. That's the point, I guess. You don't get to be fit, unless you go *hard*. (Note: You can be plenty healthy by going "long and slow" four days a week and *never* doing intervals. "Fit" is a little different.) The nicest thing about today's push is that it's up in the Berkshires again on a sweet spring morning. It is *such* a privilege to bike in country like this.

The plan for the day—after the warm-up—is to do five two-minute intervals, with three-minute rests in between. Easy-peasy. I have picked a fairly quiet, flat road for all this, the local "rail trail." And it's early so I won't kill a pedestrian.

I wait for the second hand on the watch (just a regular watch with a visible sweep second hand, taped to the handlebars, where I can see it) to hit twelve, and I stand up and hit it. In the first two minutes I don't get my heart rate up very high. My top in the first minute is a less than 80 percent of my real max. Not much. I loll along at 70 percent for the next three minutes.

Then repeat: This time my two-minute sprint—going flat out. That takes me over 80 percent. That's better. The three-minute rest still feels generous. This is not that hard a workout. Not yet. The third sprint or interval—again, going as hard as I can—takes me up to 85 percent. This is getting harder. The three-minute rest is welcome.

But by the fourth interval, I am hitting it very hard. I get up over 85 percent and am panting during the three-minute rest. Same on the fifth one. Even with three-minute rest periods, this is not easy. Well, it's not supposed to be, and the one three days from now will be worse. That's okay—that's the idea. We're *building* here.

Then a cool-down. Which just means that I turn around and head home. But—even with this easy interval piece—I can see what Riggs is getting at. It was hard to keep going flat out for two minutes. And more demanding intervals—with longer sprints and shorter rests—would be a lot harder. Sure enough, Riggs is not kidding. This is serious business. Do all eight of Riggs's interval days—over four weeks—and you'll have quite an experience. And begin to be *fit*. (Or—better idea for most of us— *never* do an interval at all. Settle for healthy and the dickens with "fit.")

Interval Day 2: A Walk in the Snow

That was a formal interval day; this is a goofy one. I am in Aspen again, early in the morning. A nutcase trainer I know—not Riggs this time—has driven us high up above the town in his truck to the McNamara Hut parking space, well up into Hunter Creek, east of town. The Hunter Creek drainage—as they sometimes call the big valleys up here—is a stunning broad valley that rises, for miles, into the mountains to the east of town. One of the most beautiful places on earth. You look down into Aspen, to the west, and up into the mountains beyond. There are abandoned miners' cabins here and there in the valley, with corrugated roofs and log walls. Mountain streams tumbling along, flashing black and fast through the deep snow. We put on snowshoes and head up the valley. This is going to be a snowshoe interval morning. Going to take about an hour and a half. Going to be a bit of a workout.

Intervals are a little different up here. The snow is some three feet deep, but other people have been up here, on cross-country skis and snowshoes, so a path of sorts has been packed down. We warm up for ten minutes; same old story. No one with a clue skips warm-ups. We take it slow on the packed trail. Get my heart rate up to about 60 percent of max, hold it there. This is a little more serious than the morning on my bike. I have a watch on an expansion bracelet, so I can wear it outside my clothes, on my left arm for the minutes. Same with the heart rate monitor on the right. I check my heart rate every few minutes. I am into this.

We pick up the pace a little. I take my heart rate up into the low 70 percents for a while. I know my companion is planning intervals—we've talked about it—but I don't know exactly what he has in mind. It turns out to be wonderfully simple. "Off the trail," he says. I follow him into the deep, untracked snow and—in twenty seconds—my heart rate is around 80 percent of max. That's my interval: going over into the deep snow. Five minutes in the deep powder, five minutes back on the trail. Back and forth. Back and forth. Snow-made intervals. Not bad.

But it is building. The path is getting steeper and before long my heart rate is deep in the 80s when we're off the path. And my companion is by no means done with me. He leads us up a steep side trail, in the direction of the Four Corners (for the few who know this area). I am huffing and puffing big time. My trainer is not impressed. "Run!" he suddenly says and he breaks into a trot. (He weighs about 150 pounds and has body fat of maybe 13 percent; this is not hard for him. For me, a little different.)

He means it. We are running—more like slogging in my case—up this steep mountain path, in fairly deep snow. In no time, my heart rate is in the 90s. What happens, I wonder, if I have a heart attack? Not to worry, I suppose. This guy could easily carry me down. But suppose it's bad? Does he have a knife? Will we be having open-heart-surgery-by-jackknife, high in the Hunter Creek hills? Or will he just say the hell with it, let me die, and lug the body down? It's a question. My heart rate is at 95 percent when we crest the last pitch. *Wowee!* That was something. I am *panting*, panting so deep it feels as if I am stretching my lungs, in a desperate effort to get more oxygen. But it is exhilarating, too. Hard, hard, hard, but kind of neat. Wonderful, in fact.

PERSONAL NOTE FROM CHRIS ON INTENSITY

These interval days are great fun, and a little addictive after a while. Intensity feels amazing and does wonderful things, fast. But I want to mention that I have lately decided not to go above 95 percent of my real max any more, even though I am in good shape. I may cut it to 90 percent when I hit eighty, which is still plenty for building fitness. Not going to hit it as hard as possible with the strength training either. Why? Because I am seventy-eight years old, that's why. And shit happens when you're seventy-eight. Also when you're fifty. Even if you're a Masters Athlete, you're more like a terrific "Classic Car," after fifty, than a new one. It does not make sense to "peel out" in a Classic Car. You crank it up and some dusty old wire may go. Some ancient gasket. So I'm going to hold it down a little. You too, maybe. Even better for lots of you: Settle for long and slow. That's plenty for lots of folks.

Now it's the long walk down. A half-hour walk, with small talk and looking at the views. Easy-peasy. The round-trip was an hour and a half, and—I hate to admit this—one of the best mornings of my life. Again, let me caution you not to try this prematurely, *if ever.* I was in super shape that day, and I was with a super-experienced guide who knew me and the hills very well. Even so it was a little scary. To do something like that alone would be nuts. Sure was fun, though.

Interval Day 3: Playing with Girls

This third one was last week in New York City and it was part of my kedge training (for Ride the Rockies). We have an apartment in town that we bought for about ten cents at the bottom of the last real estate recession. We're not in town enough to justify joining a gym, but we've found a wonderful solution in special-purpose workout places, where you can pay by the day or the week. The best of these, for me, is a spin class place called Flywheel on the East Side. You wouldn't say fancy, but it sure is serious. All too often the spin classes in normal gyms are lackluster affairs, aimed at the lowest common denominator. Too easy. Not the problem with these kids at Flywheel. They are *into it.*

Class is in a big nasty room on the third floor of a modest commercial building. It's maybe 30 by 40 feet. The windows have been painted black, and there are three wooden tiers for the bicycles, like a modest amphitheater. Sixty stationary bikes in half circles, facing the front of the room. Where Marion—the very best of the spin meisters—has her bike. And a huge music system. And a single light that shines down on her pretty head, and sweating body. Marion does not mail it in; she *leads.*

The place is packed. Hilly reserved us spots in the back, away from the speakers. Except there is no place away from the speakers. These folks did not spend big bucks on decor, but the speaker system would blow the paint off the walls, if they had any. I wear earplugs, which make it hard to understand Marion but do nothing to cut the noise. What the hell; I am deaf already. Let's go.

The knowledgeable crowd assembles, fiddles with their seats and pedals, takes swigs of water. They are two-thirds women and a few fit men. They are mostly between twenty-five and thirty-five and the women are *wonderful* looking. Alarmingly fit and beautiful. The women do not dress up for this event. Sweats and hair in buns. But never mind: There is nothing better looking on earth than a woman of just about any age who is in great shape. And these people are in really great shape.

They turn off the lights, except the one spot on Marion and a crack of light under the door. The music cranks up big time. You can no longer hear. Or think. Or do anything else but *be in the zone.* That's why we're here, I guess, and it works.

They did spend some money on the bikes and they are all wired with the latest wattage metering system. Measuring your electric output is much more sophisticated even than heart rate monitors. The gadget measures your actual power, second to second, and keeps a running total of your total power for the session. There is a little gauge on your bike that shows power, cadence, and degree of resistance. You know everything about your performance all the time. And—most alarmingly—there are some whack jobs who choose to have their names and performances posted on a massive electronic screen at the front of the room, behind Marion, so they can compete with each other, the little fruitcakes. Have I conveyed that these people are a little bit serious? Well, they are.

The Horror!

So off we go, the warm-up and then into the intervals. This is, basically, an interval class, and a pretty serious one at that. Not Hunter Creek, but not a walk in the park either. We are thundering along in the dark when I look up, in absolute horror, and see Hilary's nom-de-bicyclette (everyone uses code names) up there on the public tote board. *What* can she be thinking! She is listed as "Hil-Coop" on the big electronic sign, but it's obviously her; that's her email and all kinds of stuff. My own precious wife has put her name up on the board, in plain sight of all these crazy people.

And it gets worse. For me. Each of us knows how we are doing personally by looking down at our own little dials. Power, cadence, resistance—and, most critically, how hard you've worked, cumulatively, so far. And here's the thing. Hilly is young and strong and whatnot. But despite my vast years, I have always been in better aerobic shape. Whenever we bike or do anything like that, I go on ahead, and then wait—smugly—for her to catch up. No such problem today, of course: These bikes aren't going anywhere. But according to the numbers on the tote board—*Hilary is screaming along just as hard as I am.* And our cumulative power is almost identical. *What* is going on here?

Without making a fuss, I quietly reach down into my massive reserves of aerobic power and take it up a notch. (Show her, by heaven!) And Hilary does, too. I reach down again and tighten the resistance knob quite a bit. The power gadget keeps track of cadence and degree of difficulty. Hilly can spin her pedals pretty fast, but she is no match for my wonderful self when it comes to power. Not until this morning, anyhow. She stays with me, stroke for stroke, at the new level. Oh, Lord!

I look over to see if she is ready to pass out, but not a bit of it. She is cruising! She looks as if she could do this all morning! I stand up, crank it up, crank it down. I go nuts.

Hilary, too. She is now in second or third place, up on the big board, in total power for all the women in the room. She is first some of the time! Has she been *sandbagging* me, all our life together? Has she been living a *lie* with me so as not to break my aging spirit? It is perfectly clear, looking at her calm face: She can bury me any time she wants. She has *huge* reserves—she's barely sweating. I am sweating *blood.*

It goes on like that for the next ten minutes, neck and neck. Me going nuts and she seeming not even to notice. Talk about *intervals!* This is madness. And my own precious wife is leading the way. My life is over. I have always known this day would come. I am old, after all, and I deserve it. But *this morning! No! Too soon!*

Finally, the stinking class is over. We towel down and walk out. Hilly is utterly serene. Gives no hint of what she's just done. My face is a nasty purple and she is breathing easily. Finally, I can stand it no longer.

"How the hell did you do that?" I demand, not angrily, you know. Respectful. And a little scared to see what the rest of our lives is going to be like.

"What do you mean?" she asks pleasantly. And finally I explain. "Oh," she says with a merry smile. "I put us *both* down as 'Hil-Coop' but I didn't register in the top twenty. That was you."

I have been racing *against myself* all morning? Oh, Lord! What an idiot. What an absolutely dreadful day. In the end, I suppose it's just another metaphor for life; in the end, we're all just competing against ourselves anyhow. Literally, this morning.

So look, intervals. They are the key to fitness, as opposed to health. And a real boost for any faltering efforts to lose weight. There is nothing like intensity when it comes to exercising for weight loss. I have the greatest respect for those of you who go only to long and slow and stay there. Not easy, and it will do great things for you. But you may want to give intervals or intensity a shot one day. It's a little different.

Dinner That Night; New Relationship with New Food: FARRO!

The night of that spin class debacle, we're having eight people over for dinner at the apartment. When we bought this place, we doubled the size of the kitchen, and I went down to the restaurant supply part of town and scored this huge Montague Grizzly gas stove, my pride and joy. Six burners, two huge ovens, and a "salamander," or special grilling space, with overhead flame. *Very* sophisticated. I am not a great cook, but I am *hell* on buying gear.

One of the pleasures of living in New York is food—in restaurants and in grocery stores. There are great food stores all over the place, and a trip to one of them to shop for a dinner party is a particular joy. And one of my new pleasures is scratching around for new stuff

Farro

You cook it like any other good grain, except it cooks faster than some. Takes about fifteen minutes, with, say, 4 cups of water per cup of farro. As with any grain or pasta (or vegetable, as you now know), the trick is to taste it often as it gets close to being done. Take it out, drain it, add some scallions if you feel like it, or just eat it as it comes out of the pot. *Superb.*

to eat that fits Jen's regimen. Nothing exotic tonight: a couple of slabs of halibut, to take advantage of the salamander, great salad stuff, and fresh baby beets. Easy-peasy. The only interesting thing is the grain. I am a hound for grain and used to eat tons of white rice. Those pleasant days are over, but the surprising news is that the substitutes are quite a bit better than the original. Especially my new favorite, farro, an Italian grain that looks like brown rice on steroids.

I have loved rice since I was a little kid, but this is the best grain I have ever tasted. Very chewy, nice texture. Nutty good taste. It's my new favorite. Even better than quinoa, my last big grain discovery. Try it. Sneak a little butter on it when no one's looking. It's calorie-dense, so you can't go nuts, but *so* good for you.

Do you have trouble cooking beets? Lots of people do. They think they have to peel them or some damn thing. You don't.

Beets

Cut off the tops and the bottoms before you boil them. Then into a pot of boiling water. When they are perfect—crisp to the bite but not too crisp, like almost all vegetables—dump 'em into a colander and go to the sink. Grab a hot beet so the bigger, cut-off end is away from your hand. Squeeze 'em. The skin squirts off. Hold them under cold running water while you're doing this so you don't get burned. Now all you have to do is cut them up a little, again under cold water. Put 'em back in the pan, and warm 'em back up when you're ready to serve.

Beets are wonderful. Very good with farro, by the way. Good with a baked potato too, but we're not that kind of girl anymore. Too bad; I love baked potatoes. Still eat 'em once in a while. But the farro is even better. There you go.

For a simple all-veg meal, try this. Farro with a can (in winter) of chopped (not pureed) tomatoes poured over it, after it's cooked. Add a good salad, and you are so lucky. Gonna love it. And not feel deprived for one second. Not a bad idea to have an all-veg meal once in a while. Makes you feel as if you are moving into the veg world. Nice going.

CHAPTER FIFTEEN

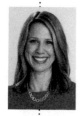

Sports Nutrition

O nce you start a rigorous exercise program—forty-five minutes per day, six days a week—you need to think about nutrition in a different way than the average person. The more that we understand what the foods we eat are doing within our bodies, especially during exercise, the more likely we will eat the Good Stuff and recognize the Bad Stuff for what it is. Beyond that, it is truly fascinating to see how thousands of mini-mechanisms involving nutrients within our bodies sync together to make the body move. This will be a little arcane, I imagine, for some of you, and fascinating, I hope, for others.

Are You Slow-Twitch or Fast-Twitch?

Y ou may have heard of slow-twitch and fast-twitch muscle fibers before, and you certainly have both. Most of us are around 50 percent slow-twitch and 50 percent fast-twitch, but the variation of percentages is great, especially across muscle groups. The muscle fibers you have dictate how you move, the speed and force that you generate, how quickly you fatigue, and the fuels that you burn. Those fuels come directly from the foods that you eat—carbohydrates and fat, for the most part—with carbohydrates the most critical for muscle movement.

Slow-twitch fibers are highly oxidative or aerobic—they are full of mitochondria and are great at allowing you to do continuous low-intensity movement. They burn glucose but mostly fat for energy. They are your marathon muscles for long and low. Fast-twitch fibers, in contrast, are your "sprinter" muscles. They are highly anaerobic and blast through your muscle glycogen and glucose for energy. They allow you to do high-intensity exercise, but they also fatigue quickly.

Each of your muscles—biceps, quadriceps (thigh), gastrocnemius (calf muscle), and so on—is made up of a mix of fast-twitch and slow-twitch muscle fibers (and to complicate matters there is a gradation of fibers that are in between the slow- and fast- twitch, but we won't go there). Some muscles have a higher percentage of slow-twitch fibers than fast-twitch and vice versa. For example, muscles involved with posture are mostly slow-twitch (like your soleus muscle that is between your calf and heel), whereas the muscles in your gastrocnemius or quadriceps are more of an equal mix.

As it turns out, your individual nerves dictate whether a muscle fiber becomes fast- or slow-twitch. Your genetics determine which muscle nerves you have, and those muscle nerves then innervate each muscle fiber, causing the muscle fiber to be either slow- twitch or fast-twitch. For example, about 50 percent of the muscle fiber "type" in your thigh is determined by genetics. Wait! That means the remaining 50 percent is dictated by *you,* by the type and amount of physical activity you get. Think of different athletes—most are born with a predisposition to do naturally well in their sports—for example, marathon runners will have 75 percent slow-twitch in their calf muscles, whereas sprinters will have 75 percent fast-twitch. You can say, yeah, they were born with it, but to a certain extent they also trained themselves to optimize the type of fiber that would benefit them the most. The marathoner needs long and slow and a steady burn of fat; the sprinter needs explosive energy but not for long. Interestingly, as we age, we tend to lose fast-twitch muscle fibers due to the loss of fast-twitch nerves. We become more of a slow-twitch endurance machine. So here you can see that by virtue of training and aging our metabolic machinery in our muscles can shift with both activity and time.

The Metabolic Pathways

L et's take a quick look back at how the body actually accesses carbohydrates and fats for fuel for use in the body.

There are two metabolic pathways in the body that use carbs and fats as fuel: the anaerobic system and aerobic system. The aerobic system, the one that is in use most of the time, dominates in slow-twitch fibers, and involves the use of oxygen to burn fat or carbohydrate mainly in the form of glucose or glycogen. Recall that glycogen is simply the storage form of glucose in the muscle and liver. The anaerobic system burns fuel without oxygen, predominates in our fast-twitch fibers, and works only with carbohydrate, typically muscle glycogen.

The anaerobic system is used much less than the aerobic system, but you use it first, in the sense that it is quickest and easiest to be turned on. Stored glucose in the form of muscle glycogen is right there in the muscles, waiting to go in an instant. It does not require the patience for oxygen to be made available, but it is only there in limited supply. If it is burned without oxygen, it can create a huge "exhaust" or ash problem. It can generate a tremendous amount of lactic acid, which quickly rises to intolerable levels during intense activity.

The anaerobic system can be thought of in two ways: (1) it burns extra-hot, and generates energy quickly, but because the system is fast, it does not generate tons of energy; (2) it is a limited system because you can run out of muscle glycogen and/or if you rely only on this system you will generate too much lactic acid, which will inhibit your muscles' ability to contract. It is the pathway to use for explosive power, the sprint or the last all-out push on the bike to the summit. You can only go "all out" using this system for thirty seconds to maybe two minutes. That's it and you're cooked. So this is a fight-or-flight fuel source that we use to run from the murderer or the lion.

The anaerobic system turns on first, but it is mostly the precursor to the aerobic system as oxygen becomes available. It gets you going. The muscles can also access this glycogen or glucose for aerobic

Phosphocreatine: The Third Energy System

The story of metabolic systems would be shamefully incomplete if I left out the phosphocreatine system. There are actually three metabolic systems in our muscles, and the third—and most amusing—is the phosphocreatine system. It doesn't play a large role in the great scheme of things, but it has a special nook, because it does not burn carbs, fat, or protein for energy. Or oxygen. A miracle.

What *does* it do? The body makes creatine—actually phosphocreatine—and uses it to create ATP, which your muscles can use for energy. It produces energy for very short and high levels of activity: two to seven seconds, tops. But for that period, you howl. This is particularly important for football players, sprinters, boxers—and those of us who are a bit more hyper, but not you. Most of us don't have to think much about it. There was a craze for creatine supplements in the 1990s. Average people (nonathletes) were buying them like crazy. Not a good idea, as usual. Your body actually can synthesize its own creatine, and dietary sources include meat and fish. That's it. Now the story is complete and I feel better.

metabolism, but it has to wait for the oxygen to be delivered to the working muscles. There is some oxygen present in muscle cells, in myoglobin, but not too much. Most has to be delivered by the circulation. The blood can deliver circulating blood glucose to the working muscle as well, but this takes longer and does not become a major fuel source until later in exercise. With the aerobic pathway, the one used predominantly, you use oxygen to burn glucose or free fatty acids to make the fire. It takes a bit longer to get revved up, but it generates enormous amounts of energy that you use all day long.

The Lactate or Anaerobic Threshold

The great decision point inside your body when you are working out is not between going totally aerobic or going totally anaerobic. The most important turning point is called the anaerobic threshold, a point that lies somewhat in the middle of using both systems. That is the point at which the exhaust from the burning process—the ashes, the smoke, the lactic acid—builds up faster than the blood can carry it away. When you reach that point, and if you don't ease up on the intensity, the end is in sight. Depending on how hard you are working and how fit you are, you may be able to go on for another half hour, maybe an hour, and maybe even longer. But you can't run from the Berkshires to Canada in this mode. The acidity in your muscles will build up and they will stop contracting. At low intensities of effort, you are able to get rid of the lactic acid and maintain a steady-state level. As you work harder, you cannot recycle it fast enough and it starts to accumulate. This is the point where lactate starts to rise quickly.

One of the great goals of serious trainers of aerobic or endurance athletes is to move the lactate threshold, or anaerobic threshold (same thing), to the right to get the runner or cyclist or whatever to be able to reach ever higher levels of work output without hitting this threshold. Basically you are able to increase your intensity and avoid going anaerobic for longer. For example, an untrained person may start to accumulate lactate or hit their anaerobic threshold at 50–60 percent of their maximum (max) heart rate. However with regular exercise and training, the point of lactate accumulation can gradually be shifted to the right at higher percentages of your max—say at 60–70 percent. That is a big part of what Riggs Klika does; it is at the heart of his art as a master trainer, and you'll hear more about it from him in later chapters. Some of the world's best endurance athletes have their lactate threshold around 80 percent of their max, meaning they can produce a tremendous amount of physical effort without going totally anaerobic. Pretty amazing.

Metabolic Realities

We are almost always using a combination of aerobic and anaerobic pathways. How your body triggers and blends the two systems and which fuels it uses are a direct result of three things: the intensity of activity, the duration of that activity, your level of fitness. And these three in combination have a great deal to do with your performance in terms of your ability to do endurance activities, on the one hand, or explosive movements, on the other. And we can train each system. For instance, the more long-distance running we do, the more effective we are at generating energy from the aerobic pathway—the enzymes work more efficiently and effectively and we are better able to burn fats and less muscle glycogen. The more sprinting we do, the more that those enzymes in the anaerobic pathway work efficiently and effectively, and our lactic acid buildup is less and we have more tolerance for it.

Intensity

This will become more interesting to you as you read more about workouts of varying intensities. Here I paint a picture of what happens to your body's fuel use in four different domains of activity, ranging from being at rest to going into an all-out sprint.

1. At rest, about 60 percent of your energy comes from fat and 40 percent from carbohydrates (i.e., your muscle and liver glycogen stores or your circulating glucose). Note: It is not all coming from fat! It is almost totally aerobic.

2. At about 50 percent of your max, the split is about 50/50 between carbohydrate and fat usage. This is a blend of aerobic and anaerobic.

3. At a little higher intensity, say 60–80 percent of your max, the zone where you will likely find yourself during much of your intentional exercise, you will really shift into using carbohydrate as a predominant fuel source—about 80:20 carbs to fat. Again, it's a blend of aerobic and anaerobic.

4. At nearly your max, 85–95 percent effort, say when you are attempting some sprints during your interval training, you will surely be burning almost all carbohydrate at a ratio of 95:5. This is almost totally anaerobic.

Here are a few things to keep in mind. You are always burning a little bit of all fuel sources, no matter what your state of rest or exercise—this includes carbohydrates, fat, and protein. We don't put much emphasis on protein as a fuel source, because it typically contributes only a trace amount, except at longer and higher intensities of work, where it can hover around 5 percent. For these reasons, we focus mostly on carbohydrates and fats.

The second thing to keep in mind, and Chris will remind you of this later, is that there is no such thing as a fat-burning zone. This is honestly one of my pet peeves. If there were such a thing, sleeping would be a fat-burning exercise. What is happening is that fat contributes a higher percentage of the total fuel used at lower intensities of work, but the calories are so much lower that you actually burn the same if not more absolute fat at higher intensities. Work harder and you burn more calories and more fat, period.

Duration

This is pretty straightforward. The longer we exercise, the more we deplete our muscle glycogen stores and have to rely more heavily on circulating glucose and free fatty acids for fuel. Blood sugar is not as important early during exercise; we rely mostly on our stores right in the muscle, especially for anaerobic activity. An hour or so into exercise the glucose from the circulation becomes more critical in fueling the muscle as the muscle glycogen stores start to become depleted. This glucose from the bloodstream can be burned aerobically or anaerobically depending on the task.

The muscles and the bloodstream together still hold a limited supply of glucose, around 2,000 kcal stored as glycogen in the muscles, or about enough for a serious ninety-minute workout. We have only minimal glucose in our blood. What next? That, for a lot of us, is the good news: The body also burns fat, from storage in your tush, your gut, or in your muscles for a major energy release for endurance activity. Aerobic, metabolism-burning glucose certainly yields a lot of energy, but oh boy, if we can burn the fat, it generates three to four times the energy. Once our muscle glycogen is mostly gone and there's not much left in the blood, it is critical to eat a ready source of glucose to maintain blood sugar levels. Remember how important blood sugar is to fuel our brain!

Fitness

With training, use of all of the systems just described is optimized. We are able to store more glycogen in our muscles, so that it is not depleted as quickly. Free fatty acids are better mobilized and made more readily accessible to trained muscles. The availability of fat as a fuel reduces the pressure to deplete stores of muscle glycogen. The enzymes in muscles that burn fat become more plentiful and more active. There is an overall "glycogen sparing," which is critical for you to maintain any muscular activity. And don't forget that your ability to move your anaerobic threshold increases, along with your ability to tolerate and clear lactic acid in your muscles. You are able to exercise longer and more intensely—and therefore burn more calories. These are some amazing reasons to think about becoming a new, fitter you.

When and What to Do with Fuel

You know what they say: Timing is everything. That is also the case with eating foods when you are going to work out. Scheduling exercise into a busy lifestyle is one challenge. Scheduling your eating around that exercise makes it more complicated. Eating too much food or the wrong food before exercise can impair your performance or cause indigestion, cramps, sluggishness, and nausea. But if you haven't eaten in six hours and try to work out, you may feel weaker as the workout progresses and you will likely poop out sooner.

Fueling Before Exercise

Your number-one goal for fueling for exercise is to have fed your body nutritious food that ensures a normal blood glucose concentration going into exercise and at the same time, making sure this food is no longer present in your stomach when you work out. You want your blood to flow freely to your working muscles, to bring the oxygen to power aerobic metabolism, and also to clear away any waste generated from the anaerobic system. Your muscles are greedy, but so is your stomach. What happens then when you have a snack or meal too close to exercising? Your blood flow is basically torn between redirecting blood flow to the working muscles or to the gastrointestinal tract where there are foodstuffs to digest. As a result of this battle your body does neither well. You are literally taking the needed pipeline of oxygen away from the muscles where it is also needed for metabolism and muscle contraction. Many times this results in a cramp, nausea, and the inability to tap into your exercise potential.

Here are some simple rules:

1. Don't eat too soon before exercise.

2. Avoid eating altogether for the thirty minutes beforehand. I don't care if it makes you feel good; it doesn't help.

3. Consider consuming some calories during exercise, if you are going to be out for longer than 60–90 minutes.

4. Stay hydrated: 8–12 ounces of water before a workout, and an hour into a workout, drink 4–8 ounces of water every twenty minutes.

5. No sports drinks except during prolonged exercise that lasts longer than an hour (useful in that situation and useless the rest of the time).

Here are more details. Another issue with eating something— especially a high carbohydrate/high sugar food—in the fifteen to forty-five minutes prior to exercise is that it causes that dreaded sugar high followed by an insulin surge and subsequent sugar low—right when you are about fifteen to twenty minutes into your exercise bout. That won't help you with anything. You know what happens when your blood sugar drops during a workout—it drops and so do you.

So what to eat and when? If you eat well in advance, I would suggest anything healthy and balanced, and you certainly can choose from our good foods list. In general, carbohydrates are easily digested, but foods high in protein, fiber, and fat will linger in the stomach for some time, depending on how much you eat. Large meals take longer to empty from the stomach, about four to six hours. Snacks (three hundred calories or less), depending on their content, take about thirty minutes to an hour to leave your stomach. Eating a high carbohydrate snack two hours before exercising can leave you ample energy and a calm stomach for a great workout. Many competitive athletes avoid food within two hours of a very hard workout, but they can tolerate a lighter snack within one to two hours of a light workout. A light workout can be preceded with a light snack, but definitely leave more lead time for an intense workout. The closer you eat to a workout, the fewer calories should be consumed.

Common sense says that during exercise, if you need to consume something, it should be readily digestible, so make it low in fat, protein, and fiber. I hate to say this, but for once foods with a high glycemic index (easily and quickly digestible) are just what you want. You want to get the glucose in there fast. Sports gels, a small banana, or bread with jam are good choices depending on the type and duration of activity. And the neat thing is that during exercise, you "get away with it," in the sense that you do not get the dreaded insulin spike that usually follows the eating of high glycemic junk. Chris thinks of this as free play with food (alas his big chocolate chip cookies on long bike rides). Your body uses sugar without needing much insulin, so enjoying a sports drink during exercise is no problem for events lasting over an hour. On a longer exercise effort, consuming thirty grams of carbohydrate every thirty minutes provides an important extra boost.

Do You Chow Down After a Workout?

I f you are anything like me, you may not be hungry after a workout and feel happy that this is one of those rare occasions when you can take advantage of not wanting to eat. Depending on what type of exerciser you are, you could be missing a critical window of opportunity to restore your muscle glycogen levels without much risk of bad effects. And your muscle glycogen has everything to do with how hard and how long you can exercise the next day. To simplify things, I would look at your workout and the types of workouts you are doing over the course of one week and categorize yourself into one of two buckets: (1) the athlete or "wannabe athlete" who works out six days per week, with several of those days including workouts that are an hour or longer where you exercise at 75 percent or higher and/or include intense lifting sessions; or (2) the "exerciser" or "recreational athlete" who never goes over an hour for a workout, doesn't go too intensely or for too many days per week.

If you are in the second bucket, you can just forget about what I am going to say next because the muscle glycogen levels in your muscles do not limit your workouts. For you, timing of snacks and meals after a workout is not critical.

If you are in the first bucket, what you eat after exercise is critical to your performance the next day because the body needs carbohydrates to restock your glycogen stores. Unlike the second bucket guy or gal, you may have dug pretty deeply into your glycogen stores; you may even have tapped them out. In that case, it's a great idea to have a high carbohydrate with some protein snack within thirty minutes to an hour after exercise. This is the critical window when your muscles are best able to take up circulating glucose to store as muscle glycogen. The receptors responsible for uptake for glucose in your muscles are primed and waiting for the extra sugar and can optimize the storage and recovery of your muscles. Even the enzymes that synthesize muscle glycogen are more active. Your muscle glycogen storage capacity is maximized during this time. Fueling your body after an hour or so is less efficient—it happens slower and not to the same capacity.

Now a bit about the protein piece of the snack. As it turns out, the muscles take up the glucose even more effectively if there is some protein consumed with the carbohydrate snack. Protein also offers the added benefit of helping to repair any damaged tissue. In both young and older adults, consuming protein after weight training has been shown to be extremely effective in helping to build and maintain muscle mass. Fortunately, there are many easy food choices that contain both carbohydrate and protein: yogurt, cereal, brown rice or pasta, nuts and seeds, beans, tofu, and legumes. Even an egg white on a piece of whole-grain toast is a great option. Chocolate milk is a recent sensation, but I won't dive into that controversy here. I will save that one for the boathouse.

Hydration Is Key

Hydration, even more than shrinking glycogen stores, may be the number-one limiter of performance. Without adequate fluid, your plasma volume—the amount of blood circulating through your body—is compromised. When this happens, your blood becomes thick and viscous, the delivery of oxygen to your working muscles becomes

DO YOU REALLY NEED THAT ELECTROLYTE BEVERAGE DURING YOUR WORKOUT?

Electrolyte beverages include sports drinks and a whole cadre of waters with added electrolytes and various amounts of sugar. Sports drinks are uniquely designed with 4–8 percent glucose that maximizes their rate of absorption, so they won't be sloshing around in your gut all day. The calories help maintain blood sugar levels and mental alertness while the electrolytes replace those that are lost in sweat and the water keeps you hydrated. This is so critical when exercising for long periods of time, especially in the heat, when muscle and liver glycogen start to become depleted and it is difficult to stay hydrated. Other electrolyte beverages, including coconut water, have been hyped up recently—full of electrolytes and lower in sugar. However, these are less beneficial to exercise performance and are not calorie-free.

Rule of thumb: If your exercise bout is one hour or less, you do not need to consume anything beyond water. However, if you exercise longer than one hour, say in the one- to four-hour range, consuming a sports drink is beneficial for your ability to sustain activity and to continue feeling great.

Note of caution: These drinks *have calories*. These are not what you want to be sipping all day at the office.

compromised, and you are unable to sweat and properly thermoregulate, meaning your internal core temperature will increase. Your heart rate increases to help push the blood to your working muscles and vital organs. Water loss from sweat of as little as 1–2 percent of body weight has a negative impact on performance.

You need to hydrate, and thirst alone is not a good indicator of adequate hydration levels. If you are thirsty, you are already dehydrated and you likely will not be able to overcome this dehydration during a workout. If your urine is yellow, you are also likely dehydrated. Ideally, it should be nearly colorless. The key to feeling well hydrated for life and for exercise is to stay hydrated throughout the day. Drink beverages that are low in caffeine and alcohol because they encourage dehydration. Drink eight to twelve ounces of water before a workout and drink four to eight ounces every fifteen to twenty minutes during a workout. Remember, water is the only beverage that is needed during workouts lasting one hour or less.

Exercise and Free Radicals

Exercise is a bit of a double-edged sword when it comes to the pesky free radicals. You may remember that they are created by the simple act of breathing. When you breathe more—as you do in exercise—you make more of them. In addition, there is some muscle damage when you exercise that also produces free radicals. Because of all that, it is so important to eat right, in the sense of eating foods with antioxidant properties. Thus it makes sense for active exercisers—like you, now— to go heavy on foods that are high in vitamins C and E but also the numerous phytochemicals that have antioxidant properties. That takes you right back to eating an abundance of fruits and vegetables.

The good news is that exercise itself foments anti–free radical molecules. Essential nutrients like zinc, copper, and selenium (which are minerals) are part of these enzymes. Here's the best news: Although exercise can stress your body in ways that produce free radicals, the positive antioxidant changes in your body far outweigh them. Net/net, exercise is the great reducer of free radicals and the great improver of your basic health. So the double-edged sword mostly cuts our way.

Other Nutrients Important to Exercise

There are several essential vitamins and minerals that play key roles during exercise. The B vitamins—thiamin, riboflavin, and vitamin B_6—are critical in energy metabolism and assist in energy release from carbohydrates and fats. Calcium is critical for muscle contraction and the transmission of signals from your nerves to your muscles. Magnesium is also involved with muscle contraction but also in glucose metabolism. Phosphorus helps to form ATP and release oxygen from red blood cells. Iron is the critical mineral in hemoglobin that allows our red blood cells to carry oxygen to our muscles and is involved in aerobic metabolism. Chromium enhances insulin function. Zinc is a key player in cell-mediated immunity and keeps our immune defenses up when we are worn out or fatigued, and it is also important in enzymes involved with tissue repair.

For most of these nutrients, there is not much evidence to say that there is an additional requirement for exercisers beyond normal dietary recommendations. Special considerations may be warranted for those who do not eat particular foods (e.g., vegetarians or those of us older than sixty-five who might be low in B_{12}) or who participate in a particular event (e.g., runners who may need to watch their iron levels); zinc, calcium, and magnesium may be lost in sweat and are often low in some individuals' diets. If diets are balanced from all food groups and if there is an adequate intake of protein, most of us can stay in a nutrient-healthy exercise zone. Again, the bottom line: Those who exercise are not exempt from having to be meticulous about eating a sound balanced diet.

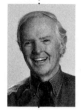

CHAPTER SIXTEEN

Aerobic Exercise: *The* Secret of the Good Life

There is no silver bullet in life, but aerobic exercise comes close. Why is it so important? For a bunch of reasons, but the basic one, I suspect, is that we were primarily designed to be aerobic creatures. Endurance predators, trotting along for hours, out there on the broad savannahs. Our niche—in the Darwinian crucible of survival—was to trail along beside a herd of antelope or elands for most of a day. Until one of them got a little tired and one of us could smack him on the head. Eat him. We were not as fast as the antelope, but we had great endurance; that and *focus* were our gifts for survival. They worked, and they run deep in our bodies.

When we get too far away from those predator roots, things get messed up. Which, of course, is where we are today: Most of us are pretty idle and pretty badly messed up. But the great news is that our idleness-induced rot is reversible, to a remarkable extent, with a relatively modest regimen of steady exercise, especially *aerobic* exercise. Getting back to serious aerobic exercise is the single best thing you can do to get back to your endurance predator roots and have your body work the way it is supposed to.

Putting Exercise into Practice:
Meet Bill Fabrocini and Riggs Klika

n the next few chapters I am going to pass along a distillation of the considerable wisdom of Bill Fabrocini (strength training) and Riggs Klika (aerobics) that they have carefully reviewed and blessed. They are very serious experts indeed, and they have been thinking, writing, and practicing this stuff—at the cutting edge—for a long time. If you'd like to be in touch with them directly, see the note about the website in the appendix.

Riggs Klika, Ph.D., has focused during his long career on aerobic exercise in particular, but he knows the whole exercise field well. He has led our Aspen Total Immersion Weeks, which you can also read about on the website—from the beginning. (Those were weeks where we "beta tested" much that you are reading about here on small groups.) Riggs and I have biked, skied, and trained together, and been friends, for twenty years.

Riggs was an all-American swimmer at Southern Methodist, got a master's at the University of Colorado and a Ph.D. at the University of Texas, with a specialty in human development and aging. A former team physiologist for the U.S. Ski Team, he has been a trainer of professional athletes—and the rest of us—all his life. He has published a dozen peer-reviewed articles in scientific journals. One of his recent ventures was establishing a *serious* exercise program for cancer survivors. He scared the dickens out of the cancer doctors, and had amazing success with his clients.

The other great expert is Bill Fabrocini, P.T., C.S.C.S. Bill is a physical therapist, but he is also a star trainer. He has trained a lot of famous athletes, including NBA MVP David Robinson, Olympic medalists Chris Klug and Gretchen Bleiler, tennis grand slam champions Martina Navratilova and Conchita Martinez, U.S. Open Women's Golf champion Jane Geddes, and NFL Rookie of the Year, Mike Croel. He was also trainer to an NBA basketball team, and he's been written up in *Outside* magazine, *Men's Health*, and *Skiing*. He's good.

But the reason I turned to Bill is the fact that he is such a creative and original thinker about strength training in general. Bill has created a comprehensive and sophisticated strength-training system that he calls Posture, Stability, and Movement (PSM), and it is the basis for *everything* we say in the book about strength training. Bill insists that he is just one guy in a long chain of people who have developed the new strength training. Could be, but my sense is that he is the star and that we are very lucky to have him.

Why Aerobics?

There are four underlying reasons: (1) It builds and rebuilds our aerobic base, the elaborate machinery that lets us *move*. (2) It fundamentally changes our blood chemistry in a way that *radically improves our health*. (3) It *improves our mood* and fights depression. (4) It makes us *smarter*. Let's take a closer look.

Rebuild Your Aerobic Base

As you know, we are internal combustion machines, big endurance predators with big complex engines. Billions of mitochondria, out in the muscles, instead of a single V6 engine in the middle like a car, but the same idea. We were *built* to move, just as surely as your car was built to move. That's what we are all about, and much of our body is devoted to it.

The aerobic system (heart, lungs, and circulatory system) is designed to fuel the engines and clear out the exhaust or waste after the burn. Our whole muscular/skeletal structure is the moving machinery. And the signaling system makes it run. It is all designed to make us *move*, which is what we are all about. When that system or any part of it gets buggered up, we can't move. And in fundamental ways, we cease to be ourselves.

For a long time, people thought that we—like car engines—literally wore out with use. We had only so many revolutions or whatever before we wore away the "piston walls" and died. But no! We are *living* flesh, and it doesn't work that way. When we use our bodies, we do not wear the system down, we *build it up*. When you do aerobic exercise, you actually create millions and millions of new mitochondria.

You grow miles of new capillaries. You *increase the horsepower of the whole machine*. Use it and it grows. Let it sit idle and it rots.

Change Your Blood Chemistry: Fight Disease

The second one is even more important. When you do serious aerobic exercise, your blood chemistry goes from inflammatory to anti-inflammatory. This little trick is instrumental in reducing—by a whopping 50 percent!—your risk of heart attacks, strokes, adult-onset diabetes, lots of cancers, Alzheimer's, and others. Talk about your miracles. There isn't a pill or medical regimen in the world that begins to come close.

The Master Mood Changer

If you happen to get as old as I am, you will realize that *grumpiness* often arrives with aging. Grumpy old man . . . crabby old woman. It's the saddest thing. Drives people away and makes you feel like an idiot. Mood in general is serious business. Depression is *very* serious business, and there are some suggestions that widely used antidepressant drugs aren't that great. At the same time we are learning that the single most effective thing you can do to improve your mood is aerobic exercise. And we are not just talking about the "runner's high." We are talking about *raising the water table of your mood* in general. We are talking about broad, deep mood change. With no side effects and no dosage problems. Only Good Stuff.

More Marbles

When you get old, you lose your marbles. Everyone knows that. Better get your Nobel Prize work done before you turn thirty-two because after that you start losing your marbles. You're sitting in the kitchen with your wife and you hear this rattling sound. What? It's one of your marbles, rolling across the kitchen floor. Not a great sound. And it goes on and on. Every year, you lose a few more. Rattle, rattle, rattle, across the kitchen floor.

But that turns out to be wrong. The body continues to manufacture brain cells, all the way out. New ones pop up and have a look around. See what's going on. Interestingly, if absolutely nothing is going on—if you are just sitting, watching daytime TV—they shrug and die a quick death in thirty days. But if you are active, engaged, and *at it* in some significant way, why, they pitch right in and go to work. Last a long time. You get smarter.

They did IQ tests on people age twenty-five and people age seventy-five. If the tests were *timed*, the young people did better. If they were not timed, old and young did about the same. And of course, the old people had a vast amount of experience and wisdom that the young did not. Here is the lesson: If you want a fast, *bad* result, hire a kid. If you want a slightly slower *good* answer, hire the older woman or man.

I forget why we were talking about this. Oh, I remember. Aerobic exercise. Slightly surprising news: Aerobic exercise is the single best thing you can do to enhance *the creation of new marbles*. How do you like that? Aerobic exercise does not *merely* keep you moving, ward off 50 percent of all serious disease, and radically improve your mood, it makes you *smarter*.

A Teeny Bit Boring

Did you like that? I thought you might—me, too. And I am going to use the momentum from that segment to *try* to pass along some information which you really ought to have but is a little bit boring. Sorry, but I am going to finish the story I started in Chapter 6 about your heart rate. Again, if you are going to be doing aerobic exercise four days a week for the rest of your life, it might not be a bad idea to have some sense of how *hard* you are working out. And to know that, you must know how hard your heart is working. It's not totally easy, but it's easier (and more important) than you might think.

Take a look at this little chart (next page). It shows some basic levels of aerobic effort (from long and slow to intervals to fight-or-flight), measured in two ways: rating of perceived exertion (RPE) and percentage of maximum heart rate. The RPE is subjective (how hard do you *feel* you are working out). And the percentage of max is scientific,

LEVELS OF AEROBIC EXERCISE

ZONE	RATE/PERCEIVED EXERTION	% OF MAX HEART RATE
Zone One (Long and Slow)	1–3 RPE	50–70%

This is a trot or a canter. You are breathing deeply but not panting. You can carry on normal conversation. You feel you could do this for hours, once you're in decent shape. Chase down that antelope. This is as hard as many of you ever have to go for health.

Zone Two (Endurance)	4–6 RPE	70–80%

Now you are breathing fairly hard. Can still talk, but you're taking some deep breaths. You could do this for a while but not forever; not at the upper reaches, anyway. If you are in great shape, you can do this for a couple of hours. Zones 1 and 2 are variations of the same thing: Zone 2 is a more intense level 1. Go there when you get in better shape and feel like it.

Zone Three (Threshold/Intervals)	6–7 RPE	80–90%

This is serious business. You are breathing pretty hard now. Talking is possible at the lower reaches of this level, but not at the upper ones. At upper levels, you are panting hard. You can do this only (at the upper reaches anyway) for a few minutes. You get to the upper reaches of this level only when you're in great shape. And your doctor knows what you're up to. This is different. This is the more serious effort you get into, for fitness. Mostly you do this level only for "intervals" sprints of one to eight minutes, with rests in between. This is fitness country. Remember: You never have to go there unless you feel like it.

Zones Four and Five (Fight-or-Flight)	8–10 RPE	90–100%

You certainly never need to go this hard. Not in our regimen, anyway; I don't recommend it for most people over sixty. This is flat out. The lion or the robber is closing in, and you are giving it everything you've got. You can do this only for a short time, say, 60 seconds. Watch it! You can hurt yourself.

based on what you learn by looking at your heart rate monitor. We'll talk a little more, but look at the chart to get an idea.

The intensity of aerobic exercise is a continuum, of course, so these lines are a little arbitrary. They do track some physiological lines. For example, the chart refers to a "threshold" level, which is roughly the threshold at which fit people start to build up residue from burning fuel in their muscles, faster than their body can clear it. Jen just talked to you about it. That's a critical phase, and most people reach it at 50–80 percent of their max. That's when lactic acid buildup starts to occur; you cannot go on forever, once you reach that level. That's a huge range. Unfit people may start the lactic acid buildup at 50 percent of max. One of the miracles of getting in shape is moving that threshold up toward 70 percent.

Now back to figuring out your own maximum heart rate. To get your own max, start with the formula I mentioned earlier. Take 0.7 times your age and subtract it from 208. (If you're in dreadful shape, use the more conservative formula: 220 minus your age.) Neither formula is perfect and both are merely estimates. The difficulty is that maximum heart rate is idiosyncratic: Riggs showed me a graph of the actual maximum heart rates of a bunch of people the same age and of the same relative fitness; the dots were all over the place. So, inevitably, no formula is going to work for everyone. There are averages for each age, and as with all averages, individuals will fall along a bell-shaped curve.

The only way to find your real max is to go to it. You shouldn't do this until you're in great shape—and have the blessings of your doctor. Then do intervals or some other craziness until you think your heart is about to burst. At the top—if you have not had a heart attack and died—look down at your heart rate monitor. Remember the very highest number you see. That is your *real* max, even if you only reach it for a few seconds. The single, highest number you see is your max. It will change over time—go down, actually—but it is good for a year or so. If you are into this stuff, you may hit it really hard a few times over the course of a few weeks.

I did it yesterday, on the back side of Wells Hill, a killer hill out our way (14 percent grade!), in the Berkshires. Damn near killed myself, which is roughly what it takes. My max is 166, which seems reasonable. By the way, notice that if I used the old "220 minus your age" formula, I would have assumed my max was 143. And my whole training effort would have been nonsense. The better formula would put me at 155. Formulas don't work. Use 'em until you get a real number.

Anyhow, do figure out your theoretical formula-based max, preferably using the 208 minus 0.7 times your age formula. Then figure out 60 percent, 70 percent, 80 percent, and 90 percent of your max with a pencil and paper. Memorize 'em or write 'em down. At some point, you may want to find your real max and figure out the percentages of it. Formulas are weaker as you get older. They assume you are going to go to hell, like most older people. But we're not!

Recovery Rate

One of the neat things you can do with heart rate monitors is figure out your recovery rate. Everyone who is interested in aerobic health wants to know how quickly your heart recovers after major exertion. If your heart beats 160 beats a minute (bpm) at your max, the question is how fast it falls to normal levels when you stop. How resilient is it? In particular, how many bpms will you drop in 60 seconds? That is the standard question. The answer to it is your recovery rate. The faster it drops (in bpms) in sixty seconds, the more resilient and healthy the heart. If it gets stuck up near the red line for five minutes after you stop, you might want to sit down. Because a slow recovery is not a great sign.

The general rule is that a drop of 20 to 30 bpms is a good recovery rate. Do you happen to remember how I checked my heart rate that day on Bash Bish? I was checking my recovery rate. It was way over forty because I am such an aerobic nutcase. I was delighted.

Here's a critical detail about when you start to count the seconds for the sixty-second recovery period. (I told you it was a little esoteric.) Let's say you have biked or run your heart out to get to the top of a hill. Your heart is thundering away in the 80–85 percent range or higher. Get off your bike and look at your monitor and look at your watch with the sweep second hand. Wait until the first down-tick (from 160 to 159) on the heart rate monitor. Now start tracking the time. See how many beats it goes down in sixty seconds. You don't want to start until that first down-tick or you'll mess things up.

As I hope you will find out, recovery rate varies a lot, depending on a lot of things, mostly, in my case, depending on whether I have been good about aerobic workouts. If I am dogging it or missing days, down tumbles the recovery rate. It is also sensitive to airplane travel. Doesn't like that. And the onset of a cold. If I am feeling puny, I take my recovery rate early on a ride. If it is unusually low, I take the hint— that a cold is coming on or I ate and drank too much last night—and take it easy. But if it's well into the thirties or forties, I may crank it up. And remind myself to tell absolutely everyone about it at supper. Warning: Even workout nuts look at you a little funny when you start to talk recovery rates. It's a great thing to know, but it does not sing at cocktail parties.

If you refuse to get and use a heart rate monitor (dumb), you can figure out your pulse, as you know, by sticking your finger by your Adam's apple (boys only) or find your pulse on your wrist. Count for ten seconds and multiply the result by six, I believe. Yes, that makes sense. Or, if you are in a fierce rush, you can count for six seconds and multiply by ten. Doesn't matter; neither number is going to be worth much. Buy a heart rate monitor!

Or you can just go with your subjective sense, your RPE. I find that mostly useless, but no less an authority than Riggs thinks it's terrific. But find a way to keep track. That's the critical thing.

Are you a little bit bored now? Of course you are. But don't tear these pages out of the book. If you get into aerobic exercise a little—as I profoundly hope—you may want to circle back some day and try this stuff out. I live by it. But hey, I am getting a little odd.

CHAPTER SEVENTEEN

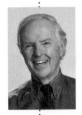

The How-To of Aerobic Exercise

The world of aerobic training is both very simple and very complicated. I am going to try to stick with the very simple version for the compelling reason that I do not really understand the complicated version. Riggs has been working with me for years (and now Jen too) trying to get me to understand how various metabolic systems cut in at various levels of athletic effort and what it means for your anaerobic threshold and to your ultimate fitness. And I still don't get it. I don't think you will either. So this is going to be simplified quite a bit. You will get some of the hard stuff—but not a lot. At the same time, you'll be relieved to know that Riggs and Jen have crawled through this chapter and say it is sound. Simple, maybe, but sound. And Riggs, of course, created the interval day regimens toward the end of the chapter. And they mostly won't kill you.

Well, they may kill you, a teeny bit. Highly unlikely but true. Serious aerobic exercise is serious business. But *not* doing serious aerobic exercise is much more dangerous. Harry, as he does so often, puts it beautifully: "The surest way to avoid death by heart attack today is to go home, lock the door, and get in bed. But the surest way to avoid death by heart attack, tomorrow and for the rest of your life, is to head out the door and do serious aerobic exercise. Four days a week. Forever. It will reduce your risk of heart attack and stroke by half in the long run. And it probably won't kill you today, either. Got it? Good. Let's go work out."

Two Views of Aerobics
Long and Slow for Health

I can't say often enough that you can get a huge part of the health benefit discussed in the last chapter by following a comparatively easy aerobic regimen—"long and slow," never going over 60–70 percent of your max. And the emphasis is on comparatively. We are talking about an exercise regimen that will seem hellishly demanding to some. We are talking about exercising a whopping forty-five to sixty minutes a day, four days a week, forever—on a bike, an elliptical machine, swimming, jogging, or whatever. Even at a relatively low, stable clip, that is a huge undertaking. But it really is not that hard. It is a major commitment of time, but the workouts themselves are not brutal. A "low stable clip" means just that: You can still talk while you're doing it; you're breathing a little harder, but you're not huffing and puffing. Your heart rate is in the 50–70 percent of your max range. Or a Rating of Perceived Exertion (RPE) of 1–3. Easy-peasy.

Do just that and you will get a huge part of the health benefits that one can derive from aerobic exercise. A huge part. You may decide to do more, but you surely don't have to. That will be a miraculous change for most people and a wonderful one.

Long and Slow: The Details
First: The Warm-Up

Warming up is key to having a good workout and avoiding catastrophe. In a sense, warming up "turns the muscles on." Warming up triggers the machinery for burning fuel, which you need during the session. It allows for hormonal and neurological changes in your heart and lungs to get them ready to pump blood and breathe. It warms up your joints too, an increasingly important step as we age. Think of this: When you are just sitting around, only 20 percent of your blood goes to your muscles. When you are working out hard, 80 percent of your blood goes to your muscles. That is a major plumbing change inside your body—lots of valves opening and closing, signals being sent, all kinds of stuff. It takes a moment or two. *Warm up.*

Here are two suggestions as to how to warm up. First and best, do the warm-up suggested by Bill Fabrocini, in the strength chapters. Alternatively (not quite as good but good enough), just do what you're going to do on a given day (bike, run, whatever) at a very moderate pace—say 50 percent of your max or an RPE of 1–2—for five or ten minutes. Bill's warm-up is better, but do whichever one you are more likely to do. And *do it,* religiously. It matters.

The Workout

This workout really is comparatively easy—a lot of time, but not a struggle. The hardest part is making up your mind. The second hardest part is probably picking the mode of exercise: biking, jogging, the elliptical or treadmill machines at the gym, speed walking, swimming, or whatever. There are two great keys at this early point: One, pick something you like. If you don't like it, you won't keep it up. Two, don't kid yourself. For most people, mere walking is not doing the job. For some it is, and if you are in wretched shape, it is a good place to start. Remember Freddy and how it transformed him. But mostly, it is not enough. Neither is golf or gardening or holding your hand up for the manicurist. Best defense against kidding yourself: Get a heart rate monitor. It is the great antidote to lying to yourself. Get your heart rate up to say 60 percent of max or you're kidding yourself.

Get into it slowly. Remember my friend Freddy, again. If you've been idle for a while, take it easy. But do follow the one big rule: Do some aerobic exercise, no matter how tame, four days a week, regardless. Don't take it easy by cutting days; take it easy by cutting minutes or going slower. Set a goal of at least forty-five minutes a day. Of

Long and Slow Aerobics Day

• Warm-up: 5–10 minutes (consider adding the Fabrocini warm-up prior to starting the workout)

• Main set: Long and slow 30–40 minutes (zone 1–3 RPE; about 55–65 percent of your maximal heart rate)

• Warm-down: 5–10 minutes

that, a total of, say, fifteen minutes can be warm-up and warm-down. Don't skip the warm-down. A sudden stop is dangerous: Blood pools and does goofy things. Ease your body out of exercise mode just as carefully as you eased your body into it. If you get thirty to forty-five minutes of exercise, apart from warm-up and warm-down, that's fine.

The Mythical "Fat-Burning Zone"

One of the benefits of Long and Slow is that it is done entirely in the fabled "fat-burning zone." The only trouble with that is that there is no such thing as a "fat-burning zone." It is a myth. The facts go like this. You burn both fat and glucose all the time. The mix of fat and glucose changes at different levels of exercise intensity. At the easier, Long and Slow levels, a higher percentage of the mix is fat, rather than glucose, but not the absolute amount. You burn more fat—in absolute calories—the harder you work out, all the way up to zone 5 and an RPE of 10! Don't make yourself nuts on the subject: You are burning plenty of fat in all zones of exercise.

Mix It Up and Enjoy It

This workout may pall after a while. Do consider mixing up the modes of exercise. If you haven't biked lately, do give that a shot. It is my absolute favorite. It's not an impact sport so you don't bang up your joints. And it's easy. That and rowing are my two favorites, actually.

But if you live in the frozen north, don't miss snowshoeing and cross-country skiing. Both are easy and both are an absolute joy. If there is anywhere near enough snow, I am out the door. And both cross-country and snowshoeing are bone-easy to learn. And you do them in some of the prettiest places in your world.

The Endurance Zone

As you get into Long and Slow, there is another whole level to enjoy, the Endurance Zone (zone 2, 70–80 percent of max, RPE 4–6). No need to push yourself in the early days—or ever, I guess—but in time you will almost certainly find yourself spending more and more time in the Endurance Zone. It is, obviously, a little more demanding than Long and Slow. You will be breathing harder, sweating more, and talking a little less, but eventually that may become your comfort zone for much of your workout. It is mine. You still need to warm up and down, but otherwise you can spend as much time as you like in the Endurance Zone.

The Rich Hours

You are going to be spending a lot of hours doing Long and Slow (and endurance) aerobic exercise, so make them rich hours. You may not think of working out as a rich time, but it is. These hours are going to be some of the best in your day, some of the best in your life. If you get into it, I predict that you will come to look forward to them as a deeply personal treat. I have spent a huge amount of time doing Long and Slow and Endurance exercise, and it is often the peak of a given day. Getting away for an hour regularly leads to endless contemplation. I write stuff in my head. I scheme, I plot, I dream, and dope-off. I am peculiarly in touch with myself at these times. If you're the type, Long and Slow is an armature for meditation. I love it.

That, in its entirety, is our discussion of the world of Long and Slow (and endurance). It ain't hard, kids. And all it will do for you is radically change your life—your health, your mood, your energy levels, your intelligence, your optimism, and your joy in life. Couldn't hurt. And do remember that's all you ever have to do. The rest is "fitness" and that's optional.

Going Hard for Fitness

Training for fitness is a little different. I have probably bored you by saying, over and over, that not everyone has to go this far, and it's true. But do read this, even if your initial thought is that it is not for you. It's probably *not* for you, and that's fine. But there may come a time when you'll want to give it a shot. I've gotta tell you, it's an awful lot of fun, if you're the type.

Training for fitness is a little more complicated than training for health, but not a lot. Basically it is a matter of introducing a bit of intensity into your workouts, two days a week. Sorry to say it, but *intensity*—in both aerobic and strength training—leads to much better results pretty fast. Two of your four aerobic days are still Long and Slow and Endurance. But the other two are now "hard days"—you *go for it.* You take it up into the threshold area, zone 3 (80–90 percent of your max, RPE 6–7). The Threshold Zone is called that because, if you're in good shape, your anaerobic threshold is in the lower reaches of that zone (80–85 percent of your max, if you're in decent shape, much less than that if you're not). You do intervals by popping in and out of the Threshold Zone. The next zone up I call Fight-or-Flight (not what trainers call it) (zone 4, 90–95 percent of your max, RPE 8–10) but only a small part of the aerobic training population goes there, *not* including you and me. Or *mostly* not including you and me.

Interval training is a matter of strengthening the body by stressing it. The heart and the whole aerobic system are being stressed and adapted. For example, your heart learns to pump more blood with each stroke (your heart muscle literally gets stronger); your metabolic system adapts so that you can go longer and harder and still be at an aerobic level (really key), the level at which your body can get rid of exhaust products as fast as you produce them, the level at which you can, in theory, lope all day. Your food metabolism becomes more efficient, and so on.

Jen has already told you about the metabolic pathways (the different fuels and the different ways your body "burns" them). That subject is almost *all* that exercise physiologists like Riggs think about. Let me hit it just once more: We burn two kinds of fuel, glucose (sugar) and fat. And there are basically two systems to consume fuel with and without oxygen: the aerobic (with) and anaerobic (without) systems. Glucose can be consumed by both systems, with or without oxygen. Fat can be burned only with oxygen. We burn both fuels, fat and glucose, and use both metabolic pathways—aerobic and anaerobic—all the time, whether we are sitting around or working out hard. Although that is true, the more interesting and important fact is that—as the intensity of your activity increases—the fuel use shifts as does the metabolic pathway you use most.

At lower intensity, you rely on slow-twitch fibers that primarily burn fat and glucose, aerobically. As the exercise intensity increases, you ask the fast-twitch muscles to jump in and help. Remember, they tend to burn predominantly glucose and they do it both aerobically and anaerobically. But as the intensity of movement increases even further, they rely mainly on glucose burned through anaerobic metabolism, with the by-product being lactic acid.

If you go hard enough, long enough, you do run out of fuel and hit the wall. Really what happens is your glucose levels fall so far the body says, "That's enough." That marathon runner we see in all the films, on the ground and desperately trying to *crawl* across the finish line, he or she has "hit the wall."

Most of us are not marathon runners, and we are not going to really hit the wall anytime soon. But the issues are there for all of us, and we reach them much earlier in the exercise process. You slow down long before you stop because muscles that are increasingly jammed with exhaust products don't function as well. You feel sluggish, then pain. You lose power; you have to slow way down or quit. Call it a "mini-wall." People who are in rotten shape hit the mini-wall very early in the proceedings. The beauty of aerobic exercise is that it strengthens the aerobic base so that we hit the mini-wall much later with intense movement. All aerobic exercise does that, most assuredly including Long and Slow and endurance workouts. But fitness workouts—stress-based workouts—will do it faster and take the process further. Fitness training gives you much more endurance and a lot of other neat things. And the only price is hard work.

The "Hockey Stick": Moving the Lactate or Anaerobic Threshold

Just a last bit of theory. Trainers are absolutely fascinated by this great dividing line inside our bodies—the *Lactate Threshold*. There is a point in a workout where the exhaust products start to build up faster than your venting system can clear them away. You start the lactic acid and CO_2 buildup. If you take the great test of aerobic fitness, the "VO_2 max test," you can see it very clearly. In that test, a physiologist or doctor stresses your body (puts you on a stationary bike or treadmill and eventually takes you close to 100 percent of your max). The gadgets measure a number of things: your heart rate, and how much oxygen you are breathing in and how much CO_2 you are breathing out.

Your heart rate goes up every time the work is increased. (In the chart on the next page, heart rate is the top line and lactate buildup is the lower line.) At lower and middle levels of exertion, the lactate is recycled and kept low. Then all of a sudden—somewhere around 50–80 percent of your maximal heart rate—depending on how fit you are—they spike. The line looks like a hockey stick: flat for a long time and then this much sharper angle. That is your lactate threshold. When you reach that point, it is a matter of time before you hit the wall and have to back off or stop. Again, if you're in rotten shape, the "hockey stick" effect cuts in earlier, say around 50 percent. A basic object of aerobic fitness is to move the hockey stick to the right, toward 80 percent.

What's happening is that, up to that point, you have mostly been burning fat and glucose aerobically. Both burn clean during aerobic metabolism, so there is less exhaust. Second, you are not working so hard so you are not burning as much fuel of *any kind* and there is less exhaust to deal with. When you are in that mode, somewhere in the Long and Slow/Endurance range, you can keep on going. Because you can clear the exhaust before it builds up. Nice.

Lactate Threshold

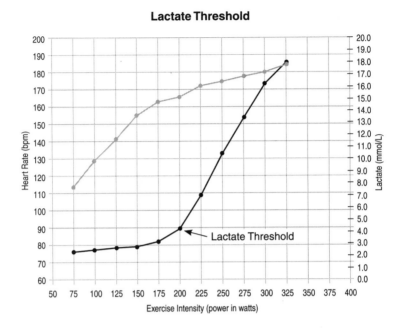

Here's another important point: In the aerobic mode, you are burn-ing, as a percentage, more fat. The thing about fat is that you have a huge amount of it, even if you're in good shape. So, in that mode, you can go on forever as long as you have a steady trickle of glucose to help keep the metabolism of fat going. Those all-day bike trips that I love? Mostly fat, most of the way. Which makes it easy. Burning glu-cose, too, obviously, but burning both at a level where getting rid of the exhaust is never a problem.

Key point: During exercise (especially fairly intense but still aero-bic exercise), the body goes straight to your gut to get fat for fuel. You will recall that your big fat belly is not your friend; that it is the pesky "open sewer" with the nocturnal rats and all that. Well, the single best thing you can do to get rid of the sewer is hard aerobic exercise. Not sit-ups, not eating kale. Hard aerobic exercise.

To get fit, we are going to go out and play in the Threshold Zone (zone 3, with an RPE of 6–7). These hard or interval days do a cou-ple of neat things. One, they move the blade of your hockey stick to the right. Which means you can work longer and harder while still burning a relatively high percentage of fat and getting rid of all the exhaust before hitting your threshold. If you can go harder longer, you can burn a lot of calories. Second, you can go longer once you have crossed the threshold. And finally, teaching your body how to do intervals will result in a quicker recovery rate after you cross that threshold. You become aerobically stronger, a more effective endurance predator.

And it's not just a matter of improving your endurance. Your efforts to lose weight take a great leap forward. Your mood is improved, your levels of optimism, and so on. All the Good Stuff. You get more of it, faster, if you do fitness training. Okay, you say (a little cranky at the news that this exercise business seems to be getting a little tougher). That's nice, but what, exactly, do I have to do to get these benefits and move my hockey stick to the right or whatever I'm doing?

Intervals

Again, the answer is stress—whole-body stress, aerobic system stress—by pushing yourself. All serious trainers and athletes agree: To build a better aerobic base and be a stronger endurance athlete, you want to create stress by doing intervals. During the interval, you really hit it. Intervals are typically between one and five minutes (with a period of rest in between) but they can be eight, ten, or even twenty minutes long. Mixing them up is part of the magic. The shorter the interval, the more intense the effort. But you would not do a ten- or twenty-minute interval unless you could do the whole thing at 80 percent of your max or above (RPE 6–7).

The design and administration of intervals can be wonderfully complex if you are an Olympic athlete with carefully tailored goals, and even if you are not. Physiologists like Riggs spend a lot of time developing interval models for athletes (and nonathletes) at various stages of their development. Riggs has over a hundred of them on his computer. The good news: We're not going there. This is going to be simple.

Let's take a look at Riggs's chart of training ranges. This is slightly different from the one I showed you in the last chapter, but mostly at the top range, where you will not be much anyway. Take a look; but

YNY Fit Training Ranges

ZONE	GOAL	INTENSITY	RPE	% OF MAXIMUM HEART RATE
1	Long and Slow	Light	1–3	50–70%
2	Endurance	Light to moderately hard	3–6	70–80%
3	Threshold	Moderately hard to hard	6–7	80–90%
4	Intervals	Hard to very hard	7–9	90–95%
5	Sprints	Very hard	9–10	95–100%

bear in mind that the descriptions of intensity are for athletes. If you're in bum shape, going 70–80 percent (if you can do it at all) is *not* going to be "light to moderately hard," as the chart says. It is going to be hell.

A quick look at Riggs's chart would suggest that you are going to spend a lot of time in the 90–100 percent of max zones, his zones 4 and 5. Uh, no. You are going to spend very little, if any, of your workout time up there. You may eventually spend a little time in zone 4 (90–95 percent of max) and, one day, you may even dip your toe into zone 5 (95–100 percent of max), but it is not going to be an important part of your training. Interval training is basically *intensity* training. For most of us, we are going to find all the intensity we need and can safely use in zone 3, the Threshold Zone. If you need more, congratulations. Zones 4 and 5 are out there.

Two Great Rules of Interval Training

The two great lessons of interval training go like this. Rule 1: Spend two hard days a week doing intervals, which (for you and me) means moving in and out of zone 3 for thirty to forty-five minutes a day, on schedules like the ones set out below. Rule 2: Do not do all your time in zone 3 (or zone 4, come to that). It feels like heroism, and lots of serious, amateur athletes find themselves doing it. Dumb idea. Turns out that almost everyone who does it gets burned out. The secret of gaining strength—whether aerobic strength or muscle strength—is *stress*, followed by *recovery*. No recovery, no gain. Spending all your time in zones 4 and 5 may not seem like much of a temptation today, but remember, you may get there. And remember this, too. It's dumb.

A Formal Interval Regimen

Take a close look at Riggs's regimen and give it a try. Riggs is the real deal.

Intervals: The Details and Some Samples

Daily Plan

On interval days you are trying to get your heart rate into the Threshold Zone (zone 3) or higher for one to ten minutes at a time. Those are the intervals in question. The rest period between the harder work is typically the same as or shorter than the intervals. "Rest" means slow down but keep moving.

Weekly Plan

Again, the basic pattern for the week, if you are going to move on to fitness, looks like this:

- Monday: Aerobics (long and slow)

- Tuesday: Strength training

- Wednesday: Aerobics (intervals, in and out of zone 3)

- Thursday: Day off

- Friday: Strength training

- Saturday: Hard aerobics (intervals, in and out of zone 3)

- Sunday: Easy aerobics (long and slow: maybe two to three hours, for the joy of it)

How you allocate the days is up to you. But there should be four days of aerobics (two easy and two hard) and two days of strength. It is best to alternate the easy and hard days. Some like to add a third day of strength, doubling up a bit on a given aerobics day, which is fine. And some keen folks like to turn strength days into aerobics *and* strength days by doing the strength exercises at speed with only thirty seconds between sets. Circuit training and variations on it, like those strength classes to music. That's a great idea—a *great* idea—if you're up for it. Especially the classes. If you can do any of this stuff in a good class, it is a great idea. Some spin classes (not many) are interval classes (in and out of zone 3, typically). I do those and love them, for some reason. You've already read about one. Being in a group and having a leader set the structure makes a huge difference.

In the same vein, having a trainer to help with aerobic training makes interval training much easier and more doable. Riggs offers a serious online version on our website.

Monthly Plan

Your *months* should be made up of weeks like this but—on the interval front—it makes sense to have a progression toward greater difficulty as the weeks go by. To push yourself a little harder, that is. You are pushing greater adaptations, over time. You are getting more fit. Riggs suggests that the monthly plan include one week of all Long and Slow—no intervals—especially when things are getting tough at work or at home or you simply can't go that hard this week. You don't stop the routine; you just wind it down for a week.

Yearly Plan

Your *years* present a slightly different problem. As we have hinted, it makes great sense to *periodize* your workouts, through the year. We are not going to try to cover that in this chapter. But the overall approach is obvious: It makes sense to have peaks and valleys in your training. Build up for a biking trip—try to "peak" as you head off to the mountains with your bike for a week. Or a ski vacation or a week's hike in the mountains. Take it down some in the weeks or even months that follow—just go on maintenance for a while. Then start a new progression with a new goal. Gotta keep yourself amused.

Four Interval Days

H ere are four interval days (good for two weeks) that Riggs has put together to get you started. They go up a little in degree of difficulty.

#1

Warm-Up	1 × 10 minutes
Workout	5 × 2 minutes (zone 3) with 3-minute rest between intervals
Warm-Down	1 × 10 minutes
Total Time:	approximately 45 minutes

NOTE: *If you can't do five intervals, do as many as you can today and simply take longer rest periods between the intervals you do.*

#2

Warm-Up	1 × 10 minutes
Workout	1 × 3 minutes (zone 3) with 2-minute rest
	1 × 2 minutes (zone 3) with 2-minute rest
	1 × 1 minute with 2-minute rest
	Perform the above set 2 times
Warm-Down	1 × 10 minutes
Total Time:	approximately 45 minutes

NOTE: *If this seems challenging, try only one set.*

#3

Warm-Up	1 × 10 minutes
Workout	3 × 3 minutes (zone 3) with 5-minute rest between intervals
Warm-Down	1 × 10 minutes
Total Time:	approximately 45 minutes

NOTE: *The extra rest should allow you to reach zone 3 each time.*

#4

Warm-Up	1 × 10 minutes
Workout	Ladder: 1-2-3-4-3-2-1 minutes with 2-minute recovery between each interval (try to reach zone 3 each time)
Warm-Down	1 × 10 minutes
Total Time:	approximately 50 minutes

Four Slightly Harder Interval Days

Were you seduced by the first four interval days? Hope so. And I hope you want more. Here it is, in the form of four more, slightly harder, interval days from Riggs.

#5

Warm-Up	1 × 10 minutes
Workout	8 × 2 minutes (zone 3) with 3-minute rest between intervals
Warm-Down	1 × 10 minutes
Total Time:	approximately 60 minutes

#6

Warm-Up	1 × 10 minutes
Workout	1 × 2 minutes (zone 3) with 3-minute rest
	1 × 1 minute (zone 3) with 1-minute rest
	1 × 30 seconds at zone 4
	3 minutes easy
	Repeat the above set 3 times
Warm-Down	1 × 10 minutes
Total Time:	approximately 55 minutes

NOTE: *First time flirting with level 4 if you are up for it.*

#7

Warm-Up	1 × 10 minutes
Workout	3 × 5 minutes (zone 3) with 5-minute rest between intervals
Warm-Down	1 × 10 minutes
Total Time:	approximately 50 minutes

#8

Warm-Up	1 × 10 minutes
Workout	Ladder: 1-2-3-4-5-4-3-2-1 minutes with 1-minute recovery between each interval (try to reach zone 3 each time)
Warm-Down	1 × 10 minutes
Total Time:	approximately 55 minutes

NOTE: *There is only a 1-minute rest between each hard effort. This is a hard workout!*

Okay, there is the general idea and some detailed instructions. Do give it a try. If it's no fun, the hell with it. But keep it in mind for later, when the Long and Slow/Endurance regimen has had some time to work its magic. This fitness stuff is certainly not for everyone, but neither is it as hard as it may seem to you at the outset.

Fast-Twitch and Slow-Twitch: Alive in the Hills

Riggs wrote a lot of stuff to help me with this chapter—some of it *slightly* technical—but my favorite piece was a bit about two different days he and I spent together—one biking and one skiing—in the West. They show how different muscle types—and fuel systems and all that—cut in at different levels, but they seem a little more real than some of this discussion. First day, early March, last year. Riggs and I are skiing on Aspen Mountain. In the chair on the way up, Riggs says, not much is going on. Whatever muscle movement there is, it tends to be slow-twitch, and the "fuel" is mostly fat then we start off on a fairly steep mogul run. Mogul skiing is very intense, like doing forty deep knee bends in a row, at speed and at goofy angles—with a lot of balance and a touch of fear. It takes tremendous force, Riggs says, and you have to be in decent shape, have decent balance, and all that. A mogul run recruits a lot of fast-twitch fibers and invokes mainly the anaerobic system but a good deal of the aerobic as well. As we go flying down the hill, we use every muscle in the body but especially the muscles in the legs and core.

After a minute of that we pull up at the bottom of the pitch. I am huffing and puffing and my legs are beginning to burn because the fast-twitch muscles and the anaerobic system have produced a ton of lactic acid that builds up inside the muscle and *stops muscle contractions.* And hurts. (Cruelly, the lactic acid buildup also inhibits the further breakdown of glucose; they're working both ends, *against you.*) There is a lot of CO_2 being made that has got me breathing hard. The body is trying to get rid of it. The slow-twitch muscles had a relatively minor role in this stretch and are not too fatigued. I have to rest a minute, maybe two, at the bottom of the run to catch my breath, let my legs come back. What is going on is that the waste removal systems are getting rid of the lactic acid in my muscles and the CO_2 in my lungs.

The next part of the mountain is much easier . . . steep but no moguls. For this "groomer," the slow-twitch fibers have the leading part. There is no need for the tremendous forces you need to work your way through a mogul run. We ski comfortably all the way to the bottom and are not tired or sore, a couple of minutes later. Because our exhaust system was well able to keep up.

Second day: Riggs, my close friend Terry (a fit age sixty-four), and I are making a hellish, six-day bike ride, our Ride the Rockies kedge, last June. Terry and I have done a bunch of these over the years, but today's ride was the hardest ever for both of us. And not just because we're so shamefully old either. We are riding from Crested Butte to Buena Vista, an eighty-five-mile pop. But it is not the distance that's hard, it is the climb over Cottonwood Pass (12,400 feet), one of the hairiest and hardest rides in the Rockies. The last fourteen miles up are *unpaved*, hardpack. We can ride it, on our skinny-tired racing bikes, but it's tricky not to get tumbled in the ruts. You would not say "restful." It adds a major additional balance problem to an already ferocious ride.

For most of the way, we use slow-twitch fibers and burn mostly fat. Which is a good thing because this is much too long and tough a day to rely solely on glucose; we don't begin to have enough stored glucose in our bodies for a jaunt like this. We add to our glucose supply by eating power bars and a few large chocolate chip cookies on the way up. Near the top, when my whole body is struggling just to keep the pedals turning and to keep from keeling over, I am standing up and pedaling hard, I am most assuredly using fast-twitch fibers, too, and tons of muscle glycogen. Everything but the kitchen sink on a day like this. It was as hard as anything I have ever done. Hundreds of riders wound up in the "sag wagons" that day, like ambulances leaving a battlefield. Not us, though, because Terry and Riggs and I had trained pretty hard. Never hard enough, but not bad.

We burned over four thousand calories apiece on that eighty-five-mile ride. Got a lot of it back pretty fast, though, drinking beers and eating burgers as we rejoiced in a terrific cowboy bar in Buena Vista. Few margaritas too; they make a hell of a margarita in some of these little mountain towns. Stop in Leadville, some time. This was one of the great meals of my life. We were worried when we walked in that we looked too geeky to be welcome. This *was* a cowboy bar, and we *were* men in tights, after all. And it was the middle of a Saturday afternoon, so the young people at the dark bar—who got around in junker-pickup trucks, not $5,000 bicycles—were *not* having their first drink of the day.

But I strode up, full of myself as usual, and told 'em all we'd just biked over Cottonwood Pass, by heaven, and we were *thirsty*. And damned if they didn't light right up. They were locals and they *knew* about Cottonwood Pass. They put their glasses down and gave us a ripple of applause, grins all around, a couple of handshakes. I got a kiss on the cheek from a pretty girl. Sweet moment. We ordered drinks for everyone and a double round for ourselves. We'd been hydrating but never mind—we were *dry*. And hungry. I was practically licking the salt off the taco chips. Pretty good saloon. Pretty nice people at the bar. Pretty good day.

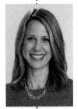

CHAPTER EIGHTEEN

Muscle as the Grand Negotiator of Body Signals

M uscle is big. It constitutes about 45 percent of male body weight and somewhat less for women, about 35–45 percent. As we all know, muscle has everything to do with letting us walk, run, pick things up, and write—basically any and all movement. What is less well known, even in scientific circles, is what we say in the title of the chapter: Muscle is the grand negotiator of signals in your body. That is a very important concept, about as important, I believe, as anything in the book. The study of muscle has been my life for some time, so I may exaggerate, but I don't think so.

Muscle has a lot to do with why it makes sense to do all the exercise we recommend. It's why exercise creates such profound and positive changes inside your body, and even with how you perceive your body on the outside. I believe healthy muscle, to a surprising extent, is the key to bodily health. In certain parts of academia, you could get an argument about that—or bland-faced expressions of surprise— but I have no doubt about it. I think a heavy and more pointed focus on muscle is warranted here, where I hope it will serve as further inspiration.

Muscles Send Signals

M uscle biochemistry is one of my science loves and once you "go deep" into muscle, you learn that muscles are at the heart of a complex signaling network. They are integral with the brain and the signaling system. Muscle acts in response to signals from the brain, billions and even trillions of them. Every muscle cell, every fiber, has its own wire from the brain. Muscles are therefore nothing without signals: no signal, no movement, no action and muscle shrivels up and dies. It goes away. The stimulus must be consistently there to keep your muscle alive.

On the flip side, mechanisms underlying muscle physiology also demonstrate that not only is muscle on the receiving side from the nerves, but it is on the sending side, too—muscle actually communicates through a variety of molecules with other organs. It is a complicated system that scientists are still trying to tease apart and understand, but the basics are clear. Muscle signaling does three great things: It *sends signals to consume sugar* and *burn fat*, and, best of all, *it sends signals that are anti-inflammatory*. This is how exercise becomes so *key* to muscle (and signal) health. That is a big deal.

The Tide of Aging

A s you age the default is to decay; you lose muscle mass at 1 percent per year starting as early as age thirty, and the loss escalates from there after age sixty. Literally, the "soup" that your muscle bathes in changes over time—there are lower levels of hormones that stimulate muscle growth (including growth hormones and testosterone); there is greater free radical production and the muscle encounters more "oxidative stress" (don't ask); and "pro-inflammatory cytokines" increase. This soup is not growth promoting—it is destructive and leads to a dysregulation of several signals that would otherwise enable a muscle cell to survive and grow. Finally, beyond the soup, muscles start to lose their lifelines, those motor nerves from the brain to the muscle that make everything work.

That's a little grim, I know, but there is some very good news too, which I think is quite neat. And it goes like this. There *are* counteractive forces that oppose the armies that promote sarcopenia and decay. Those forces are (1) maintaining a vigorous level of physical activity, (2) eating healthfully, and (3) reducing the amount of fat you're carrying around. These factors are within your control. It may be difficult for some and requires effort for most, but they are still completely manageable. We've already gone into detail on sound nutrition—a balanced diet adequate to "build" muscle takes all components, not just protein. Healthy carbs and fats fuel exercise and keep muscle cell membranes healthy, antioxidants decrease stress (especially if you are overweight), B-vitamins promote energy metabolism, and so on. If even one of these elements get out of check, exercise will not be quite as beneficial.

Of those three things, the first line of defense to offset the sarcopenia of aging is *regular* exercise—it's the easiest to implement and offers significant results in fairly short order. Consistency and frequency are key for exercise to work its magic because it's the only way to build sound muscle mass. It makes the good systems work better and attacks the bad systems. Muscle movement and signal recruitment by exercise are critical to keeping you moving, maybe even keeping you alive.

It is not just a matter of muscles getting bigger through exercise. They also get smarter and more efficient. Neural connections stay intact and get stronger with use. They send signals faster, and with more efficiency and precision. The *connectivity* between nerves and muscles is enhanced. That step alone means you'll have more muscle force and effectiveness even before any change in the muscle itself takes place. The "soup" that the muscle bathes in changes, growth signals return, and the muscle becomes healthier.

It is not so much muscle *size* that matters—even for strength, to say nothing of coordination. It is signaling efficiency that counts most. You can improve and preserve signaling by sending more—and more complex—signals. The best way to do that is by exercising frequently, and with as much variety as possible. We'll explain in depth about this later in this book: Listen to Bill. It is a good idea. But in short, consider cross-training or taking up new forms of exercise as often as possible. Switch your routine daily or weekly. Don't just go to a spinning class day after day for a year. Besides, the same routine gets boring, and that could become a seductive excuse to give up.

Muscle Gulps Up Sugar

Muscle is the supreme controller of your blood sugar. Between 80 and 90 percent of the carbs that we eat end up in our muscles. That's true for the idle as well as the fit. If you exercise, the sugar simply gets sucked up faster. We can use it for energy, but importantly, we start to store more glucose in the muscles—as opposed to converting it to fat elsewhere. Remember that your muscle *changes*. Enzymes that assist with energy metabolism increase and work more efficiently. Oxygen delivery is enhanced, and exhaust removal improved. With all of these changes, we also respond differently to the foods that we consume, especially sugar.

Why is the exercised muscle better at taking up glucose? When you are physically active and get fit, you are less likely to have sugar highs because the sugar in your bloodstream gets funneled quickly to the muscles; the sirens for a surge of insulin, to get rid of the sugar, *do not go off.* There is no need, as the little receptors in the muscle, which take in the glucose, have already popped up to the surface, ready to wolf down the sugar. Insulin is still needed but there is no nasty insulin spike. Great news. And during exercise itself, the contraction of your muscles alone will cause the little buttercups to come to the surface of the muscle to chow down on glucose. You barely need insulin when you are exercising to get the glucose in the muscle!

The combination of fewer blood sugar spikes and less insulin floating around means there isn't enough insulin to do the dirty business of storing excess glucose as fat. Congratulations! Thank your muscles.

Muscle Over Insulin

As you may already have guessed, your muscle can also take charge of insulin. Healthy muscle makes insulin behave by helping the entire metabolic system to work faster, cleaner, and more efficiently. Muscle dictates how sensitive you are to insulin, and muscle contraction itself, as I just mentioned, can wipe out the need for insulin to move glucose into the muscle. If less insulin is needed, there is less insulin floating around, less insulin surge, less soaking up fat and putting it in your belly, and less of a drop in blood sugar that makes us ravenous. It does more of the good work: making glucose available to the muscles. And less of the bad: putting fat into storage in your gut and in your muscles.

The sugar-burning process also works much better with exercise. Without constant mega insulin surges, you are far less likely to have a breakdown in the ability to make insulin or a rising demand for *more* insulin from the muscles. Short version: Muscles burn more sugar, more efficiently, with less insulin. You need less insulin and are more sensitive to it. So the risk of sugar spikes, insulin spikes, and a disastrous breakdown of the insulin system is much, much less likely. Diet still matters, but you can start to see exercise is the great antidote to adult-onset diabetes.

Here is another terrific thing about insulin and exercise. It helps store glucose as glycogen in muscle cells for a ready source of fuel for movement. Insulin also stimulates muscle protein synthesis, which is to say *muscle growth*. Hooray. The bad news is that—as we get older—the power of insulin to promote muscle growth weakens. The very, very good news is that with exercise the ability of insulin to promote muscle growth is restored.

Healthy Muscle Burns More Fat

We have talked about how exercise grows new mitochondria and miles of new capillaries to increase muscle strength and effectiveness (and, incidentally, burn more fat). It may be obvious, but that growth multiplies tremendously in response to exercise. The extra network of capillaries that increasingly surrounds each muscle fiber ensures that oxygen and nutrients reach the muscles. And ensures that the exhaust is taken away quickly. You know about the increase in mitochondria, but you probably do not know that there is a sharp increase in enzymes that assist with metabolism, *and* they work more efficiently.

Here is the payoff: With exercise, the production of energy becomes more efficient and, *in particular*, you are better able to rely on fat as a source of energy. Fit, active people burn fat whereas unfit idle people are burning more glucose. Those who exercise are much quicker to dip into the fat stores—including your dangerous gut—than the idle.

Getting fit is the *fast road* to losing that gut. Your muscle helps and *that* is worth everything.

Here's how it works: There are signals (various molecules, cytokines and hormones, for the science buffs) released from fat and from muscle that talk with one another. What they say to one another changes with exercise. Do you remember the Pac-Man enzymes (lipases) that chomp off free fatty acids from your fat cells? They are the critical enzymes that free fat from its hiding places and make it available as *fuel*. Exercised muscles send more signals for more Pac-Men to be made and to start chomping on the fat globules, especially in your gut. In that way, muscle signals—but only *exercised muscle signals*—promote the burning of fat and the reduction of your gut. It is one of the most important health, weight loss, and fitness benefits of having healthy muscle mass and exercising it.

Here is another interesting tidbit. Remember how we tend to lose our fast-twitch muscle fibers with age and become somewhat of a slow-twitch endurance machine? Well that may sound like a drag, but recall that those slow-twitch fibers love to burn a high percentage of fat. That is the good news. Here is the bad news. When we don't exercise our muscles at any age, our aerobic fat-burning, slow-twitch fibers tend to suffer the greatest loss in size—meaning our ability to burn fat is compromised! On top of that, obese individuals tend to have lower percentages of slow-twitch fibers. They have less slow-twitch muscle fiber area with less mitochondria to burn fat. A major double whammy—having more fat to burn, but less able to do so. This low slow-twitch profile in obese individuals may actually underlie one of the mechanisms by which they develop type 2 diabetes. Chew on that for a minute. Two more great reasons to stimulate your muscles through exercise and keep the extra weight off!

Healthy Muscle Is Anti-Inflammatory

Bad or chronic inflammation is a major force for the *evil* inside your body: the great promoter of heart attacks, strokes, adult-onset diabetes, cancers, and Alzheimer's. It's more complicated than that but not much. Here is what you need to focus on for this discussion.

1. Fat cells, especially around your gut, send messages, which are inflammatory.

2. Well-exercised muscles send messages that are anti-inflammatory.

3. Chronic inflammation kills.

The fat around your gut, you will surely remember, is *the great* repository of inflammation-issuing fat cells. More bad fat—the kind that interlards unhealthy muscles—hides in the muscles themselves, if you are idle. It "lards" the muscles, as in the CT scan of the older woman's thigh muscle in Chapter 3. In idleness and obesity, your muscles, and other organs, are being suffocated by inflammatory stimuli that are released into your circulation from the visceral fat and by the fat that has invaded and marbled the muscle itself. The inflammatory stimuli—inflammatory cytokines, free radicals, and the like—lead to muscle damage and atrophy, and to many of the gravest diseases.

The Biggest Payoff of All

f you are physically active, your muscle dramatically changes from being the receiver of inflammatory stimuli to being the sender of anti-inflammatory signals. You change the muscle biochemistry, just as you change your blood chemistry, and it is just as big a deal. Healthy muscles, well-exercised muscles, are anti-inflammatory engines. They fight atrophy and disease. Fat cells throw out inflammatory signals that are disastrous for your health.

Fat cells and muscle cells are at war. One side (muscle) wants to stamp out inflammation. The other side (fat) wants to promote it. Who wins? Well, it depends on two things: one, how many fat cells you have, and two, how healthy, which is to say, how well exercised your muscles are.

Depending on who wins that battle, you are sick or healthy. So here's that tip we keep giving: Work out hard, six days a week. You're not just getting in shape; you're throwing resources behind the good guys in a battle over inflammation, the battle for your health. Again:

fat cells spew out all sorts of bad inflammatory signals that make you weak and sick. Healthy muscle throws back positive anti-inflammatory messages. It is as clear and as simple as that. This is why we are drilling the exercise message in. It really matters.

I am sorely tempted to go on and explain in detail just how the muscle releases nitric oxide, which prevents damage to our muscle cells. And to tell one and all that nitric oxide is a great vasodilator of our blood vessels, meaning it enhances blood flow and will have a great impact on the extent to which certain diseases progress.

I could then go on to talk about certain cytokines, namely interleukin (IL)-6 and IL-15, which are released from the muscle in response to exercise. Both of them promote the breakdown of adipose tissue, especially the toxic visceral fat around your gut. Internally, they also positively influence fat metabolism within the muscle cell. These muscle signals chomp away at our midsections. They clear out the swamp, empty the sewer in your body, which tries to kill you by releasing a ton of inflammation and free radicals. But I won't bog you down with endless details.

Just bear in mind that maintaining and exercising lean muscle mass is even more important than you have read so far. There is a war going on inside your body, basically between muscle and fat, and you have a huge stake in who wins. You have powerful resources to throw into the battle: Lose fat (visceral fat), eat sanely, and exercise a lot.

Just a Little More Good News

Exercised muscles send signals to promote the generation of growth hormone and testosterone, which help stem the tide of aging. Exercise enhances immune factors and increases endorphins. You are less likely to get sick and you feel *good*. Cognition is improved and your focus is better. So let those muscle signals roll! Scientists are still learning more, but the overall message will not change. Muscle is the grand negotiator of signals inside your body. Exercise makes the muscles work. Exercise is the flywheel of the good life.

CHAPTER NINETEEN

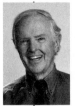

The Astonishing Importance of Strength Training

could read that last chapter of Jen's all day. *Such* good news. I have been hearing this from Jen for a while. But I just read an article that bears nicely on what Jen says.

A recent study began with the grim statement that, in the normal course, people lose 10 percent of their muscle mass a decade after age forty. And that it gets worse after seventy. You lose muscle mass *and* suffer a serious accretion of fat into the muscles. But here's the great news: They took a look at cadres of serious athletes in their forties, up to their eighties. The muscle loss didn't happen to them. "The athletes in their 70s and 80s had almost as much muscle mass as the athletes in their 40s, with minor if any fat infiltration." There was some drop-off at age fifty, but not much. And there was little further decline after that. "The 70- and 80-year-old athletes were about as strong as those in their 60s." Other studies support the same conclusion. That, kids, is amazingly good news. Is strength training hellish for many of us? You bet. Is it worth it? Oh, yes!

That was a study of serious lifelong athletes. Will it work if you're starting later in life? Less clear, but yes. What studies there are say it certainly will. And Jen says, absolutely.

So there you sit, asking uneasily if you are really supposed to toddle off to the gym two or three times a week in costumes that do not flatter and pick up heavy metal or nasty machines till you drop. And the answer is. "Umm, yeah, you are." Oh boy.

A Personal Note

I was thinking about all this very early this morning, the gray light just coming into my study where I'd fallen asleep. I was thinking about how to persuade you that such a serious strength regimen is really worth it. I found myself looking at a picture on the wall of my father, the dear man. He was standing on a steam launch, in a white straw hat and a big American flag in the background. It was probably 1915 or so, when he was nineteen. And I had the sudden realization that he was exactly my age now (seventy-seven) when Mother and I decided that a series of strokes had so ravaged his body and mind that he had to be put in a nursing home. He was too gaga and too dangerous to stay at home—he was lashing out at the nurses. So unlike him, the poor creature.

And I thought how wildly lucky I am at seventy-seven. Because, in a little while, I am going out on my usual twenty-mile bike ride, even though it is a freezing fall morning. Then breakfast with Hilary and chat about the details of our hectic, pleasant lives. Then work on this book. Email about lectures and stuff. And I am not going to a nursing home today. Not today, not tomorrow, and maybe not ever. Because I do these damned exercises, six days a week, like a crazy person. Including the weights, two days a week. Sometimes three. Because I want *so much* to be myself, if I *possibly* can be, all the way out to the waterfall. And not be like Pa.

I remember the morning we took Pa to the home, almost forty years ago, with piercing clarity. Oscar the handyman and I are wheeling Pa, a frail, dazed old man, out the kitchen door. He's not lashing out now, just sitting there. Oscar is in back with the handles of the wheelchair; I am in front with the wheels, my face inches from Pa's face as we lift him down the big granite step into the kitchen-garden through which he had passed almost every day for forty years. Mercifully, he has no idea what's going on today.

But suddenly he has a lucid interval . . . senses exactly what is going on. And he gives me this furious look. Astonishes me by saying, with all the old force, in his old, frightening growl: *"This* is a bum's rush!"

Break your heart. *Break your heart.* Because it *was* a bum's rush. At the end of a good life, a bum's rush. On the way to three dreadful years in a nursing home.

I don't want that, man. Not totally nuts about strength training but love it *so much* more than the bum's rush. I don't want that at the end of life. Bet you don't either.

Quality of Life

Jen talked about the serious new science of muscle-messaging. Let me talk for a minute about the slightly more familiar but still miraculous "quality of life" reasons for strength training.

There are four separate, hugely important things that strength training does for you, *in addition* to the things Jen talked about.

First, it makes you stronger. Duh! But it does, and it does it remarkably fast. And that is more important than you might think. You can have a 35–50 percent increase in strength in just six months. And that makes *such* a difference. Not just to get out of the chair, climb the stairs, all that, but to avoid *falling*. Falls are one of the great interrupters of Third Acts. The curtain comes down, and it may not go back up. (Not on the same play, anyhow.) After age fifty, a fall can alter your life. Maybe end it. Hard to believe when you're young, but true. And there are few things as important as plain strength, especially strength in your legs, to prevent falls and keep you mobile in general. In the absence of serious strength training you will lose some 10 percent of your strength a decade after fifty; that's the default-to-decay business at work. Gotta send *grow messages* over that signaling system, kids. Gotta overcome that tide. Few things matter as much as simply avoiding sarcopenia, the loss of muscle mass and muscle signaling with age.

Second, strength training grows new bone. One of the worst things about the tide of aging is that it is sucking the bone out of your bones. All of us lose bone mass at the rate of up to 1 percent a year. Women, during and after menopause, lose bone mass at the rate of up to 2 percent a year, with terrifying results. Listen to these numbers: Woman falls down after sixty and has the traditional older woman's injury, a broken hip. Fifty percent of the women who have that break will never walk unaided again: It is the cane, the walker, and the chair. And 20 percent will be dead within one year. Those are *appalling* numbers. And it is all because of osteoporosis, silent bone loss with aging.

The *only* thing that prevents bone loss is serious consistent strength training. Calcium with vitamin D helps a little, but it doesn't help much. The only real answer is serious strength training. You may think you don't look great going to the gym in your Lycra? Tough! You aren't going there to get dates, for heaven's sake. You are going to *save your life*. Just do it. Two days a week. Especially the legs. And hips. We'll tell you how.

Third, strength training is the single best thing you can do to refresh, renew, and strengthen your internal signaling system, and thus to restore and refresh your *balance, proprioception, and coordination*. In the normal course of aging you lose balance, proprioception (your sense of where you are in space), and coordination at the rate of some 12 percent a decade. Much like muscle mass. And it is brutal. The cumulative effect bids fair to make you into a ridiculous stumbling old man, an absurdly fragile old woman. Not the star of the Third Act.

Balance is so important, and you can radically improve it with strength training. Do it right, the way Bill and Riggs teach, and you do not have to be a stumbling fool in your fifties and beyond.

Fourth, it relieves pain. It is the great anodyne, the reliever of pain that is already here, and the armor against pain to come. It is not perfect. Pain will come with age. But it does more than anything else to hold it at bay. You will not know until you get there, but pain is the great handmaiden of aging, and it is a curse. A relatively little bit of chronic pain soaks up your attention, cuts you off from others, and gives you a nice solid push into becoming a busted-down old guy, a pathetic old girl. It slows you way down. It makes you walk funny. You want to talk about it all the time, which is a *real* curse. For everyone. It transports you into the land of the fragile old.

Good strength training will do more than anything else to fight off and reverse chronic pain—arthritis, bursitis, sore joints of all kinds—and your wretched sore back. Oh my! Strength training done badly can make things worse. But the kind Billy teaches will do more to fight off and reverse pain than anything else. That's worth tons.

We Live in Glass Boxes

Years ago, Bill was struggling to explain to me what he felt so strongly and what I was not getting: the enormous importance of compound whole-body movement. It was early days, and his message wasn't sinking in.

Look, he said, standing up, we all live in glass boxes. And their size and shape are defined by our ability to move—our balance, our range of motion, the soundness of our joints and muscles, our proprioception and coordination, all those things. He balanced himself, his feet well apart, and moved as he talked. He moves constantly when he talks about this stuff because he is so into it. Can't stay still.

He twisted his hips sharply from side to side—reached out to the sides with his hands, toward the back, out toward me, over his head. It's not having powerful biceps or quads or whatever that matters in the end, he said. It's how well they work together with your signaling system and the little muscles and joints to *reach out*! Which he did. And up. And he reached way down to touch the floor, outside his right foot, and way up over his head and to the left with his hands, stretching as high as he could.

He went on for a while, and it began to resonate: We live in these glass boxes, all of us, all our lives. And they set the outer limits of our ability to move: from side to side, and back and forth, and up and down. Range of motion, flexibility, sound joints. As we get older and lose balance, strength, and mobility—as our joints go—the glass boxes get smaller. When we are very old, the box tends to get very small indeed. Not much bigger than a coffin really, one of those old wooden jobs, without much elbow room.

Do nothing, and that glass box starts to shrink in your thirties. And by the time you are sixty, it can be pretty tight. The quality of your life has everything to do with the size of your glass box, and it can get awfully darn small.

But it doesn't have to. To a surprising extent, the size of your glass box, all the way through life, is in your own control. Balance is trainable. Proprioception is trainable. Coordination is trainable. Strength is trainable. Fundamentally, the whole signaling system and the combination of signals, small and large muscles, and ligaments can be refreshed and strengthened by the right kind of strength training.

To get a better sense of it, Billy says, think of a great skier—Bode Miller, for example. Look at him during a race. He is cantilevered way out to one side, almost touching the snow, as he goes screaming around a gate at sixty miles an hour over an icy rutted surface. The next gate comes up in a heartbeat. With amazing force, he swings up and over to the other side. Boom! All those horrendous g-forces, still at sixty miles an hour, screaming down the hill but on the other side now. Different muscles, different joints, different cascades of signals. And still canted out so far to the other side, he almost touches the snow. He flips back and forth like this again and again in a single race while making astonishing micro adjustments in the angle of his feet, the degree of lean, the cant of his hips, so that he is faster at this than anyone else in the world. Quite a trick. Bode Miller lives in a glass box, just like you and me. But his is enormous.

Or think of a great shortstop. A ball comes flying into the hole between third and short. He races right, stretches almost flat on the ground to snag it, rights himself in an instant and throws to first in a single movement. He lives in a glass box too. It is huge.

Okay, now think of a little old lady I know on the street outside my apartment on 57th Street in New York. She has one of those canes with four little rubber-tipped legs on the bottom. She is concentrating with all her might and she is scared to death, right here on this flat sidewalk on a nice October morning. She takes tiny steps, only four or five inches, very carefully. And feels her way the whole time with that four-footed cane. She can't look at you or me as she walks along. She can't look at anything but the ground because she broke her hip a while ago, and knows that if she tries to take bigger steps or lifts her eyes or puts her cane wrong, she will fall down. And with her porous old bones, she could break something again. And never get up. Small box. Very small box. And before a hell of a long time, you think, there will not be any box at all. Just the bed. And then nothing.

She is a human being, just like you and me, by the way. A wonderful human being, in fact. At one time she was a great beauty and great *fun*. You would have done anything to be her friend. I know this because I knew her back then. She is just like you and me—more amusing than you and me, at one time. But not today. Today she is very busy. Today she is out for a walk. In her little glass box.

Keep her in mind. You're going to meet her again at the end of the book. She is going to be transformed. Nice story.

In many of the exercises we are going to do, you will be stretching your glass box as if it were made of Saran Wrap, not glass, and you could literally push it out and make it bigger. It can be done, no matter how old you are, no matter the size of your glass box. And it's a great idea.

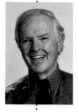

CHAPTER TWENTY

Train Movements, Not Muscles: Whole-Body Movement and the Three Little Pigs

Modern strength training grew out of the old model of the body building movement of the 1960s and 1970s when Arnold Schwarzenegger and the movie *Pumping Iron* were all the rage. But it also grew out of the development of modern weight-training machines, especially the Nautilus machines. Nautilus machines were a brilliant invention by a genius named Arthur Jones that used complex cams and pulleys to maintain even pressure on muscles throughout a given exercise.

And very importantly, they promoted muscle stress over a "full range of motion." For reasons you'll understand in a bit, that is a big deal. The new Nautilus machines—and their progeny and competitors—were great gadgets, and they pulled people into the gyms. Partly because they were kind of fun, partly because they were more or less safe, and partly because they were easy to use. And they did build muscle, as millions know. Anyhow, Nautilus and its rivals and successors have been at the heart of the conditioning movement for the last forty years. You see them, wall-to-wall, in every gym in the country. I go to the occasional fitness industry convention in places like Las Vegas, and one of the treats is to walk into some vast exhibition hall and see miles of absolutely *amazing* new fitness toys. Boys love toys, and fitness boys love fitness toys. Girls, too. Makes sense. Fun counts.

The New Model

But there are problems. Problems with the machines, and serious problems with using body building as a model for strength training. Bodybuilders are wonderful looking, if that's your taste (not mine, I confess, but hey), but their bodies don't work very well. They don't *move* very well. And they don't last well over time. Huh, you'd think we'd have focused on that over all those years of using the machines. But somehow we didn't.

Bill tells this interesting story. He had a client out in Aspen who had been a great success in life *and* who had been very serious about his weight-lifting regimen. At seventy he was built like a bull: bulging muscles and he could bench-press almost three hundred pounds. Trouble was, he was falling apart. Hideous back pain, terrible shoulder joints, awful knees and hips, everything. He couldn't sleep for the pain. What had happened, Bill said, was that decades of isolating and lifting had worn away his joints and ruined his posture. He couldn't move normally and his balance was atrocious. When you took the support of the bench away, he was weak. Really weak. His coordination was terrible, and he struggled to lift anything that required whole-body movement, which is most things. And he was looking at serious neck and other joint surgery.

Bill took him under his wing. It took a while—two years. Two years of emphasis on the joints and whole-body movement. But in time his joints stopped hurting, his posture improved radically, and he could *move* freely. The doctor who had been discussing surgery was shocked and delighted at the change. Today, surgery is off the table, he is stronger than ever—*stronger in motion*—and he does not hurt. Happy guy. He ought to be.

That is an isolated anecdote, but it makes profound sense because of the bodybuilder's focus on muscles, not movement. They don't *move* very well. As far as Bill (and this book) is concerned, movement is the whole point. We train to *move*, not to strike poses for the cover of *Men's Health* or the judges in the Mr. Peoria contest. And that leads to Bill's fundamental point: *Train movements, not muscles.* I say this is our insight, and it is. But it is also a concept shared by all the best trainers and fitness people in the country, say the top 1 percent.

Listen, machines are terrific. I don't use them as much anymore, and most of the leading experts do not, but I still use them and I like them a lot. That's the big thing: People like them and use them. Any weight-training devices that get used are good ones. I still use mine as part of a combined whole-body and machine workout (not all the machines anymore but the best of them). My primary exercise is *whole body*. But when there's time, I'll often slip off and do some machine work, just to build strength in particular muscle groups.

But the great revolution is mostly a revolution *away* from machines. You do not have to get over machines, and you certainly do not have to drop them completely from your strength-training regimen. But you should know about the alternatives, the much better alternatives and what's so good about them.

The miracle of the new strength training is *complex adaptation to movement*. Training creates muscular and—even more important—*signaling* adaptations to improve movement. You literally tear down and rebuild the muscle cells and rewire the neurotransmitters that control them. That's how you adapt. That's how you avoid the tide of aging. In this book, we are training you for *life*. *Your life*. For a life of lifting stuff off a shelf, riding a bike, getting out of a chair, skiing the bumps, walking to work, paddling a kayak, picking up a kid, hitting a hell of a golf drive. Training for life. A long one. Sounds a bit doctrinaire and bookish when you first hear it, but don't worry. It makes profound sense. And it *will* sink in. Give us a few pages.

Life and Movement in Three Dimensions

L ife is movement, and movement is very different from muscle-isolation training, the kind of training you get on machines. Movement does not involve muscles in isolation and a single plane. It involves muscles—and bones and sinews and the amazing signaling system—working in elaborate concert, in three dimensions and three planes, in depth (like *you*). The great focus of machines and body-building is on isolating and building specific muscles. You sit down at the bicep curl machine, you put your elbows on the pad, and away you go: You *isolate* and strengthen your biceps. Or my favorite, the leg press machine: You sit down, after putting on a ton of weights, and push. With your quads. Terrific. I have quads of steel because I use that gadget all the time. Goody. (Caution from Bill: This machine may be risky for folks who have lost some hip mobility.)

But life is not like that. It is not a matter of using isolated muscles. Quite the contrary. It is muscles and joints and signaling systems in groups, all working in sync. Think about any athletic move. Think about a tennis serve or a golf drive, for example. Your arms and hands do the last bits, but tennis and golf are not hand and arm sports. They are whole-body sports, like just about everything else.

All the power, for example, comes roaring up from the great muscles in your legs, then from the fierce torquing of your whole body, and only toward the end is it your shoulders, arms, and hands. The power comes from the legs. The *effectiveness* is mostly a matter of transmitting and enhancing that power through the *core*. Transmitting it, with the least *loss* or "spill," up to the shoulders and beyond. Again, golf is a whole-body exercise. Skiing is a whole-body exercise. *Living* is a whole-body exercise—a compound, complex exercise in three dimensions, often involving significant rotation. If you are training for sports, or for life, you are training for complex movement. If you are training for complex movement, *do* complex movement. Which mostly means using free weights, or your body, or elastic tubes or gadgets, which put a premium on balance and whole-body coordination. And do not spend *that much* time doing muscle-isolation exercises on the machines.

As I said before, a lot of people have come to love and use machines. Me, too. And I mean to keep using them to *supplement my regular whole-body training*. But quite a lot less. As I get better with the free weights and the whole-body gadgets, I defer more and more to those. But I recognize that it is hard to get used to doing the free weights and so on correctly. It is harder than the machines. And it may become a deterrent to doing strength training at all. That would be the worst possible result. It is our hope that you will keep working at the free-weight, whole-body approach because it really does do a much better job. But for heaven's sake, do not drop machines entirely, if doing so is going to keep you from doing strength training at all. The beauty of machines always was the fact that people used them. So keep them in your life, if you like. But as you get further and further into the subject, see if you cannot get deeper into the whole-body workout. It is better for you.

Signaling in Three Dimensions

Think for a second about the signaling system that supports all movement. As you now know better than most people in the gym, the body's signaling system is the key to movement. Every muscle fiber— not just every cell, but every fiber—has its own neuro-connector that tells it when to fire, the *sequencing* that is the key to coordination, to everything. And there are billions of them. And those signals are coordinated body-wide. It's one grid. The integration of those billions of signals is of the essence. It is what movement is all about. So start with this: Strength training is signal training. Not one signal at a time either. Or even a million at a time; all of them. They work together; that's the deal.

And that has some strong implications for how you train. You train for integrated, *instinctive* movement. You cannot make up your conscious mind to move this muscle cell and *do* it. It doesn't work that way. Ultimately it is a matter of muscle-group memory. Of remembering and recruiting *the movement, not the muscles*. It is a whole-body affair. Strength per se is *relatively* minor. You want strength and you must have it; you surely must have substantial lean muscle mass. But signaling comes first. Signaling actually *is* strength to a remarkable extent. You can beef up the raw power of the cells, but signals come first, always.

And signals work on a whole-body basis. The power grid of the body is an integrated one, or we could not move the way we do. That is what grace and coordination are all about—the well-tempered signaling system of the whole body. Bill's basic point begins to be obvious: We do not live in a two-dimensional world. Ever. And our muscles do not work in isolation. Ever. We use our muscles in concert, and only in concert. Concert is a good word for it, as a matter of fact. Muscle movement is *music*. And it is not solo music. Not a bicep solo or a quad solo. It is a concert every time. Bode Miller screams around a gate on skis; he uses every muscle in his body *in concert*. Train the orchestra, not just the bassoons. Do the bassoons get a little separate training once in a while? Sure. And the violins and the drums? Of course. So use the isolation machines some of the time to strengthen certain muscles. But remember it is an orchestra you are running here. Train the orchestra.

A Special Blessing for Those Who Rot!

Compound whole-body exercise makes sense for a bunch of reasons, but one of them is particularly important if you happen to be over thirty-two. Or forty. Or seventy. Remember the warning from early in the book? The stuff you don't use *rots*. Muscles that are not used *rot*. Sinews that are not used *rot*. And most important of all, signaling systems that are not used *rot*. You can use machines that isolate and strengthen some muscles all day long, and *rot* can still be going on in the supporting muscles (and signaling systems) that are being carefully *excluded* from the exercise. The whole point of most machine exercise is to isolate and exercise and build muscles while, obviously, *excluding others*. Well, the poor little guys who get excluded have their revenge. They *rot. And when they do, they take down the big boys, too.*

Let me give you an example from life that has been curiously underreported in the popular press: The gripping story of my bum hip. I have been a good kid about exercise, having spent zillions of hours on my bike and done a lot of old-fashioned weight lifting, especially on leg-press machines. (I actually own one, in my home gym, as I mentioned someplace: No one has his own leg-press machine.) It worked in the sense that my legs were very strong. I can leg press four hundred pounds all afternoon. Weird. But here's the funny thing. The muscles like the psoas and the gluteus maximus that support the hip and the signals that run through them—those muscles were not being worked out enough, or correctly. And sure enough, they *rotted*. Just a little bit. Just enough so that my hip joint got a teeny bit *out of alignment*. And slowly, slowly, over time, things started to chew on themselves in there. And one day, on a strange squat machine, I tore my labrum. That's a sort of cartilage cuff that helps hold your hip joint in place.

That's the mishap Bill eventually diagnosed and that was fixed in an operation. The operation involved a lot of pain and expense and rehab. And the hip is much better but still not perfect. Never will be. All of which I might have avoided if I had done more whole-body exercise. Like free-standing squats and lunges. To look after the support muscles and the wiring.

Balance

This is obvious by now, but one of the great things about free weights and whole-body exercise is that they are terrific for your balance. The great flaw in the machines—and the reason they are easy to use—is that they do not require much balance. The machine does the balancing so you don't have to. You don't learn how, and you don't develop the exquisite networks of muscles and signals that make balance possible. Squats are hard because you have to balance. Lunges are hard because you have to balance. And here's the deal: Balance is *trainable*. You can improve your balance radically, at any age, by doing exercises that require *balance*. After forty, training and developing your balance is *huge*. One of the great keys to the good life.

Boomers and the Shrinking Margin for Error in Movement

The advice in this book—and the exercises in the next chapters—will work like a charm for everyone, whether twenty or fifty or seventy. They are as close to universal as we can make them. But the advice and the exercises are much more important for men and women who are no longer twenty. Or even twenty-eight. They are hugely important for boomers and beyond.

Think about a couple of things. Your prospects now, your upside, is greater than you had dared to dream. Much greater than it was when you were twenty. True. But it is also true that you are not twenty anymore. And there are consequences. A lot of you, as many as 80 percent, have had some loss of mobility: a bum hip, a bum shoulder, a bum knee. Some pain, some loss of flexibility. And you are a bit more vulnerable. Your "margin for error in movement" has shrunk a little. Work out more, not less, and you will improve the margins. But do it wisely. Because the margin for error is narrower.

After forty, doing strength training *right* matters more and more. Doing it at all matters the most of all, of course. That is the great key to a good Third Act. But you are not bulletproof. When you were a kid— like most of the trainers in most of the gyms—you could jump on any machine without warming up and bang out however many reps, and be fine. And you could use them any old way. Form mattered less because you had such a huge margin for error. Today, it is more important to warm up, the right way. It is more important to set your core before you lift. It is more important to rotate your hips, not your lower back. The margins for error have shrunk. The price of doing things wrong has gone up. Much of our focus in the next two chapters is on doing strength training correctly. So you can keep on moving forever. And not get hurt.

The Three Little Pigs and the Importance of Posture

All right, now let's talk about something that may strike you as dull but has everything to do with *increasing* your margin of error and making life safer for you. More fun for longer. Let's talk about *posture.* Actually, let's not talk about posture. Let's talk about "The Three Little Pigs."

You will perhaps recall the heartbreaking story of the three little pigs who had such a harrowing time with the Big Bad Wolf. Two of the little pigs—the two *fun* ones, it always seemed to me—slapped together crappy houses out of straw and twigs. Didn't take any time at all, and they were delighted with themselves and their shoddy houses. But sure enough, the Big Bad Wolf came around and simply blew 'em down, and ate the two nice pigs. Awful.

The third little pig—who always struck me as a bit pompous—had warned his brothers but to no avail. So he sanctimoniously went off and—with great care—built his house out of brick. The Big Bad Wolf came around, made ugly threats, which the third little pig was pleased to ignore. And then the wolf huffed and puffed—no luck. Strong house. Wolf was screwed. He eventually had to go off to McDonald's or something. Ate crap and died. The third little pig, the smug and sanctimonious one, lived to be ninety-five, was married three times, and had 1,037 piglets (he was a pig, after all). I hate to use the smug little pig to illustrate a moral, but I have no choice. He was absolutely right.

You will be relieved to learn that I tell this ancient story for a reason. Turns out, there is a Big Bad Wolf in all of *our* lives. A big, dangerous sucker and absolutely ravenous. And about 80 percent of us—maybe 90—live in straw or stick houses. Not a good idea in a wolf-infested neighborhood like ours. Mercifully, the wolf does not actually eat us anymore. But he does cause little problems. For example, let me ask you this: Does your back hurt?

Of course, your back hurts, you dope! I do not mean to be smug, like that third little pig, but of course your back hurts. *Your back hurts like crazy because you live in a house that is a dangerous, tilted wreck, slapped together out of sticks and straw. Your posture stinks, you don't even know the terms stacking or alignment. Your core is weak, you don't know how to move—or lift or twist or crouch—so you're doomed to a life of serious back pain that is only going to get worse. The wolf is contentedly gnawing on your backbone. And he will not stop, no matter what you do, until you rebuild your damned house. Out of brick this time, for God's sake.* Pills won't help. There are no guarantees with back surgery either. You gotta rebuild the house. Even if you wind up needing surgery, you *still* have to rebuild the house sooner or later. Better to do it sooner.

The pleasing news is that Bill—who has been such a help to me and thousands of others—is going to show you how. It is not going to be easy, and it will take a lot of change. But it will work and be worth it. A bit technical in places but very important. Because the junk pile you live in now, well, it just isn't safe.

Geologic Forces

B ill likes to talk about the "geologic forces" at work on your body. We all recognize that geologic forces—wind, rain, and gravity— can cut huge canyons through rock and bring the mighty mountains down. Time, pressure, and shear, Bill says. That's all it takes, lots of pressure and lots and lots of time, to reduce the mountains to rubble.

Same for you. Bill says that there are forces at work on your body that are like that. There's basic gravity and there are all the twisting, compression, and shear forces we generate in daily life. Bending, lifting, and twisting a few million times intensifies the influence of those forces on our bodies. Those forces don't amount to *that* much on a given day or over a year. But over a lifetime, they have astonishing and sometimes deadly consequences. They can turn your backbone into rubble.

Built Like a Brick House

B uilding a good brick house is a three-step process. The first one is architecture, structure. You have to get the walls and the support beams generally in place. And they have to be straight. For you, that's simple. It's good *posture*. You have to stand up straight. Easy-peasy.

There is a certain amount of geologic wear and tear, no matter what we do. There is aging, after all. But it is made much worse if we do not take decent care of ourselves. The original sin of bad self-care is bad posture. Rotten posture opens the door for the big bad wolf. Rotten posture—and especially rotten posture in motion—brings us low.

What Is Good Posture?

A chieving good posture is a bit dodgy, if it is not natural to you. The great trick is to have what's called a *neutral spine*. And to have your body properly stacked. What in the world does that mean?

To get an idea, look at the picture on the next page. See the curve of her back: That's perfect. It is a complex series of curves that they call

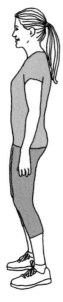

the neutral spine: shoulders back, head up, chin tucked in slightly, weight straight up and down on hips, knees, and feet. Perfect. See the very slight arch of the lower, or lumbar, spine. That's the key part. You don't want to be hunched over, which eliminates or flattens out that curve. You certainly don't want to be swaybacked, which exaggerates that curve and thrusts out your butt. And you don't want your head thrust forward. You want to be just right. When you have it right, your weight is aligned, as if with a plumb line, down from your head, to your hips to your feet. Spend some time on this. Look in the mirror. If you have a trainer, get him or her to drill you on this. Getting this right is a critical step in making the rest of your life a pleasure. Weird but true.

Your spine, a miraculously powerful but flexible structure, is made up of a stack of bones (the vertebrae), intermediate washers or shock absorbers made of sponge-like gristle (discs), and a bunch of wires (sinews). And a powerful network of muscles and fascia tissue. The whole business—everything but your arms, legs, and head—are your core. It is an elaborate structure and works remarkably well. But it is not bulletproof. About 80 percent of the people in this country have back pain bad enough to have sought medical help. Avoiding a bad back is a key to a good Third Act.

Your back is designed to tolerate remarkable loads when it is aligned properly, when you have good posture. You have to stand up straight. You have to sit up straight. You have to do exercises with a neutral spine. Just as important as posture is stability, the second leg of Bill's stool. *Stability* is a matter of having your core or the girdle of muscles that holds your back steady, *strong and engaged.* Engaging or activating them is a simple matter of tensing your core muscles slightly—as if to get ready for a light tap on the belly—before you use them. The goal is safe, successful movement, in three dimensions, with force, and without getting hurt. It is a matter of having good posture supported by good core stability. That, of course, is what Bill's PSM is all about: posture, stability, movement. Think PSM all the time when you work out, and you are headed for a lifetime of effective, injury-free movement. Takes a little work but it is so worth it.

Stability

People tend to think of the core as just the abs, the so-called six-pack you see on the covers of magazines. It is a lot more than that. In fact, it is a set of several overlapping bands of muscles that run all over the place, from your front to your back and all the way up to your neck. The abs are just one—and a rather minor one—out of a bunch. You need your whole core to be strong. The exercises in the next chapters are heavily focused on that. Gotta have a stable core. So you can stabilize your structure and move with power and safety.

Things Going Wrong

That's a quick outline of PSM. To bring it home and make it real, the best thing may be to show you what happens when you exercise *wrong,* when you ignore good posture or don't have good enough stability. Let's look at just a few people who—like so many you see every day in every gym in this country—are busily, virtuously, *blindly* making a wreck of their bodies.

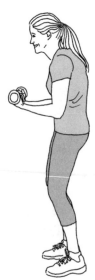

First one, look at this woman picking up dumbbells with her back all slouched. When you slump like this woman, you put *more pressure* on the front side of the discs. When you slump *and* lift weights, like this poor devil, you put horrendous pressure on the front of the discs. Eventually, the pressure is going to take all the resilience out of the discs and flatten them on one side so they can't do their job. And in the longer term, she is going to tear the discs, the dreaded ruptured disc, and she is going to be in serious trouble. Then she is going to go to work on the bone segments themselves, the vertebrae. And some surgeon is going to start lecturing her about the magic of a spine fusion. Hint: The real magic is not having this problem in the first place. The real magic is doing exercises with a neutral spine and an engaged core. The real magic is training movement, not muscles. The woman in the picture is a virtuous, hardworking dope. Hate to be mean, but it's true. And the gyms are full of people just like her. Don't be one of them.

Critical Lesson: Do Not Bend, Lift, and Twist with Your Back

You should know that your lower back, your lumbar spine, is not designed to rotate. Your upper back and your middle back can rotate some, but not your lumbar spine. It was not built for that. If you learn nothing else in these exercise chapters, learn this: *Do not bend, lift, and twist at the same time with your spine. Lots of compound motions are great; this one is disastrous.*

Your upper and middle back can do some rotating but—even if you are mostly using your upper back—the bend-lift-twist move *from your back* is not a good idea. *Always rotate with your hips, not your back.* It is inevitable that you will bend, lift, and twist in any good exercise regimen. But the great trick is to *rotate your hips, not your back.* Lower back rotation with weight is suicidal. Here is the mantra one more time: *Do not bend, lift, and twist with your back! Ever.* It will make a mess. *Rotate with your hips.*

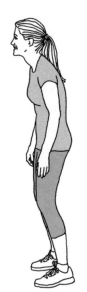

Last One: Heads-Up!

Okay, last one. Look at the picture of the woman on the right with her head slouched forward. Very, very common mistake. Lord knows what weird psychological forces of primal shame and guilt are at work that lead people to carrying themselves that way. But here is something we do know. Your head, with good posture (not slouched) weighs about twelve pounds on your neck and spine. Your head, when you slouch like that, *weighs about 37 pounds on your neck and spine.* That is a *huge* difference. It is, for sure, the difference between a healthy neck and spine and a badly tortured one. Over decades, carrying your head in a slouch is almost guaranteed to cause serious pain. Get a new self-image. *Hold your head up high!*

Don't Slouch!

If you slouch and let your shoulders fall forward and let your lower back go flat, you put much more pressure on your lower or lumbar spine, which is where almost all back pain begins. That is true when you are just standing there. And it is *really true* if you exercise vigorously with that lousy posture. You multiply the pressure on your lower back radically. In vigorous movement, such as heavy lifting, with rotten posture, pressure on your lower back can be as much as two to four thousand pounds. Ruinous. Exercising with bad posture and a weak or unengaged core is much worse than not exercising at all.

A Word to Athletes: Good Posture Is Stronger

A properly stacked body—a body with a neutral spine and a solid, engaged core—is as much as 40 percent stronger than one with bad posture. Good athletes have good posture because it works. And good athletes work hard at the core strength, which is the bedrock of good posture. Tiger Woods had his problems but not with his core. He spent thousands of hours doing *core* exercises. He is famous for it. Want to be a better golfer? Strengthen your core. Want to be skiing downhill in your eighties? Strengthen your core. Want to be on your feet and not on a walker or a chair, all the way to the waterfall? Strengthen your core. And watch your posture. PSM. It will see you through. On to the exercises.

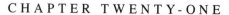

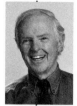

CHAPTER TWENTY-ONE

The Warm-Up, or "Preparation for Movement"

Okay, now we finally get down to what you actually *do* when you get to the gym or out the door or right in your living room. Not a minute too soon. We start with the warm-ups, which are quite a bit more elaborate and more substantive than most of us are used to. They are carefully designed to promote and preserve joint mobility and range of motion, and they are a million miles from the old "jump on the elliptical machine for five minutes and then we'll begin." In other words, there's a reason why we have devoted a whole chapter just to the warm-ups.

I hope you'll read all the way through this and the next chapter before you jump in. This is a new way to exercise, and it is not intuitively obvious, even if you already work out a lot. Doing these wrong can mess you up.

It is my notion—more than Bill's, I suspect—that most of us don't *begin* to know *what the devil we are doing* when we get to the gym. I know that I personally have been going to gyms forever, and I *never* know what I'm doing. Never. I mean, I have a clue. I have had a few hundred training sessions over the years. But now everything is changing.

The old rules turn out to be stupid. *I* turn out to be stupid. What machine or other gadget should I use? What movement? How long? How hard? And how do you *do* this stuff? And am I making a fool of myself? Am I just too old and pathetic to be here in the first place?

These next two chapters, my friends, are going to end all that. Immerse yourself in this *slightly* arcane material and—for the rest of your long life—you will know exactly what to do. And how to do it. And *why*. That last one is the most satisfying and important of all: Once you know *why*, it all comes together—and *sticks*.

No Special Toys Required

There are a bunch of different ways to skin these cats. There are a number of different approaches, using different devices, some of them new to you. Don't be alarmed. All the exercises can be done with basic gear—very basic gear like elastic expansion bands and free weights. We do not spell that out, but I think it will be fairly obvious. Expansion or elastic bands (hollow rubber tubes with handles on each end) are wonderful gadgets. They come in different strengths (degree of difficulty), and you can buy three of them and have a decent gym. I'd add other toys myself, but I am an equipment junkie. Do think about the two TRX devices we mention here; they are useful and fun but by no means indispensable. And a set of weights is always a good idea. Maybe a BOSU ball (a balance-improving gadget: flat on one side, rounded on the other). And a big "Swiss ball." But that's about it. This is not about money; it's about technique. A gym membership (or one at the local YMCA or community gym) is always a great idea, if there's a decent one nearby, and if you don't just *hate* the gym (some people do). And a few sessions with a trainer is a great blessing if you can afford it and you can find one that understands the new whole-body techniques. Not always easy.

We illustrate each exercise (especially the substantive ones) using what we think of as the best equipment for it. But a moment's thought will make it possible to do almost all of them with some combination of elastic bands and free weights. Sometimes we show gym machines, often the body alone, and other gadgets. Use 'em if you got 'em, but use elastic bands and free weights if you don't. Doesn't matter *that* much.

It's easy to put together a "home gym" for peanuts, if you like. And a "gym in a bag" for travel, if you need that, and it won't cost much. We'll try to give you some guidance on the website. I spend a fortune on gym gear and other sports stuff because I am a child, but you don't have to. Trust me, the toys are not going to be the limiting factor. *You* are going to be the limiting factor. And even you, poor bugger, are not going to have any excuses after you read this.

One Size Does Not Fit All

We are deeply mindful of the fact that you are not all the same age or level of fitness, not all blessed with the same familiarity with or passion for the subject of strength training. And we know your own needs will change over time—your need for variety, for harder or easier stuff. Whatever. Individual trainers are sharply focused on those differences. Books cannot be.

What we *have* done is focus, hard, on the basics of movement that really are equally important to all comers, regardless of condition, experience, and so on. Then we offer the twenty-five sacred exercises, Bill's cull of twenty-five strength training exercises that will form the base for all you will ever need to know on the subject. Learn these, and you'll be set. Later, you may want to learn more, but you won't need to. These are comprehensive. These will teach you how to move.

The Warm-Up: A Quick Intro

Bill calls this "movement preparation." Bill does this warm-up himself, every single day, no joke—I've seen it. Because he knows—from thousands of hours spent looking at men and women who have made a hash of their joints—how important it is. This is a whole-body warm-up but with special emphasis on your joints. Especially your hips. And your poor back. And your ankles. Oh, and your knees. Do please remember that 80 percent of the people in this country have impaired movement in their hips and bad backs. The difficulty frequently starts with the ankles. And guess what? These unpleasant phenomena are closely related. Step 1 on the road to *preventing or reversing* loss of hip mobility—or ankle mobility or shoulder mobility —is this set of "preparations for movement." The first time, the warm-up alone may take half an hour or more. Who cares—you're learning. When you have it, it will take ten minutes or less.

General Rules

Here are some general rules for all these warm-up exercises:

1. Do ten to fifteen reps of each warm-up exercise.

2. Move at a slow to moderate speed (except for the footwork piece).

3. Do these "pain free" other than some discomfort from the stretch on a few exercises. A little muscle pain is okay—joint pain is not.

4. Slowly increase the range of motion for each exercise with each repetition.

When you are told to tense your abdominals or gluteals, use light to moderate force. There is no need to use maximum effort and certainly no need to hold your breath. Be gentle yet focused on these muscles. *Think* about the muscles involved.

Equipment

The only equipment needed for the warm-ups is a mat and either a bench or a chair. The warm-ups go in this order: (1) Start on your back; (2) roll over on your stomach; (3) roll up on your side (both sides); (4) get up on all fours; (5) stand up. That will help you remember.

ON YOUR BACK

The Bridge

Why Bother?

Like all the warm-ups, this one is primarily designed to loosen and warm up your joints, in this case your hips. And it's especially good for your glutes, which are your dominant *hip extensors*. This is a critical muscle that goes with aging, reducing your hip mobility. Good hip extensor function is key in doing squats, lunges, and a lot of other things. This one also is great for your core and your lower back.

Step 1:
Lie on your back with both legs bent. Tighten your abs and squeeze your glutes. (If you like, you can put a pillow or a ball between your legs and squeeze it.) Lift your butt off the floor. Hold for five seconds.

Step 2:
Relax to floor. Repeat. Do ten to fifteen of these. Go slow.

Make It Harder:

Progress to a one-legged bridge (hold other leg as straight toward ceiling as you can manage with foot flexed).

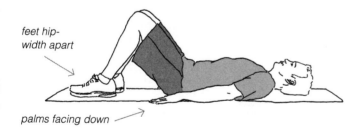

feet hip-width apart

palms facing down

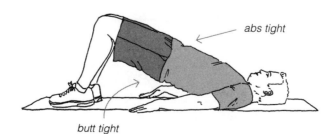

abs tight

butt tight

Leg Raise

Why Bother?
This one is good to get the hip flexors and core activated, and get the hamstrings and calf muscles lengthened.

Step 1:
Lie on your back, with one knee bent, foot on the floor, and the other leg straight. Tense the quad and flex the foot of the straight leg, then lift it upward, flexing at the hip until you feel a hamstring or calf stretch. Like a rubber band, it will "recoil" your leg back to the floor.

Step 2:
Repeat ten to fifteen times, then switch sides and repeat.

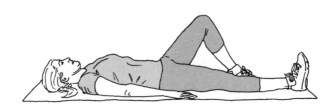

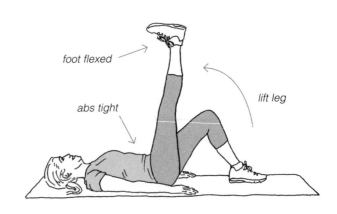

foot flexed

lift leg

abs tight

Shoulder/Overhead Reach (Dry Backstroke)

Why Bother?

This one is great for mid back and shoulder mobility. It stretches your pecs (the chest muscles in front that tend to pull you round-shouldered). Shoulder mobility is critical in life. Work on it or it goes away.

Step 1:
Lie on your back with one or both legs bent. Reach over your head with one arm as far as you can, touching the floor, if you can. (Imagine a swimmer, doing the backstroke.) Return arm to your side. Keep your lower back quiet by tensing your abs.

Step 2:
Do the other arm and continue to alternate between left and right arm ten to fifteen times each.

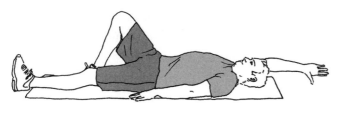

keep neutral spine

Bill Says:

There are variations you may want to try. One, do this with a foam-rubber roller vertically placed under your back; look around the gym or Google foam rollers. Two, try "snow angels" as an alternative.

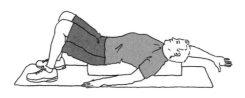

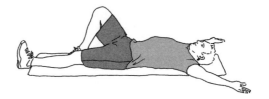

ON YOUR STOMACH
"I's" and "T's"

Why Bother?

These enhance shoulder stability and mobility. In particular, they target the rotator cuff.

Step 1 ("I's"):
Lie on your stomach on the floor or a workout bench. Your head can be supported by a rolled up towel or a small calm dog (just kidding). With arms at your sides, palms down, you are making the letter "I" with your body.

Step 2:
Pinch your shoulder blades back and down. Then lift both hands up until your arms are just above parallel with the floor. Hold for three seconds. Slowly return arms down until hands touch the floor. Repeat ten to fifteen times.

Step 3 ("T's"):
Put your arms out to the side, making a letter "T" with your body and head supported as described in step 1. Pinch your shoulder blades gently back and down; turn your arms so that thumbs point upward. Then lift your arms until they are just above parallel with the floor. Hold for three seconds. Slowly return arms to the floor. Repeat ten to fifteen times.

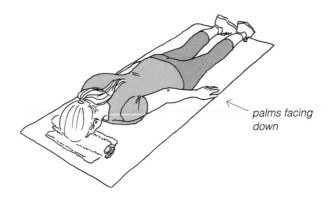

palms facing down

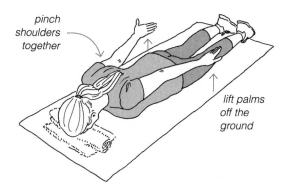

pinch
shoulders
together

lift palms
off the
ground

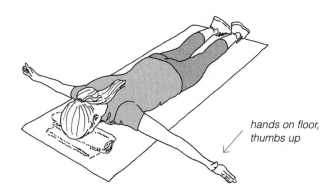

hands on floor,
thumbs up

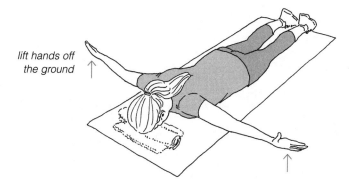

lift hands off
the ground

SIDE LIE

Side Leg Lift

Why Bother?

This one activates your outer hip muscles and improves hip mobility.

Step 1:
Lie on your side with both knees fully extended, feet flexed (pull toes up). Squeeze the glutes and tense the abs. Lift your top leg about a foot off the floor. Hold five seconds. Keep your body straight and do not bend from the hip. No need to try to lift the leg too high; the goal here is merely to activate the outer hip muscles. You should feel it right above your hip.

Step 2:
Lower leg and repeat ten times each side.

*legs straight,
feet flexed*

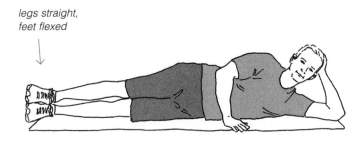

butt tight

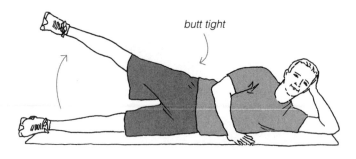

ON ALL FOURS (AS IN A CRAWL)

Cat and Camel

Why Bother?

This one lubricates, warms, and loosens all the many joints in your back.

Step 1:

Get on all fours like a crawling baby. Slowly round the low and mid back by tilting the pelvis. Hold for a couple of seconds (camel).

Step 2:

Reverse into the opposite direction until the back is arched (cat). Hold for a couple of seconds.

Bill Says:

Be gentle with your movements here.

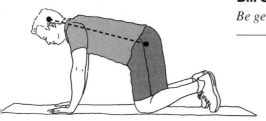

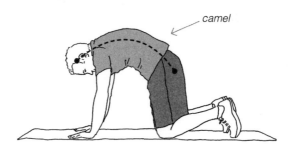

camel

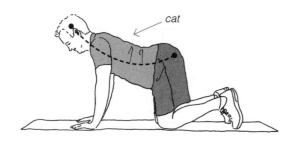

cat

Heel Extensions

Why Bother?

Most of us are imbalanced with tight hip flexors on the front of our hips and weak gluteals on the backside. This exercise helps rebalance the length and activation of these muscles. If you have lost some hip mobility already, do more of these.

Step 1:

Still on all fours, extend the heel of one leg (with knee flexed to 90 degrees) to the ceiling. Keep your lower back still by tensing your abs. Do ten reps at slow to moderate speed. No jerky movements on this one. Switch legs.

Bill Says:

If your hip is tight from years of sitting at a desk or from doing exercises (like biking) that emphasize the flexed position, you truly need this one.

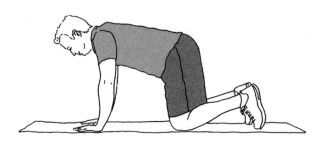

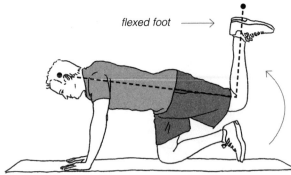

flexed foot ⟶

lift heel up so that bottom of your foot facing the sky

Opposing Arm and Leg Reaches

Why Bother?

This addresses hip and shoulder mobility, core stability, and balance. A great exercise, and a little harder than it looks. Really reach for it, in both directions.

Step 1:
In crawling position, tense your abdominals and keep your low back quiet. Then reach way out with one hand and reach way back with the opposite foot. Hold for five seconds with each reach. Activate all those muscles of the core, hip, and shoulder girdle.

Step 2:
Return arm and leg to floor. Attempt to keep back still. This exercise is best done switching back and forth, not doing all one side and then all the other.

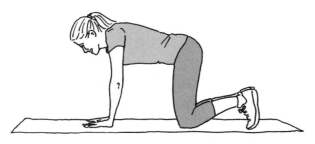

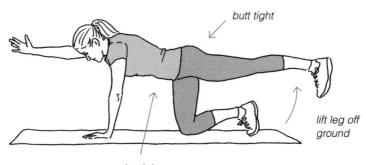

butt tight

lift leg off ground

abs tight

Middle Back Mobility Turns

Why Bother?

This will loosen your mid back, an area where everyone tends to stiffen as they age. This is designed to offset the evil consequences of *slouching* your whole life.

Bill Says:

Mid back mobility is essential for both good shoulder mobility and to take loads off our low back. Decades of slouching diminishes mid back mobility. This is a must *exercise.*

Step 1:

Start on all fours; then drop your butt down to your ankles. Put your left arm behind your head. Turn your upper body slowly to the right, then to the left.

Step 2:

Repeat with your right hand behind your head.

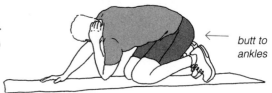

← *butt to ankles*

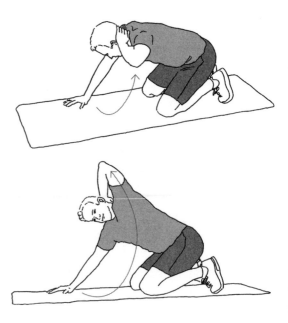

Hip Circles

Why Bother?

This is one of the great defensive moves in the struggle to maintain the glass box.

Step 1:

Still on all fours, kick one leg back in a circular pattern. Increase the size of the circle over time as your mobility improves. Do ten clockwise, on one side; then ten counterclockwise. Keep the low back still.

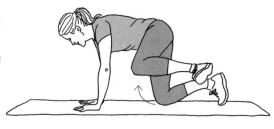

Step 2:

Repeat on other side.

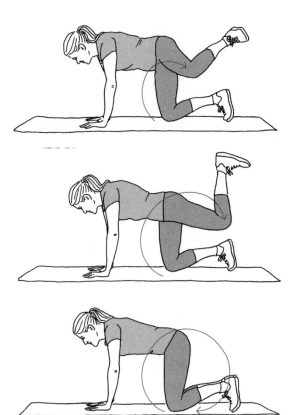

HALF-KNEELING

Half-Kneeling Stretch

Why Bother?

This one does it all: hip and shoulder mobility, core stabilization, balance, and stability enhancement.

Step 1:

Kneel down with one knee on the floor and the other leg and foot out in front. (You may want to put a towel or pad under the knee.) Tense your abs and glutes and shift your weight forward onto your front leg while lifting your arms overhead. You should feel a stretch on the front of your rear leg. Hold for three to five seconds.

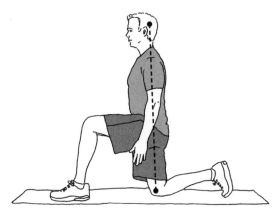

Step 2:

Bring arms to side and shift weight to rear leg. Do ten reps on each side.

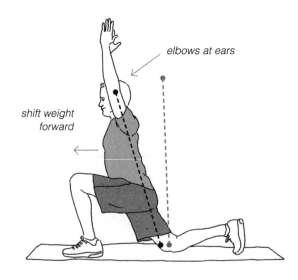

elbows at ears

shift weight forward

STANDING
Ankle Flex

Why Bother?

This is a key exercise to prevent or reverse limited ankle mobility. You need good ankle mobility to do squats, lunges, walk down the stairs—everything. And when it goes, it raises hell with everything else.

Step 1:

Stand, facing a wall. Bring one foot to within six inches of the wall. Bend that knee slightly. The back leg should be about a foot or two behind the front leg (which is the one being stretched and mobilized). Put both hands against the wall. Try to drop most of your weight onto the flexed front foot. Flex the knee farther by driving the front foot toward the wall. Do not let your heel come up or slide inward; keep your feet facing straight ahead. Drive the knee over the center of the foot. Do fifteen reps.

Step 2:

Switch sides and repeat.

Bill Says:

Don't be surprised if one ankle is more mobile than the other. You want to correct or at least improve that asymmetry over time, because it can lead to a whole host of musculoskeletal problems.

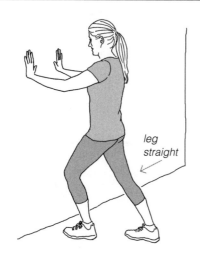

leg
straight

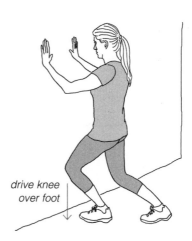

drive knee
over foot

Balance on One Leg

Why Bother?

Balance is one of the things we lose as we get older. But we can do something about it.

Step 1:

Stand tall; activate your quads, glutes, and abs. Pull your shoulders back ("military posture," if that helps). Spread your arms out wide and pick up one foot a few inches off the floor and try to maintain your balance about fifteen seconds. Repeat with other foot.

Step 2:

When you can do fifteen seconds, challenge yourself some more. First, drop your hands to the sides. Next, try closing your eyes. For the ultimate balance challenge, try swinging the lifted leg back and forth and from side to side. Your balance *will* improve.

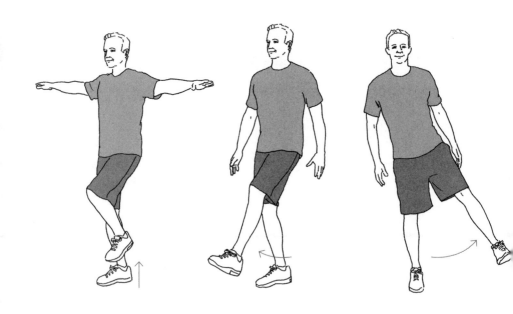

Squat and Reach

Why Bother?

This is the time to get your body working as a unit and to groove some of the basic movements.

Step 1:
Stand tall, with your feet shoulder-width apart or slightly wider. Now *reach* to the ceiling, with your arms, as high as you can go. *Really reach.*

Step 2:
Now bring your hands down, bend your hips and knees, and move into a nice squat. Touch the floor with your hands, but only if you can do it without rounding your back.

Step 3:
Stand tall again; reach to the ceiling and squat again.

Bill Says:

When squatting, do not round your lower back, no matter what. Look straight ahead and keep your chest up (military posture again). Drop your butt back and down. With each repetition, try to go a little lower, without compromising your posture.

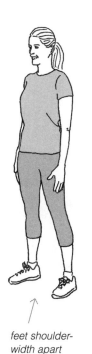

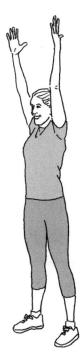

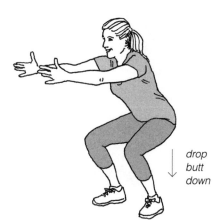

feet shoulder-width apart

drop
butt
down

Squat with Weight Shift

Why Bother?

In the process of shifting your center of gravity you fire up your hip and knee muscles, enhance balance, and improve your hip mobility. Great for skiers, golfers, and all of us who simply need to expand our range of movement.

Step 1:

Stand with your feet as much as twice shoulder-width apart. Squat down halfway; then begin shifting your weight way over either to the left or right leg. As you shift your weight over to one leg, bend that knee and hip farther while keeping feet facing forward and the knee closely in alignment with the foot. Reach forward with both arms at the same time and sink your butt slightly backward.

Step 2:

Shift your weight way over to the other leg, now bending that knee and reaching forward with your arms. Then reach out to the side with your arms, over the foot onto which you are shifting your weight.

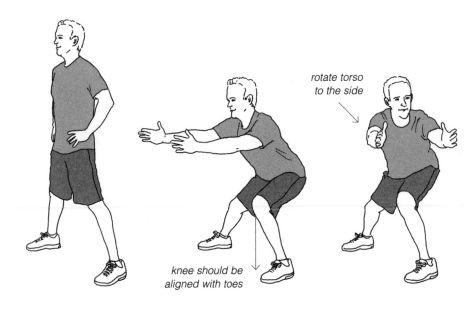

rotate torso
to the side

knee should be
aligned with toes

Fast Footwork

Why Bother?

You may look a little like the monster in *Young Frankenstein* dancing to "Puttin' on the Ritz," when you start this. But remember his joy, and keep dancing. Foot speed and coordination are key in the good life. Olympic athletes spend a huge amount of time on footwork; you should, too.

Step 1:
Start with simple marching in place, for ten seconds. Lift your knees high. Pump your arms. Start slow; get fast.

Step 2:
Do this same high stepping for another ten seconds, at speed. Go for it. As you get more at home with this, add a little bounce to your step until you are jogging in place.

Step 3:
When you really get into it (if you do), consider *springing* from side to side (see illustration, next page). Someday, we hope, your feet are going to be *flying.*

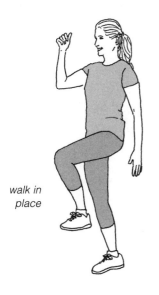

walk in place

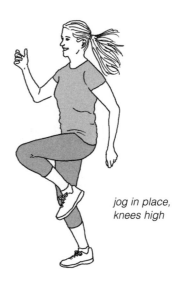

jog in place, knees high

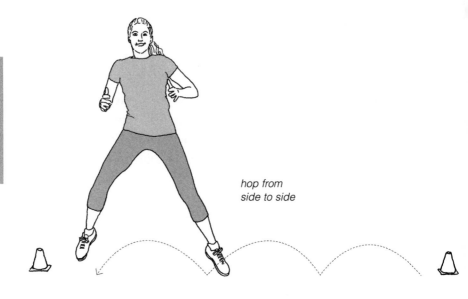

*hop from
side to side*

Bill Says:

This exercise takes advantage of the remarkable springlike quality of muscles. They are rubber bands: You stretch them and they give you a pop *of energy and propulsion. You do not get this as effectively on a treadmill or elliptical machine. Eventually, you will want to inject some side to side motion into these steps. Try laterally shuffling a few yards back and forth like a tennis player, on the baseline. Great for all types of sports and life in general.*

Okay, you are officially and fully warmed up. Catch your breath. Turn to the substantive exercises. You are *so* ready.

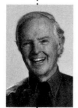

CHAPTER TWENTY-TWO

A Day in the Life:
A Cold Day in Hell

used to think, "It'll be a cold day in hell when I start doing serious strength training for pleasure." This, it turns out, is that day.

It is a cold day, barely twenty degrees, and I am carrying ski poles as I walk across the ice-covered yard, early in the morning, to the little barn I have made into a workout place, fifty yards from the house. (Unlike some of you, I like gyms, but there are no good ones up our way, so we put together our own. We went a little bit nuts, but I justify it by saying that we are "in the business" these days. Frankly, we should all be "in the business" these days; strength training is part of our *job*, if we have our heads on right.) This is a cozy spot. A small New England barn from 150 years ago, with a row of green-shuttered six-over-six windows on the outside, full of gym gear, boats, bikes, and a huge old-fashioned TV on the inside. A busted down easy chair to collapse into at the end.

There is a space heater that makes it toasty in ten minutes. There are white-metal "factory" lights hanging down from the ceiling, which is plain barn wood, like the walls and the bare splintery floor. Bare rafters, too, of course. And hanging from them, a 1964 George Pocock wooden single scull, as beautiful as a cello. On the floor under it is another wooden boat, a Whitehall skiff, a copy of the ones from the turn of the last century, with a wineglass stern. So lovely. In the middle of the room are two elliptical machines (one doesn't work, but it's too heavy to move). To the right, an industrial-strength leg-press machine and enough weights to choke a rhino. Machines, man. Lots and lots of machines. But also a TRX Suspension Trainer and a TRX Rip Trainer. Strewn around the room are other "whole-body" toys: a BOSU ball, a big Swiss balancing ball, kettlebells. If I am in lousy shape, it's not because I don't have enough toys. The walls are lined with road and mountain bikes.

Warm-Up

I t took a while, but I finally drank the Kool-Aid on warming up, Bill's way. I have gotten so I actually enjoy it, to tell the truth. Which I did not at first. In the early days, these warm-ups seemed both too hard and too easy. And mildly annoying, for some reason. Mostly because they were "new," I suspect. Old boys and new tricks, man: It's an endless battle to make yourself *open up* to new stuff. I have come to revel in the "whole-body" feel of these warm-ups, the satisfying sense that I am pushing back on the walls of my own glass box. So I now go at these warm-ups with real purpose.

Then, I go through a cull of the sacred twenty-five routine. But I'm only going to talk, for a minute, about a couple of them: squats and especially *lunges*. I have always known—thank God—that keeping your legs strong was a key to movement and the good life. What that has mostly meant for me, in past times, has been lots of sessions with the big leg-press machines and the leg-lift machine. And they have worked reasonably well. My legs are wonderfully strong in my dotage, which helps tremendously with everything.

But there are problems. Those gadgets were great but they did not do enough, it now seems clear, for the *support* muscles around my hips. And, sure enough, those started to rot, with serious consequences, including a torn labrum, which was a bear. An operation, the works. I still use those machines some—I am slightly addicted to them—but I rely increasingly on the whole-body variations, the lunges and squats.

Lunges Count

I didn't *like* lunges when I began. I *knew* my legs were strong because I could do a lot of weight on the machine. Looked great, I thought as if anyone noticed, or cared. But I looked like a dope, doing lunges. How could that be? The answer, of course, was that although my major muscles were okay, the support muscles and my *balance* were less so. Doing lunges correctly—with a neutral spine and your chest up and looking straight ahead—is not so easy. Not so easy at all. I kept tumbling awkwardly to the left or the right—"falling off" the lunge. And I didn't like that. Wanted to go back to my machines, which I could do, because they're *easier.*

But Bill convinced me (slowly) that strength without balance did not amount to much. He persuaded me that *usable strength* meant whole-body strength. The kind you actually use when you ski or row or climb a hill. I needed more range of motion and better balance. So, this morning and most mornings now, I spend a lot of time doing squats to warm myself up. And then lunges. I finally got so I could do them right. I do a bunch of them. I mean a *bunch*, sometimes carrying weights. My modest point: For those who have already lost some hip mobility—and that is most of us—learning to do lunges may be hard and a little humiliating. But it is so worth it. They are a key to leg strength, balance, and coordination. Which is key to everything else.

The Day Five Miracle

This morning's workout is my fifth *straight* day doing Bill's strength training regimen (not the normal or correct pattern, by the way, but I was getting them down for the book). And at last, the exercises are starting to feel natural and comfortable. Especially the warm-ups, which I have focused on pretty hard. And suddenly—and this is the miracle part—they didn't hurt as much. When I began, there were sharp twinges in my hips and shoulders as I did this and that. Not major pain but twinges, to tell me that I had not been using these joints, this way, enough. Now those twinges were going away. *The pain had eased already.* I could reach way up and way down, more easily. Even a bit gracefully, I thought. And almost no pain. And not only in the gym. I had begun to notice, in my regular life, that I didn't have as many twinges either. My joints felt better. I felt better just doing stuff. Hard to believe—I mean, five days? C'mon.

I called Bill, seven o'clock Aspen time, because I was so curious. I told him what I just told you and asked, "Can that be right? Can I feel quite a lot better, in motion, after just five days of these things? Especially the warm-ups? Or is it just the *placebo effect*?"

Bill is a wonderfully even-tempered, calm guy. It is astonishing that we are collaborators at all. "No," he said, evenly. "That is not surprising at all. It is typical, in my experience, that the sense of improvement cuts in at about that time. The fifth time through. Don't be confused: It's not a cure-all. There are things that take a lot longer, and things that don't ever get better. But an awful lot of the people over forty I train have an appreciable sense of real difference, starting about there, in five sessions. That's normal."

"*Normal!?*" I say. "Why didn't you tell me?"

Bill paused for a second, not quite getting it. Then, "Because I assumed you'd see." That was it.

"Everyone?" I asked. "Everyone you've trained with the new warm-up and the new exercises?"

"No," he said, "Of course not. But a lot of people. That's why I do it. That's why we all do it. It, uh, works."

"Aha!" I said. "I see. You do it because it works. Well, well, well." Pause. "In five days?!"

Bill paused to think *that one* over. Then, "Yes. Five sessions, not five days. It's the sessions that matter. But I'd say it starts, noticeably, in five sessions of workouts for a lot of people—greater mobility, less pain, and greater flexibility. It keeps getting better, of course, for a long time. And you certainly have to keep it up. But, yes. Five sessions and you are on the way. Did you like it?"

Did I like it? Yes, I liked it. The combination of the massive weight loss I've had (just kidding, but that does count, those fifteen pounds, more than you'd think) and the new training regimen is making a significant difference in an already pleasant life. I am nuts about Billy's new model. Is it a little harder than the old way? Yes, but you'd expect that when you think how much more you're doing for yourself. You bet I like it. I love it.

There you go. Hard to get a sense of it from a snippet, but there's the seed.

What We Ate

Breakfast and lunch were more of what you've seen. No need to talk about them. Dinner's a little different now. With the weight loss in hand, we are not changing the way we eat back to the way we ate before. If anything, we're getting deeper into the eating vegetables and new stuff, like farro. I have gone back to a second glass of wine. I do love that pesky wine. But not a half a bottle. Can't do that anymore and I finally *know it*. Interestingly, the way we eat—the avoidance of Dead Food and the emphasis on veg—has "taken." It feels natural now and does not "bind" anymore. It's just what we do.

Tonight, for no particular reason, we are having an all-veg meal. We have fallen into doing that a day or two a week. Tonight we're having what has become a staple, one we default to the way we used to default to burgers and white rice.

Some nights that same meal is done in a wok on the top of the stove, with a heavy dose of Asian sauces—fish sauce, soy, ginger—other stuff we find. Often some strips of "very firm" tofu get thrown in.

All-Veg Meal

We cut up some onions, fresh peppers, beets, and a little broccoli, and spread 'em out in a roasting pan. Sprinkle them with salt and (not much) olive oil, and broil them for fifteen minutes or so. That and a green salad, and some very good white wine. Maybe some whole-wheat bread. It's that new relationship with vegetables we talked about. Getting there.

Tofu doesn't taste like much, but it's a great sponge for spices and sauces. Good for you, too. Some nights, brown rice, too. Or quinoa. Or farro, one of the major joys in my life these days. Lots of nights, I toss in shrimp or fish, some chicken. But often it's just vegetables. There you go.

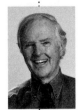

CHAPTER TWENTY-THREE

The Twenty-Five Sacred Exercises

Our goal here—Bill's goal, I should say—is to show you how to do "the twenty-five sacred exercises" that will be the foundation of *all you need to know* on the subject of strength training, *for the rest of your life*. You may want to learn more eventually, but this will be the rock on which you build any regimen. Learn to do these right, and you will know all the basic movements. Learn to do these right and you will be able to walk into any gym in the country and know exactly what you're doing. Learn to do these right, and you will get into great shape and stay there. You can do these on your own perfectly well, and without much gear.

Drill yourself a little on these; repetition is of the essence. But once you get them grooved—once they move into your *muscle memory*—you will have them forever and they will seem easy, automatic. And they will do all the amazing things that Jen and I have said will come to you with serious strength exercise. You're going to go through the exercises a number of times before you get them; it's taken me a while. But I did get them and you will, too. And here's an extremely curious thing: It gets to be fun, after a while. Weird but true.

Bill has a couple of rules of general application: Rule 1: Do these exercises for several repetitions—ten to twelve typically—but always stop at "failure." But here "failure" has a special meaning. It means do them until you fail to do them right. Then stop. If you can't maintain a neutral spine on a squat—if your knee starts to buckle on a lunge—if your head pops forward or your shoulders hunch on a pull-down—stop! That's the new failure. Go on to the next exercise. Or do an easier version of this one. But don't do them wrong; that's less than useless. You can get hurt.

In traditional strength training, "going to failure" meant lifting heavier and heavier loads until you just couldn't do another rep because your muscles hurt too much. It was a sound idea. You build new muscle by tearing the old ones down. When they are rebuilt, the muscles are mysteriously "remodeled." They grow back bigger and stronger. Going to failure in the old-fashioned way. But Bill wants you to see failure in a different light.

Here's Bill on the subject: "I cannot tell you how many clients I've had who got in trouble by ignoring good form and going to failure, the old-fashioned way, but with their bodies in poor alignment. It was as if they were deliberately hurting themselves. I have seen serious weight lifters with severe degenerative backs, worn-down knees, dreadful hip problems all from doing strength training with bad alignment. *Never overload dysfunction.* In other words, if you can't perform these exercises with good alignment, don't add more weight or try to do them with speed. It is painfully common. Our joints and backs are engineering miracles. But they will not stand up to decades of off-center pressures that come with bad posture and faulty movement. Bad strength training is much, much worse than none at all."

Rule 2: Use full range of motion (or try to) on every exercise. I think of this as the glass box rule. Reaching all the way up, all the way down . . . squat until your thighs are parallel to the ground. Those are the moves that are going to preserve full range of motion in your joints. You may not be able to achieve full range of motion on a lot of these exercises at first. Or maybe ever. But *trying* to do so keeps the glass box from shrinking. Full range of motion—or the closest you can get to it—is always the goal.

Why Range of Motion Matters

ere's an interesting thing about range of motion I got from Riggs. I was whining one day about my beloved leg-press machine. I started out boasting about what a hell of a guy I was because I could do so much weight on it. And Riggs said, smugly, "Yeah, but your range of motion is not great. Instead of going down to ninety to one hundred and ten degrees, you are going down to about seventy."

"So what?" I said, angrily. "I'm doing it in *my range.*"

"Yeah," Riggs said, "but that is not a good plan. Muscles," he said, "are a collection of fibers, strung together. The fibers a little like a bundle of elastics from inside a baseball, only stretched out. A typical muscle is a torpedo-shaped collection of fibers, thickest in the middle and tapering on both ends, to the place where it attaches to the bone or whatever. Here's the point: Think of your bicep doing a bicep curl. Different parts of the torpedo are recruited for different parts of the curl. The fat part of the torpedo—the real meat of your bicep—is what you recruit in the middle of the lift. But toward the end of the lift—when the weight is almost all the way up to your shoulder or down by your side—it's the fibers on either end that are doing the work. If you just do bicep curls—or leg presses—in the middle range, the middle of the muscle gets strong. But those fibers on the ends never get stronger. At all."

I had a ready answer to that: "Who cares?"

"You should. Think about skiing the bumps . . . in effect doing a series of squats, at speed. When you ski the bumps, do you ever go really deep like doing a really deep knee bend? A ninety- to one hundred and ten-degree angle at the knee?"

"Of course. Not any more than I must, but sure."

"Well, all your hours with the leg-press machine will do *nothing* to make you stronger and better able to ski the deep bumps when you have to power all the way down. Down to the right-angle point. I've watched you ski, and the fact is that you do *not* go all the way down to ninety degrees. You stand up surprisingly tall, in the bumps. Which is not stable, not a good idea. And the answer, almost certainly, is that you're not strong enough to do it right. Despite the considerable strength of your quads in the middle range. See?"

I sputtered, but I did see. And he's right. I am simply not strong enough to ski correctly in steep bumps. I cannot get down all the way, turn after turn. Two ways to go: Stay on the groomed trails; or learn full range of motion.

Now let us assume, just for fun, that you don't give a rat's ass about skiing the bumps. Why should you care about full range of motion for, say, your quads?

The answer to that is painfully obvious. Think falling down. When you fall down, you get full range of motion in your quads, in a heartbeat. You go all the way down to a right angle and beyond. And if you don't have strength in your legs, in that range, you will keep on going down till you crash in a heap. Maybe a painful heap because you did not have good range of motion.

Riggs was talking about range of motion in terms of muscle strength. More important, most of the time, is range of motion in joint mobility. Eighty percent of people over fifty have lost significant mobility (range of motion) in their hips or their ankles. Eighty percent have lost mobility in their back. A vast number have lost mobility in their shoulder joints. Good range of motion matters for all kinds of things. If you lose mobility in your shoulder, you will not be able to reach all the way up on the shelf, get the vodka bottle down. If you lose mobility in your ankles (a painfully common thing), you simply will not be able to walk right. And your hips will start to get funny. And your back. It's not all a matter of being able to ski the bumps. It's a matter of getting the cereal off the shelf, walking naturally. Range of motion counts. Joint mobility counts tremendously. The glass box counts.

All of which segues nicely into our first exercise, squats. Doing squats looks easy and obvious. It is neither. It is hugely important to do them correctly (especially with a neutral spine and with good alignment) *and* to achieve a "full range of motion" eventually. Squats are truly basic. Squats are key. Learn to do 'em right, and do a lot of them—with or without weights—for the rest of your life. It will keep you moving with strength and a touch of grace, forever.

General Rules for All Exercises

Do two or three sets of reps, ten to fifteen reps per set. Except where it says otherwise, do them slowly, in both directions. As you get used to the exercises, add resistance, add weight. Until you can only do, say, eight reps on the third set. This *is* strength training, in the end. This is the war on sarcopenia. This is building and maintaining muscle. And you do not do that without *resistance*. Learn to do these right. Then gradually but steadily *push yourself* with added weight. But not right away.

It is not the plan to have you do *all twenty-five* substantive exercises every strength-training day; it would take too long. You should do all the warm-ups every strength-training day, but you can do a selection of the twenty-five. A forty-five-minute (total) strength day is plenty. You may pick and choose within the exercises listed here. Or you may do all of the first dozen exercises on one day and all the remaining exercises the next. But do all of them at some point every week. They are designed to work together.

Once you learn to do these correctly *and* get into decent shape, you may want to do some of them (especially the advanced compound exercises) with more speed. Doing those exercises—which recruit a large number of muscles—at speed is a tremendous aerobic and weight loss workout. Engaging a whole bunch of muscles means a whole bunch of mitochondria—a huge *burn*. Get to this point (and eat sanely) and the weight will fly off.

Don't Make Yourself Nuts

Two things that I have learned may interest you. One: these are easier than they look when you read about them. I started that way (reading), and it was harder. (Another shameless commercial plug: Look at our website.) Two: Some of 'em are hard. For heaven's sake, don't feel compelled to do all of them, from the get-go. If some defeat you at first, *fine*! Skip 'em and go on to the others. Twenty-five exercises like this turns out to be quite a few. Do not force yourself to learn 'em all at once. Pick your way through, get into it gradually. You are not preparing for an exam next week, you're preparing for life. Take your time. Learn to do the easier ones correctly. Go on to the rest in time.

Big lesson: These are a little harder than the old machine exercises (if you're used to those) because they are so much better for you. Supplement the new workouts with the old (machine) stuff, if you like. But learn the new way. It is *so* much better.

A Word About Intensity and Difficulty

We focus hard in this chapter on technique and on showing you how to do these right. There is less emphasis on taking up the intensity, after you learn how. The fact is that the way you get stronger and more fit *is by stressing your muscles.* You do that by making the exercises progressively harder over time. Once you really learn how to do these exercises, you will want to turn your attention to gradually increasing the *degree of difficulty.* That is how you build strength, balance, and coordination. It is slowly increasing the difficulty or intensity that makes this work.

How do you do it? You increase weight. You increase challenges to balance. And you increase speed. For example, Bill spends a long, long time showing you how to do squats and lunges correctly. Eventually, you are going to want to make them harder by holding weights when you do them. Or doing squats on uneven surfaces (a BOSU ball, for example) to make them harder. You will not want to add speed to these.

Eventually, Bill is going to show you some complex *rotational* exercises, using either a medicine ball (great device), machines (the cable machine in the gym is a "good" machine), or the TRX Rip Trainer. It takes a while to learn to use the Rip Trainer correctly. But eventually, one of the joys of this device is that you can use it *hard and fast* to do basic movements. And give yourself a serious strength *and* aerobic workout at the same time you are expanding your glass box. Do it slow till you get the technique just right. Then (when you're in shape) do it as hard as you can for, say, thirty seconds. *Killer!* We spend less time on intensity than on getting the movements right. But eventually, you should focus on cranking it up . . . on stressing the body more and more. By adding weight or speed or by challenging your balance.

This has to get hard to work. Like life, I suppose. Annoying.

Don't Try to Do All of These from the Get-Go

S tart with the easier ones (marked with an asterisk). Having just said that you'll want to go hard eventually, may I say that that is a terrible idea at the beginning. This is a pretty serious strength-training regimen, and it is going to take a while to get comfortable with it. Hell, it's going to take a while to be able to do it at all. One suggestion is just to focus on the *relatively easy* ones first. Then work your way into the others. Start with the starred exercises. Stay with them for a week or two—whatever suits you. Feel your way. Even experienced trainers find some of these hard at first. Don't make yourself crazy. Last tip: Read these strength chapters over again, from time to time. *I* do and I wrote the damn things. Different points will matter to you, as you actually do the exercises. Same in aerobics, actually.

NUMBER 1

Squats*

Equipment Needed:
None, really, but a bench or chair would help.

Why Bother?
This superb exercise is splendid for strengthening your balance, your core, the big muscles in your legs (your quadriceps), and the support muscles that hold your hips in alignment. This is one of the basic movements in life. Do a lot of them.

Step 1:
With core tightened and back straight, squat down until your butt just touches the bench or chair, about eighteen inches off the ground. Flex hips and knees; hinge from hips. Shift slightly backward, as if sitting in a chair.

Step 2:
Stand up straight again, with opposite action. Do three sets of ten to twelve.

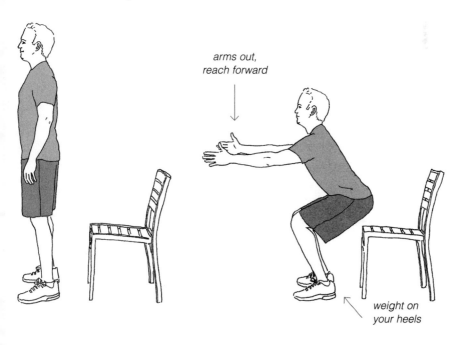

*arms out,
reach forward*

*weight on
your heels*

Do It Right:

When your spine starts to round or your knees wobble or your head pops forward, stop. *You have done it to failure.*

Too Difficult?

Don't go all the way down—just go as far as you comfortably can. You may go deeper, with good posture, if you can hang on to something. Wean yourself from it once you can do a good squat.

Too Easy?

Hold a ten-pound weight or kettlebell or medicine ball, in both hands, up under your chin, or hold dumbbells in both hands at your sides. Eventually, "go to failure" the old-fashioned way: Do as many reps as you can until you simply have to stop because your muscles hurt so. Typically, your posture will fail before your muscles do.

Bill Says:

Doing these right is difficult. Concentrate hard on doing them perfectly. Then add weight, not speed.

NUMBER 2

Split Squats*

Equipment Needed:
Same as Number 1.

Why Bother?
This version adds a touch of asymmetry and demands more balance. Billy thinks it is *the* great strength-training device. This is great for hip stability, loss of which leads to many ills. Ditto, of course, for balance.

Step 1:
Put one foot about eighteen inches ahead of the other. Stand with weight more or less evenly balanced. With the front leg, flex hips and knees; lower butt until your front thigh is parallel to the floor. With your back leg, flex it toward the floor.

Step 2:
Ascent: Drive upward with bias on front leg. Follow the same instructions regarding posture, making it easier or harder and so on.

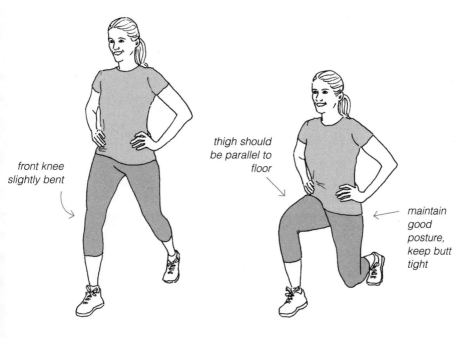

front knee slightly bent

thigh should be parallel to floor

maintain good posture, keep butt tight

STRENGTH TRAINING

NUMBER 3
Single Leg Squat

Equipment Needed:

None, unless you are a mere human, in which case you may need something to hang onto. The wall, the TRX Suspension Strap, whatever.

Billy admits that "top athletes struggle with this one." Few will be able to do an unaided, single leg squat for quite a while, if ever. But that's okay. The slightly-sissy version is also great for you.

Why Bother?

It leads to amazing hip stability and body weight control, *and ferrets out and corrects imbalance*. Being out of balance is serious, and masking it and compensating for it makes it worse. Asymmetrical exercises—especially extreme ones like this—correct weakness. No way to compensate for a bum hip when you're standing on one leg. Learn to do these. They are hard but wonderful for you.

Step 1:

Standing in front of a bench or chair, lift one foot slightly off the floor. Dip down, bending your knee and hip so that your butt moves back and descends as close as it can to the bench or chair. Note: Very few will be able to do more than a shallow squat. But the goal is the same.

Step 2:

Ascend as before.

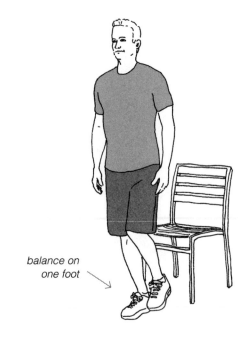

balance on
one foot

STRENGTH TRAINING

Do It Right:
The injunctions about the neutral spine and alignment are as stringent as before. Be extremely careful not to let your knee buckle inward toward the midline. Only do as much as you can do correctly.

Too Difficult?
Tap your raised foot on the floor, as needed. You can also do these near a wall with your hip descending and moving backward until it touches the wall, for support.

Too Easy?
If you think this is too easy, you have stumbled into the wrong book. But you can crank it up with weights.

Bill Says:
There is nothing like asymmetrical movement to improve hip stability, balance, coordination, and strength of the stressed leg and of the core.

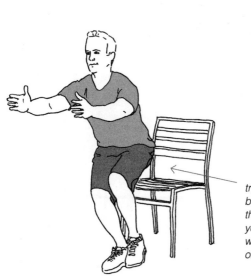

try to get your
butt as close to
the chair as
you can
without sitting
on it

STRENGTH TRAINING

NUMBER 4

The Lunge*

Equipment Needed:

None. (You may want to use the TRX Suspension Strap for balance in the early stages, maybe a pair of ski poles.)

Why Bother?

I personally think this is the single best exercise in the book. Great for hip stability, leg strength, core strength, and balance.

Step 1:

Stand with feet in fairly narrow stance, keeping a neutral spine and good alignment. On the descent, step forward approximately two feet (less if you are short) and drop body weight as in the squat. Goal: Keep the upper leg parallel to the floor. It may take a while. Do the best you can.

Step 2:

On ascent, drive up with hips and knees. Maintain neutral spine and upright (aligned) posture throughout. You can do *walking lunges*—lunge all around the gym, around the yard. Or you can lunge in place. Suit yourself.

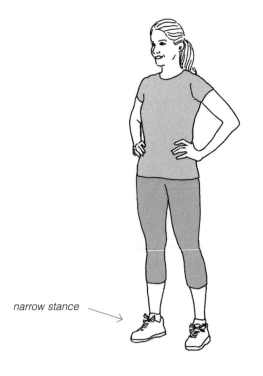

narrow stance

Do It Right:
It is of the essence in this exercise to maintain a neutral spine and good alignment. And to quit when you cannot maintain a neutral spine or your knees start to wobble or buckle. You have gone to failure; stop.

Too Difficult?
Don't drop down as deep. Use devices to steady yourself: a pair of ski poles, the TRX Suspension Strap, whatever.

Too Easy?
Add weights—either dumbbells in each hand or a single weight (dumb-bell or medicine ball) in both hands, held up to just under the chin.

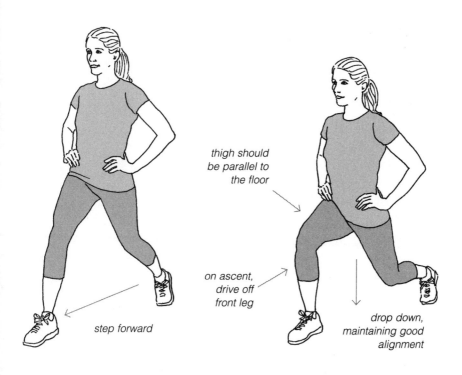

thigh should
be parallel to
the floor

on ascent,
drive off
front leg

step forward

drop down,
maintaining good
alignment

STRENGTH TRAINING

NUMBER 5

Lateral Lunges*

Equipment Needed:
Same as Lunge.

Why Bother?
This one has added benefits in terms of hip stability and unilateral leg strength, which you need all the time. Side-to-side movement is key.

Step 1:
Start with feet in a fairly narrow stance. Step to one side, as far as you comfortably can, shifting your body weight to that leg (a couple of feet is fine). Keep feet facing forward, not to the side. Hips will shift backward a bit during descent.

Step 2:
Push back up, primarily with the laterally placed leg, and stand back up in a narrow stance.

Do It Right:
As ever, it is critical to maintain neutral spine and good alignment.

Too Difficult?
Hang on to something, in the early stages. Do not drop as deep.

Too Easy?
Add weights, as in the regular lunge.

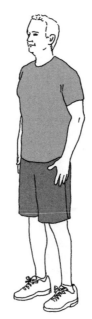

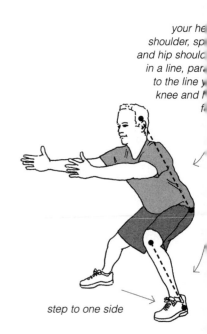

your he
shoulder, sp
and hip shoulc
in a line, par
to the line y
knee and I
f

step to one side

NUMBER 6

Pulldowns*
(with Machine)

Equipment Needed:
For this, you mostly need a machine; a tube will work.

Why Bother?
This one helps to strengthen your shoulder girdle muscles and enhances your back stabilization. I tell Bill that I don't like these and I don't care if my upper body goes to hell. He says that's stupid. It is.

Step 1:
Set weights at a light level. Feel your way toward a level where doing ten to twelve reps is demanding—impossible, in fact, on the third set. Sit down at the machine, seize bar, with palms facing away, hands shoulder-width apart (arms fully extended over head). *Slowly* depress your shoulder blades and pull the bar down all the way to chest.
(Variations: wider or narrower grip; palms facing inward; this may be easier if you have a history of shoulder problems.)

Step 2:
Slowly return bar, till arms stretched fully, overhead—*controlled* movement all the way. *Reach* at the top of the range. This is a range-of-motion improvement exercise.

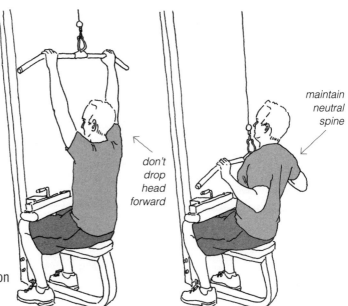

don't drop head forward

maintain neutral spine

NUMBER 7

One-Armed Dumbbell Row*

Equipment Needed:

It's a great help if you have a gym bench for this one, but any chair or bench will do, plus a set of dumbbells, suitable for you.

Why Bother?

This one improves your one-arm pulling strength, enhances the strength of your shoulder girdle, improves your core *stabilization* and strength, and teaches you to control rotational strength of your body.

Strive to create a balanced body. Unbalanced exercises like this one help.

Step 1:

Kneel, with one knee on a bench and the other foot on the floor. Lean down to grasp dumbbell.

Do It Right:

Maintain a neutral spine throughout the movement. Keep shoulder girdle depressed (don't hunch).

Step 2:

With extended arm grasping the dumbbell, pull shoulder girdle back, then drive elbow toward the ceiling. Pull dumbbell upward, just above the hip.

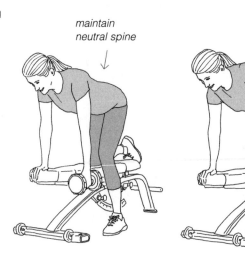

maintain neutral spine

keep elbow close to body

NUMBER 8

One-Armed Cable Row* (Cable Machine)

Why Bother?

The cable row machine is one of the best in the gym because of two things: the *angle* of the pull and the ability to increase or decrease weights easily. And you can move through a fuller range. (Tube works.)

Cross-Linkage:

The body is naturally "cross-linked" to facilitate movement across the body, lower right to upper left and vice versa. Think golf swings, tennis strokes, slap shots in hockey—all kinds of rotational movements. You need strength on the opposite ends of your body, but especially at the core.

Step 1:

Set cable machine with grip close to the floor. Start with a light weight and feel your way. With one leg forward in split squat, grasp handle with the opposite hand; if your left foot is forward, use your right arm. Depress right shoulder girdle and pull the handle to your side in a single-arm rowing fashion. Pull until hand is just above right hip.

Step 2:

Slowly return to starting position. Use controlled movement.

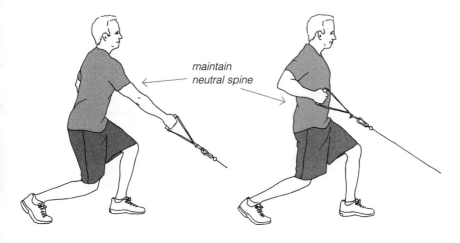

maintain
neutral spine

NUMBER 9

Chest Press (Bench)*

Equipment Needed:

A padded gym bench is great but any bench will do.

Why Bother?

This one enhances your shoulder girdle and your core. There comes a time in life when you have to *push back*! This helps.

Step 1:

This is, in effect, a push-up off a bench. Lean over the bench, arms on bench fully extended and your body rigid. The more vertically you stand, the easier it is to do. Slowly lower yourself until upper body almost touches bench.

Step 2:

Push up until arms are straight again.

Do It Right:

Doing this one (or the full push-up alternative) incorrectly is particularly deadly. The fact that you used to be able to do a hundred of these on your thumbs does not matter today. Do 'em right or don't do 'em at all.

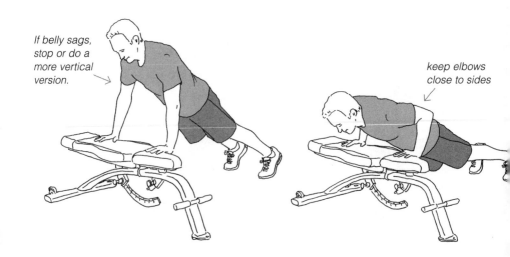

If belly sags, stop or do a more vertical version.

keep elbows close to sides

NUMBER 10

Single-Arm Dumbbell Press*

Equipment Needed:

A padded, exercise bench is more or less indispensable for this one. You can probably cobble one up at home—a regular bench with some padding. And dumbbells.

Why Bother?

This one enhances your "push strength" and core strength and enhances your shoulder girdle stabilization. Also good for your "lats," the big muscles that run down your back in a pleasing "V." The unbalanced feature does the usual, wonderful things.

Step 1:

Lie on your back on a padded bench, feet spread wide on the floor. (You may need a box or other "lift" so low back does not overarch.) Hold dumbbell in one hand, slightly away from your body, at shoulder height.

Step 2:

Engage abdominals, depress shoulder girdle. Push or drive dumbbell upward, straight over the shoulder toward the ceiling.

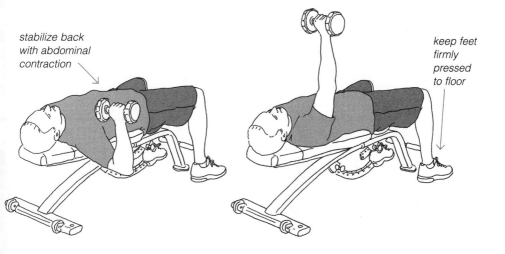

stabilize back
with abdominal
contraction

keep feet
firmly
pressed
to floor

NUMBER 11

Single-Arm Cable Press*

Equipment Needed:
Cable press machine. Note: You can do a version of this with an elastic tube.

Why Bother:
This one has a bit more of the *cross-linkage* than the dumbbell press. It is great for shoulder, hip, and core stabilization, and trains rotational movement.

Step 1:
Anchor cable at height midway between waist and shoulders. Stand in split-squat position (see Number 2), facing away from the machine. Load the machine appropriately (start light, as always).

Step 2:
The movement is like throwing a punch. If the right leg is forward, take the cable in your left hand (back) at shoulder height. Push or punch forward with the left arm in a horizontal path and shift your weight onto the front foot. Return to starting position by bending your elbow, bringing your hand back to shoulder height.

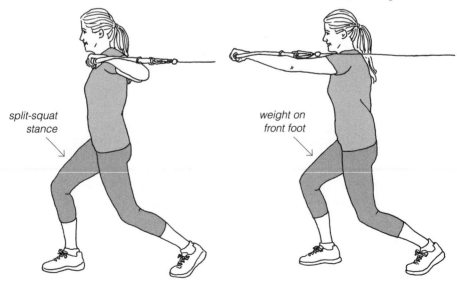

split-squat
stance

weight on
front foot

NUMBER 12

Split-Squat Overhead Press

Equipment Needed:

Dumbbell or other weight.

Why Bother?

It's great for the core.

Step 1:

Assume the descent position of the split squat (see Number 2), with hip and knee bent, while holding a dumbbell at shoulder height. If right leg is forward, dumbbell is in opposite (left) hand.

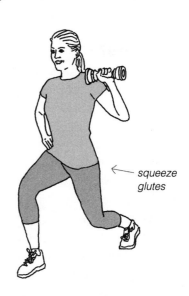

← squeeze glutes

Step 2:

Stay in the split-squat position while thrusting dumbbell straight over head. (A little upward thrust from the legs to create momentum is fine.)

Step 3:

Return dumbbell to shoulder.

Do It Right:

This, like all asymmetrical exercises, is designed to throw you off balance. Don't let it.

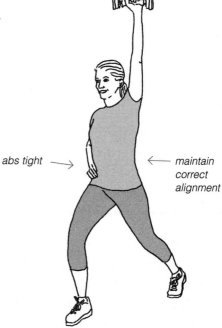

abs tight ——→

← maintain correct alignment

NUMBER 13

Rotation/Chop with Medicine Ball

Why Bother?

This is one of my favorites. If you worry about the shrinking *glass box*, this is a great exercise for you.

Step 1:
Start with a light (for you) medicine ball or no weight at all. Stand with your feet shoulder-width apart or slightly wider. Hold the medicine ball out in front of the body, arms slightly bent. Engage the abdominals. Begin squat position, moving down and to the right, bringing the ball around to the right. Squat and lower ball as close as you can get to the floor, *without losing the neutral spine.* You may not be able to get much past your knees when you start. *Your body must move as a unit, facing the ball as you swing it to your*

right or left. Rotate your hips, not your lower back. Your belly button follows the ball!

Step 2:
Slowly swing the ball up to your waist and, without pausing, straight around to the left and over your shoulder, as high as you can reach. The ball basically follows a diagonal path, moving from outside your right foot to over your left shoulder or vice versa. *Rotate your hips, not your lower back. Your belly button follows the ball, same as on the way down.* Return to starting position.

Do It Right:

More than almost any exercise in the book, do this one right or do *not* do it at all. You can get hurt if you do this wrong. The great trick is to *rotate with your hips, not your back. This is one of the fundamental lessons of this book. Rotate with your hips, not your lower back. And maintain a neutral spine throughout.*

Too Difficult?

Use less or no weight. Do not go as deep. Most of you will not be able to put the ball all the way down to the floor without losing the neutral spine. Don't! Feel your way. If you're never able to put the ball all the way to the floor, fine. It's still a superb exercise, as long as you are reaching. Feel your way.

Too Easy?

Add weight, go deeper (touch the ball to the floor) but only if you can do it with a neutral spine.

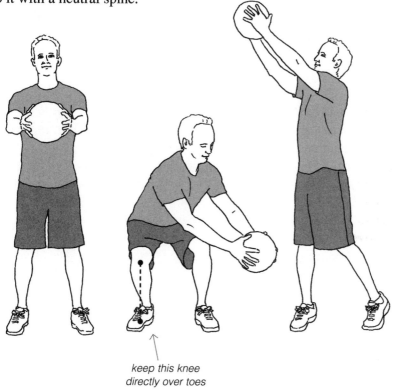

keep this knee
directly over toes

Bill Says:

Feel your way with this one for a long time, starting with no weight and focusing heavily on rotating your hips, following the ball (or your hands) with your belly button. Learn to move instinctively in this manner, and you will have done yourself a profound favor for life.

STRENGTH TRAINING

NUMBER 14

Rotation/Chop with Cable Machine

Equipment Needed:
Cable machine (or tube, in a pinch).

Why Bother?
This is a variation of the medicine ball chop, obviously, but the *force or resistance* is applied at an angle directly through the rotational arc of movement. This is what's neat about the cable machine.

Step 1:
Set machine with light weight; set base near the floor. Stand sideways to the machine with handle in both hands, your body (your whole body) turned toward the machine. Drop as deeply toward the anchor point of the cable as you can without losing your neutral spine. Have belly button follow hands, same as with medicine ball.

Step 2:
Raise handle up to waist, then—in a single continuous movement—raise handle up to your left and over your opposite shoulder, as high as you can reach. Maintain neutral spine. Have belly button follow your hands.

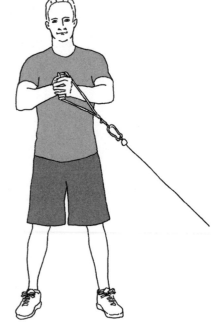

Too Difficult?

Use less (or no) weight. Do not go down as deep.

Too Easy?

Add weight.

Bill Says:

It takes a while to get used to this movement. Don't worry about weight until you really have it down. And never *go deeper on the down swing than you can go with a truly neutral spine or you can get badly hurt.*

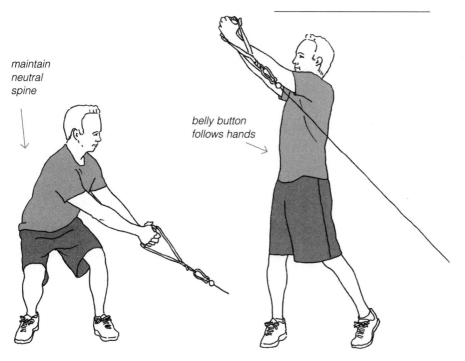

maintain
neutral
spine

belly button
follows hands

STRENGTH TRAINING

NUMBER 15

Squat Single-Arm Overhead Press

Equipment Needed:
Dumbbells.

Why Bother?
This one is all about the critical **transfer of force**—from the legs to the arms, from the lower to the upper body. It seems easy and obvious, which it is: It is what you were built for. But it helps develop the core (in rotation) and your unilateral (one-armed) coordination.

Step 1:
Start with feet shoulder-width (or slightly farther) apart, holding dumbbells (one in each hand) at shoulder level, palms facing forward. Descend into squat position while maintaining neutral spine, knees in close alignment with toes.

Step 2:
Once you reach the low point of your squat, forcefully ascend back upward. As momentum builds, drive one arm (holding the dumbbell) directly over your head. Finish by returning arm and dumbbell to shoulder level.

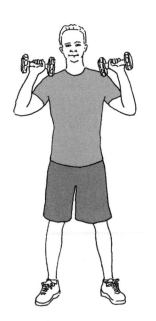
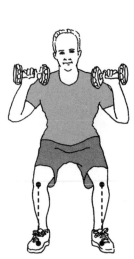

*knees aligned
with toes*

Step 3:
Repeat squat sequence again, but this time, on ascent, drive the opposite arm toward the ceiling. Finish by returning arm to shoulder in standing position. Repeat this sequence, alternating left and right arm thrust over head.

Too Easy/Difficult?
Adjust weights.

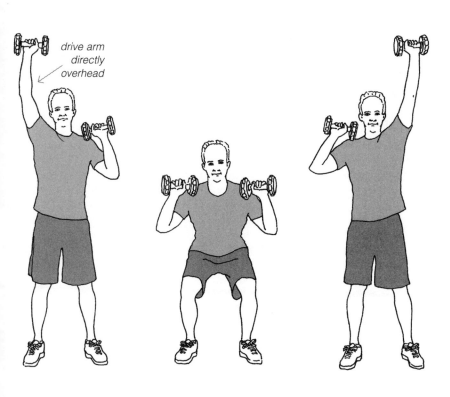

drive arm
directly
overhead

NUMBER 16

Back Step Lunge Row

Equipment Needed:
Cable machine or elastic tube.

Why Bother?
This is real whole-body stuff. Once you learn how, you'll enjoy it.

Step 1:
Set cable with anchor near floor, using modest weight. Stand in split squat facing machine. Place your left foot forward, take cable handle in right hand, fully extended toward the machine.

Step 2:
Begin by stepping forward with your back (in this case, the right) foot. Do the step by driving upward with the front or right leg. Simultaneously, as you lift your body upward, pull your right arm toward your side, just above the hip. Finish standing in a narrow stance, with your right arm by your side, in a "row" position, shoulders back and elbow bent.

Step 3:
Return to the start position by reaching forward with the right arm as you lunge back with your right foot, resuming the original split-squat position. Repeat on other side.

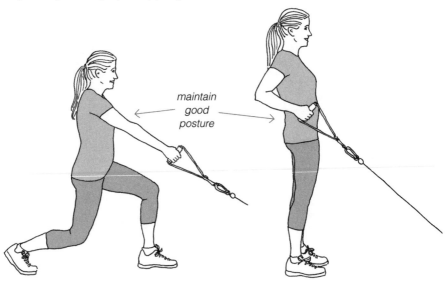

maintain good posture

NUMBER 17

Squat, Arm Curl

Equipment Needed:
Dumbbells.

Why Bother?
What Bill has done here is to combine the arm curl, sometimes called the "bicep curl" with a squat to get us all away from the temptation to do this the old-fashioned way: by muscle isolation.

Step 1:
Stand with feet shoulder-width apart, holding a pair of dumbbells down at sides. Descend into a squat with arms extended, dumbbells in hands, moving toward the floor. Palms can be facing forward or inward, whichever is more comfortable. As you rise out of the squat position, curl your arms (from your elbows) so the dumbbells move toward your shoulders. It is okay to use some momentum to swing the weights a bit on this one. But do not let your body buckle from side to side or get out of neutral alignment.

Step 2:
Slowly return weights to your sides.

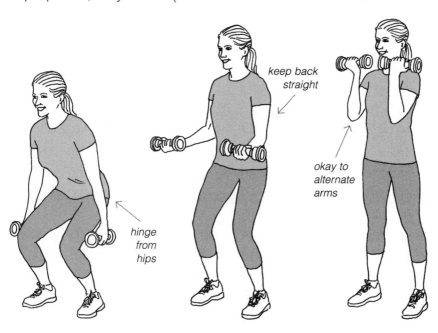

keep back
straight

hinge
from
hips

okay to
alternate
arms

STRENGTH TRAINING

NUMBER 18

Bend, Pull, Overhead Press

Equipment Needed:
Dumbbells.

Why Bother?
This is a basic lift. We pick stuff up off the floor, raise it to counter or waist height. Or raise it to an upper shelf, over our heads.

Step 1:
Bend over and grab two dumbbells off the floor. Remember to hinge from your hips and maintain a neutral spine. The movement of bending over is less of a squat and more of a bend from the hips. Your knees can bend slightly, but the object is to keep them straighter. If you have very tight hamstrings, you may not be able to reach all the way to the floor without rounding your back. In which case, place the dumbbells on a box or something so you do not have to bend over as far.

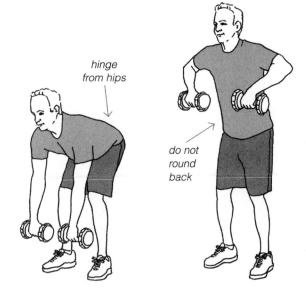

hinge
from hips

do not
round
back

STRENGTH TRAINING

Step 2:
Straighten yourself back up while lifting the dumbbells off the floor. Be careful not to round your lower back. Simultaneously pull the dumbbells upward to shoulder height. Without pausing—and using the momentum already created—push the dumbbells directly over your head.

Step 3:
Return the dumbbells to shoulder height; then bend over and reach down with arms until the dumbbells touch the floor again. Repeat the entire sequence.

use momentum to push dumbbells directly overhead

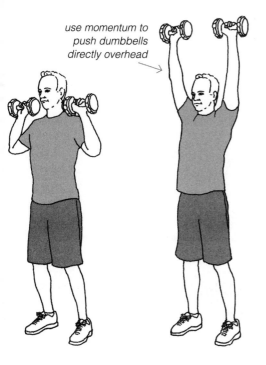

Bill Says:
This reads harder than it is. Look at the pictures, and try it a few times. Not bad.

STRENGTH TRAINING

NUMBER 19

"I's" and "T's" with Dumbbells*

Equipment Needed:
Dumbbells, a padded bench to lie on.

Why Bother?
These are great for your shoulder girdle, mid- and low-back stabilization, and strengthening your rotator cuff. Similar to the warm-up but much harder.

Step 1:
Lie on your stomach on a padded bench, head and chest just slightly off the bench. Hold light dumbbells in both hands. For the "I's," lie with your arms at your sides and palms down. For the "T's," lie with your thumbs up and your arms out to the sides.

Step 2:
Gently lift chest slightly off the bench, extending from the mid back, shoulders depressed (not hunched). Do not arch from the low back. Lift both arms (from the floor) to just higher than parallel with your body. Hold for three seconds. Return to start.

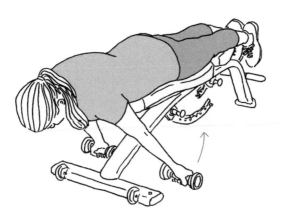

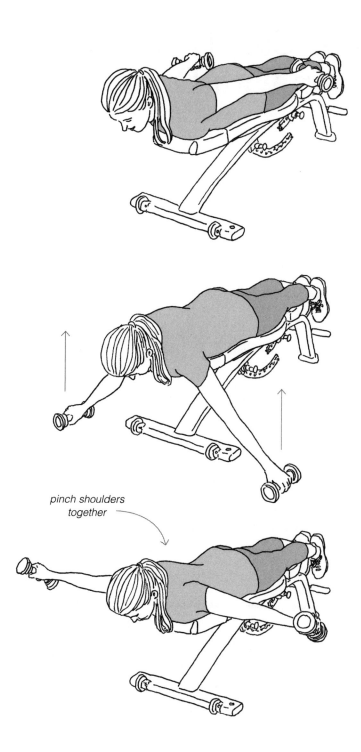

pinch shoulders together

STRENGTH TRAINING

NUMBER 20

Rotator Cuff External Rotation with Dumbbell*

Equipment Needed:
Dumbbells, pad.

Why Bother?
This one is a beauty to build rotator cuff strength and enhance shoulder girdle stability.

Step 1:
Lie on side with hands as shown, left or weighted elbow at ninety-degree angle, forearm across body. Grasp weight (start very light) and very slowly raise toward ceiling.

Step 2:
Lower weight to starting position, slowly, over a four or five count. This is very important to build strength. Repeat.

Make It Harder/Easier:
In time, try to add resistance and lower the reps until you are only able to do, say, eight reps.

slow, controlled movement in both directions

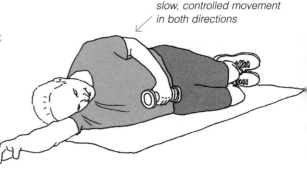

tension should be felt in upper shoulder

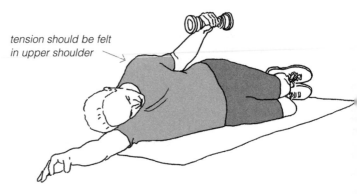

NUMBER 21

Hip Extension Lift*

Equipment Needed:
Pad. Chair or Swiss ball to rest your heels on. Or, for the very advanced, use the stirrups of a TRX Suspension Trainer.

Why Bother?
Most of us, after forty or fifty, lose hip extension strength because we spend so much time in a "flexed" position. That is, sitting at a desk. This exercise is a must for those with atrophied glutes (which is a nice way of saying "sagging butt.")

Step 1:
Lie on your back with your knees at a ninety-degree angle, heels on a chair or Swiss ball. Engage your glutes and abs. Drive your heels down on the bench or ball—keeping your feet flexed—and lift your butt off the floor. Hold for three seconds. Return.

Make It Easier:
Use a lower bench or simply don't lift your butt as high. Feel your way.

Make It Harder:
Hold for five seconds. Use TRX Suspension Trainer stirrups (to add balance component).

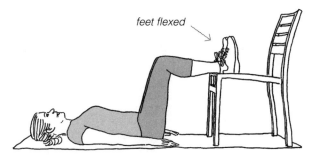

feet flexed

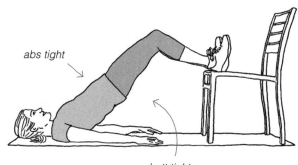

abs tight

butt tight

STRENGTH TRAINING

NUMBER 22

Plank*

Equipment Needed:
Pad.

Why Bother?
This one enhances hip, shoulder, and core stabilization, especially the core. Better and much safer than doing conventional sit-ups.

Step 1:
Lie on your stomach, up on your elbows. Engage your glutes and abs. Depress your shoulders. Lift butt and knees off the floor. Keep back and hips level (stiff). Hold for ten seconds. Only do three of these to start and focus on maintaining the contraction of the core muscles. It is much harder and more effective that way.

Make It Easier/Harder:
Try fewer reps and a shorter hold. Or if you are really struggling, don't lift your knees off the floor.

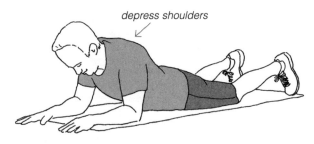

depress shoulders

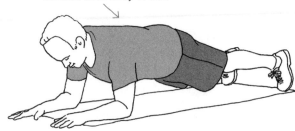

don't let back sway or bow

NUMBER 23

Side Plank

Equipment Needed:
Pad.

Why Bother?
This enhances lateral hip and core stability. Worth having, especially if you have knee or low back problems.

Step 1:
Lie on your side, up on one elbow. Engage your abs and glutes. Lift hip and knees off the mat. Hold for ten seconds. Repeat only three times.

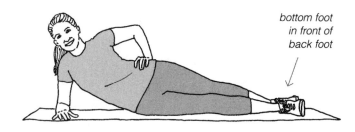

bottom foot in front of back foot

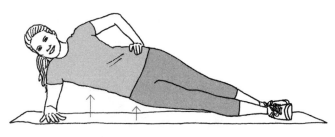

engage core, lift hips and knees off floor

NUMBER 24

Crunch*

Equipment Needed:
Pad.

Why Bother?
This is the safe version of the old military sit-up or full sit-up, which is not safe. Great for building abs.

Step 1:
Lie on your back with one knee bent, one hand behind the head, supporting neck. Lift shoulders slightly off the floor (about four inches) without flexing neck. Hold for three to five seconds. Relax. Do three sets of ten reps.

Do It Right:
Do not lift all the way up. Lift your shoulders slightly off the floor and hold for three to five seconds, then slowly return to the floor. The full power crunches of yesteryear were dangerous for your back.

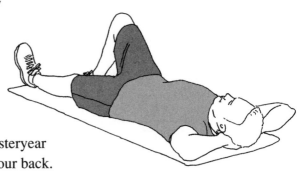

Bill Says:
Do not *do sit-ups with a twist. The twist comes from the lower back, just what you do* not *want. The only safe sit-up is a shallow one, like this.*

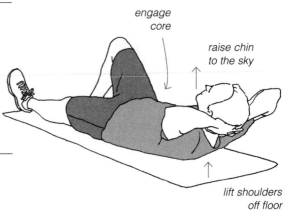

engage
core

raise chin
to the sky

lift shoulders
off floor

NUMBER 25

TRX Rip Trainer "Drag"*

Equipment Needed:
We show this with the TRX Rip Trainer but you could do it as easily with a cable machine (anchored at waist height) or rubber tubing.

Why Bother?
This looks too easy to bother with but it's not. In fact, it is a nice, stable way to exercise your whole body, one last time for the day. It particularly enhances mid- and low-back strength, endurance, and core stabilization.

Step 1:
Stand, facing anchor point (anchor at mid-level), holding TRX Rip Trainer bar in both hands, knees slightly bent, arms straight out, some tension on the bar.

Step 2:
Depress shoulder blades and pull back bar until it touches your chest. Hold for thirty seconds (up to a minute). Repeat with cord on opposite side. To make it more serious, step back farther and increase the tension.

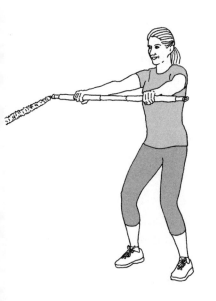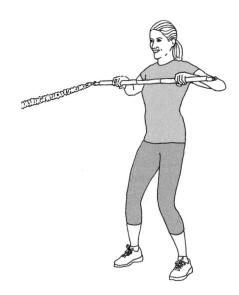

The Weight Loss Side of Strength Training

A broad tip: We talk about aerobics as the great exercise for weight loss (and they are terrific), but Bill points out that the very best way to lose weight may be to do whole-body strength exercises with a focus on resistance, some speed, and short rest periods. DO BOTH. Think about it: Nothing engages *more muscles* than compound weight exercise. The more muscles you engage, the more mitochondria you use, the more *burn*. Bill, who is not exactly a little fat piggy, says he occasionally puts on a few extra pounds, and his *standard cure* is to hit it, pretty hard, on strength-training exercise. "Pretty hard" means with enough weight to make it a real challenge, with a short (thirty-second) pause between sets, and doing some sets (only the ones that lend themselves to it) at speed. Obviously he is right: more muscle, more burn, more weight loss. And he has proven it, with himself and others. It is not a cinch, but it surely will work.

Bear in mind you must have these exercises down pat before you either add weight or go fast. But once you reach that point, you have a wonderful resource for weight loss. Give it a shot.

Another good tip: The point of modern strength training is to build strength and balance and coordination and the ability to do compound movements correctly. But a major part of it is strength, building muscle mass. To do that, you eventually have to *stress* the muscles. Take all the time in the world to learn to do these right; that is of the essence. But when you really have them down, begin to add stress. The two basic ways to do it: Add weight and, where appropriate, add speed. And cut down the rests between sets. Do not do this at the expense of technique and sound posture, ever. But the day will eventually come when you can really do this stuff. *Then* feel free to add some stress. If you are still carrying some extra pounds, they will *fly* off.

This is the weight counterpart to doing intervals in aerobics. More *intense* exercise does all the good things better. Listen, if you are doing this stuff at all, you are a great American. But if ever there comes a time when you want to do more—once you really know how to do them and are in good shape—go for it. You'll get cuter faster.

The Rhythm of These Sessions

These sessions are designed to have a certain rhythm. Not on day 1 or even day 20, when you're still feeling your way. But in time. For example, the warm-ups are intended to build a little, over their course. By the end—certainly by the time of the fast footwork segment—you want to be *going for it* some.

Same pattern, in a way, with the substantive exercises. They're all comparatively hard; they can all have you breathing hard, depending on how you do them. But they too are designed to *build*, over the course of the workout. Begin to work pretty hard when you begin with the squats. Be working hard by the time you get to the lunges. Build a little during the latter pull-and-push segment. And really go for it some in the rotational exercises and, especially, the compound exercises. The latter really lend themselves to a vigorous workout, with more resistance, less rest, and more weight. Only go to failure (quit when you aren't doing them right, every time)! But over time, you can build to quite the little workout on these babies.

Then taper off as you get into the special-purpose exercises: the weighted I's and T's, the planks and the crunches. Take it down. But toy with that rhythm as you really get into all this. Makes it more fun. And burns a *ton of calories* while it is doing all the magic of strength training.

What About Static Stretching?

A lot of you were trained to do some pretty serious static stretching over the years, and I often get questions about it on the road: Where did stretching go? The short answer, from Bill, is that old-fashioned static stretches—with a thirty- to ninety-second hold, like the good old *runners' calf stretch*—are not done as much anymore because there are other options. Dynamic stretches, like the ones in our warm-up, are more effective. Watch a ski race today, and you'll see the skier kicking his or her legs vigorously back and forth and from side to side, dramatically. Same for runners, same for everyone. Dynamic stretching is the modern model.

Having said that, static stretches still have a place, especially where a joint or muscle group has gotten proportionally tight on one side. For example, I have one bum (limited mobility) hip, and, sure enough, Bill has given me some static stretches to help restore its equilibrium. If you are going to do static stretches—for special situations like mine— it's best to do them *after* your workout. Or, if you're really stiff in a particular spot, do a static stretch before *and* after, but integrate it into the relevant dynamic stretches. That way you minimize the principle negative of the static stretch: a certain weakening of muscle tone in the immediate aftermath of the stretch.

The warm-up exercises in this book are primarily dynamic. That is, you move in and out of the stretch over several repetitions rather than holding it statically for too long. Think of the heel extensions, the straight leg raises, and so on—constant movement to lengthen the tissue, repetition after repetition. They are great for joint mobility, coordination, muscle activation, and signaling. And they do not undermine muscle tone, the way static stretches do.

Okay: You're done. Nice work. Do those exercises (or some of them) two or three times a week, and you will be amazing looking in a few months. And as for good health, energy, optimism, and ferociously healthy internal signaling? You cannot imagine. But you'll feel it soon enough, and then for the rest of your life.

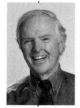

CHAPTER TWENTY-FOUR

The Third Element in the Third Act: General Grant, Scott Fitzgerald, and the Need to "Care, Connect, and Commit"

ff There are no second acts in American life." That's Scott Fitzgerald talking, perhaps the greatest American novelist and one of his most famous lines. Famous, perhaps, because it has such resonance. It scares the hell out of all of us because it just may be true in this youth-crazed society. And if there are no second acts, what are our chances of a third act? One dreads to think.

The good news, I think, is irrefutable: Fitzgerald was right about himself but wrong about America. Certainly wrong about America today. Fitzgerald, an alcoholic and a fast burner, was pretty much done in his late thirties, dead and mostly ignored at forty-two, after being such a *rocket* as a young man. Scary.

I am crazy about Fitzgerald, but may I gently suggest that you forget about him for a moment and think about a man who was more *right* about America, all the way through. Think for a minute about Ulysses S. Grant, of all people.

In Fitzgerald's last completed novel, *Tender Is the Night*, the rich and beautiful Nicole talks about her ex-husband, who is now living in bleak obscurity, a doctor in a tiny town in upstate New York. *She* has moved on with her glittering life and turned her back on him. But she thinks of him sometimes, with a careless rich girl's affection. He is not doomed, she says, he is just waiting, like Grant waiting in Galena. Such a wonderful image.

Do you know the story? Probably not, but everyone knew it when Fitzgerald was a kid. One of the great stories in American life: Grant, waiting in Galena.

After West Point, Grant was a bit of a star in the Mexican War. But he was less good in peacetime, and he drank a fair amount. He was washed up by the late 1850s. He had tried various things, most recently had been an unsuccessful storekeeper. And now he was living off the charity of his in-laws and selling firewood on a street corner in Galena, Illinois. A fellow officer (I think it was Longstreet) saw him, in his shabby army coat, on a corner with the firewood at his side, mumbled an embarrassed greeting, and hurried on.

Then came the war, of course, and Grant was reluctantly given a modest command. Anyone with any military training was in demand, even Grant. He was distrusted and kept under close watch by lesser men. But slowly his gifts as a stunningly bold strategist and a fierce decision maker became clear. And he *seized* these utterly unexpected victories. At Forts Donelson and Henry, on the Ohio. Then Vicksburg on the Mississippi. And finally Lincoln, ignoring the advice of steadier men, put him in charge of all the Union armies. And he simply won the war. Became president. One of my great heroes, I confess, and a much better man than early histories suggest.

But now think of this: After two terms as one of the best loved presidents, he lost everything to a crooked financier who had lured him into a partnership, to use his name. The Bernie Madoff of the day. Grant lost absolutely everything; he was stone broke *all over again.* Only now he was dying of mouth cancer, from all the cigars he had smoked, maybe the booze. He had no pension and he was sick with worry about his wife, Julia, whom he adored.

With extraordinary courage and in the face of terrible pain, he sat down in the last months of his life—this simple *soldier*, you know, doing something entirely new—and wrote one of the best books that would ever be written about the Civil War. One of the best histories by a commanding general since Caesar's *Commentaries on the Gallic War.* His friend Mark Twain published it for him on generous terms. But the book sold itself. And the dying Grant made a fortune for Julia, about whom he had worried so much. Gotta love Ulysses S. Grant, man. A great American. And a stunning Third Act. Grant believed in American possibility the way you and I should believe in American possibility: with all his heart and all the way out.

And here is the obvious point: Those of us who were forty or fifty at the beginning of *this* millennium had better take Grant as our model, not Fitzgerald. Because we are going to live for a long, long time. And if there are no second acts, this is going to be a long dull play. And there may not be enough to eat.

It is not Grant's *success* that I, at least, admire so much; it is the fact that he just kept on going. Always. Did new stuff without regard to his age or the string of careers behind him. There are photos of him in his final days, with a goofy little cap on his head. He does not look great. But here's the thing: He is sitting there, a few days from death, working over the proofs. Still *at it*, all the way.

That was his gift as a general, by the way: Where others were shocked by losses and broke off engagements, Grant just kept on going. Pretty hard, too. There's a wonderful story about him after the Battle of the Wilderness, shortly after he took command of the often defeated Army of the Potomac. The Union Army had taken a terrible pounding, and the veterans assumed they would retreat, as they had so many times before, over this same ground. And the next morning as they were packing up and getting ready, there came Grant, with a handful of officers. Quietly riding south.

The soldiers could not believe their eyes and broke into spontaneous cheers. It was the turning point of the war. Ulysses S. Grant, my friends: Think about him sometimes when things get ugly in the Third Act, as they are bound to do. Get back on your horse if you possibly can. Ride south.

All right, you have created this terrific *you.* What the hell are you going to do? I mean actually *do.* What's your job? How do you *use* all that energy and fitness and charm? I don't know. That's not my job. But I do think about it and talk about it with people of your generation all the time. And I do have a couple of thoughts that may interest you. May orient you, I should say.

The Limbic Brain

et's start someplace odd. Let's start with your limbic, or emotional, brain. Because—I boldly submit—the limbic brain is going to be terribly important in the Third Act. It always was, but now, more than ever. Because of the growing risk of isolation, of getting separated from the pack, which has deadly consequences for mammals like you and me.

I mentioned this in the first chapter, and now we're back. We have three separate brains, all beauties but very different. The ancient or reptilian brain is the smallest and sits at the top of your spinal column and regulates all movement. Lets your heart beat, your lungs breathe, lets you walk, go off the high board. It sits down there in darkness and lets us do all the graceful, coordinated things we do.

Next in time came the limbic, mammalian or emotional brain. Only mammals (like us) have it, and it was our *great* edge in the Darwinian crucible of survival. It let us mammals *care* about one another. The limbic brain is primarily concerned with conveying and receiving emotions. It induced us to care more about and spend more time raising our young. Best of all, it let us cooperate and work together in herds and packs and law firms. Wonderful.

Finally, there was the *human* or *thinking* brain. That's the big three-pounder that sits on top of the other two and lets us think and write constitutions and symphonies and health books. We tend to think that it is the all-important brain, which it is in a way. It makes us human. And that the others don't matter much. But that last part is a deeply mistaken view. The three brains are exquisitely, endlessly wired together, so that every single thing we do, think, smell, or feel has a profound emotional or limbic marker or spin on it. There is good reason to believe that the limbic brain controls far more decisions in life than the thinking brain. Think about it this way: We can consciously focus on about forty incoming stimuli in our thinking mind. But we simultaneously receive several *million other stimuli* that only the limbic and reptilian brains gather, especially the limbic brain.

Because of the limbic brain, we are hardwired to be connected. We are *built* for it. There is a terrible risk of isolation, with retirement and failing energy and so on, in the Third Act, and one of your primary goals should be to stay involved. To connect to and care about others. We are not just talking about enriching or ennobling your lives, which will happen. We are talking about not getting sick and falling to pieces. The *great* machine you have—built with solid exercise and brilliant nutrition—will fall apart in isolation. The wheels will come off. Exercise *stimulates* your appetite for and gift for limbic involvement and commitment, but you have to make it your conscious focus, too. It makes a huge difference.

When you had a regular job—whether you loved it or hated it— you lived in a *limbic stew*. There were people all over who cared what you were doing, what you thought, and where you were. You were part of the *pack* and that was very, very good. Huge numbers of stimuli for a limbic brain, which hungers for them. More and more of us work alone these days, but the generalization is still true: While you have a regular job, you are in the limbic stew. Some days you may get sick of it, but you are connecting in ways you were designed to do. In retirement all that goes away, and you have to think differently.

Orienting Idea: Relationships Trump Jobs

When you were younger, the great priority was *the job* and getting ahead. Succeeding. Everything was subordinated to that for most of us. It was nice to see the spouse, you loved the time with the kids and the dog and the garden. But frankly, they all ranked lower in your priorities, most of you, than the job and success. *Relationships were secondary.* They were often seen in the context of the job. This or that woman or man was important to my work, to my climb up the dear old ladder, *which was everything.* Others were not and they did not matter. Relationships as relationships were secondary.

In this next part of the play—when you have already had most of the success you're going to have and when your *limbic* connectedness is threatened—*relationships are going to be primary.* Relationships are going to define the good life. And what you actually *do* for a living or to fill your day is going to be secondary.

Here are a couple of quick stories about how you *see people*. My pal David Bliss talks about the electrician who is helping redo his house. Good guy and whatnot, but—in David's old life, where his job dominated everything—he would have been more or less invisible. The electrician was not part of David's world so he *did not matter*. Nasty, maybe, but true. That's just how it goes. But after *Younger* and in semi-retirement, David suddenly saw the connection in a different way. Relationships come first now, he had already decided, in his analytical, intellectual way. And he noticed that the electrician was a hell of a guy. And that they had a lot of interests in common: exercise, biking, the outdoors. So he recruited him as a serious friend. They have become important pals.

Walter, the Homicide Cop

In the same vein, I met an oddly charming guy in a sports equipment store a few years ago. He was selling me weight lifting gear, but we got talking. It was clear in a heartbeat that he had a ton of charm and was great fun. He was a former Boston homicide detective, of all things, a star in that field and a great storyteller. He had a hellish commute and was living most of the week in some hotel. This is a little odd sounding, but we have a lot of space in our house, and I suggested that he might train me some in our gym, and spend a night or two a week at our house. Which he did. Never trained me, as it turned out, but he spent a lot of time at the house and we became close friends. It would not have occurred to either of us in our old lives. But it's different now, when relationships dominate—and they can come from any direction. And they matter like crazy. Default to connect. Walter's a joy.

Wetting the Felt . . . Being *You*

When I retired, young, from my law firm, a brilliant young acquaintance—a guy I wasn't that close to but someone I admired and who apparently liked me—gave me some advice. It was odd: He was an associate and I was the partner, but he sat me down and gave me this advice as if our roles were reversed.

"Felt," he began, mysteriously, "is wonderful material. You can crumple it, stomp it, leave it folded and twisted for years. And—if you soak it thoroughly and *let it sit* for a week or so—it will resume its original shape." Uh-huh. Where's this going?

"We are like felt," he said. "We can regain our original shape. Your long life as a lawyer in a firm like this, twists and turns and changes you as you adapt to their ways. So, as you retire, it makes sense to sit and do nothing for a while, six months, say. While you recover from all those adaptations and regain *your own shape*. Like an old felt hat."

And when he was finished with his little lecture he just sat for a minute, obviously thinking, while I waited for more. "Come to think of it," he said, "that's all wrong for you. You were one of the lucky ones. You never *did* adapt your shape to suit the firm or the expectations. Unlike [a prominent partner] who is such a chameleon, you stayed exactly the same, all the way through. So forget what I said. You do not need to regain your shape." I tell the last part of the story because, in my bottomless vanity, I like it so much. But the generalization is true. Most of us adapt *plenty* to become this or that in the corporation or whatever. And we need to regain our true shape.

And one of the solid joys of the Third Act should surely be that that bullshit is over. One of the *great premiums* of the Third Act is that you can be utterly yourself. Your best self, one hopes, but yourself. David Bliss tells me that he counseled a lot of top CEOs about retirement. One of his best lines was to tell them that, in this part of the story, *the part of you will be played by you. Your own true self.* And that— despite all the loss of perks and limos and flatterers—may be the most satisfying part you'll ever play. I too have seen a lot of wildly success- ful men move into retirement and, mostly, they don't do well. Because they have gotten so very far from their true selves that there are only dumb "learned" parts to play. Parts no one wants to watch anymore. Felt, kids. We are like felt. Go soak yourselves; then sit for a while. Resume your true shape. Not bad.

This is a variation on a point we make elsewhere: One of the great pleasures of the Third Act is that the part of *you* will be played by *you*. The real you this time . . . not the fat piggy and not the conformist. The real you. It'll feel good.

You're Not on Vacation

One of the neat things about retirement is that pleasure, sheer "play," takes on new, legitimate importance. Like kids, now it's okay to play. It's okay in this Third Act.

Personally I think that just plain fooling around—doing stuff because you love it—is just fine in this act. Do as much of it as you enjoy. But it may pall after a while, like a meal of desserts. So it may be a good idea to think of play and pleasure in a different way . . . take it to a higher level. A lot of people make what I think is the terrible mistake of seeing retirement as a long vacation. Or a sabbatical. That ain't gonna work. You're going to be doing the next thing for twenty or thirty years. It has to be substantive or you're going to go nuts. Play is good, but all play, at the low end, is not going to work. Do some of that—travel, golf, whatever—but find something where the pleasure runs deeper, is more demanding and serious. Pleasure is the goal, all right, but at the high end. Writing books and giving lectures is that way for me: play, basically, but play at the high end. Serious pleasure takes some work.

Living More Than One Life

I retired, on purpose, at fifty-six—pretty young. And people always ask me, don't you miss the law? Why did you retire so young? And I always say what is true: Yes, I do miss the law, every day. I loved the practice, really loved it. And I was very good at it: I had the lively sense that—whatever happened next—I would not be anywhere near as good at the next thing as I had been at the law. That was one of the givens in my decision. Why, then, did I quit? Partly I was getting a little sick of it; my mind was starting to wander. But the real reason was this: I wanted to live *more than one life*. Even if the next one were not as important or satisfying as the last one. In my view, this life is all there is, and I wanted a *broad* life, even at the expense of doing something smaller, something I was not as good at. Because I wanted to live more than one life. Which I have done. And I am so grateful.

The Other Side of Your Brain

have a number of pals who, in the Third Act, have put creativity at the center of their lives, after a lifetime of much more focused work where it had been ignored. Sometimes it does not work. Or is an embarrassment. Often, those who put their creative side on hold for thirty years discover that it has atrophied. Or that it didn't amount to a hell of a lot in the first place.

I submit that's fine and still worth doing. It is a matter of living a second life, which is always worthwhile. And there are a few who have rekindled those creative flames and who have done awfully well. For example, I do not know Louis Begley very well, but we are from the same world, and I know that he was a world-class lawyer. And then, fairly late in the day, he began writing serious fiction (*Wartime Lies*, *About Schmidt*, etc.). And was superb at it. That's the true win-win situation. But I submit that you have to start in on that life with no assurance that you have a real flair. To say nothing of a commercial flair (which is so rare that it's not worth thinking about). Do it anyway, is my advice. It is using the different gifts that is the point. And its own reward.

A pal in Boston works like a lunatic designing and making very high-end furniture. A very disciplined guy, all his life, he is disciplined about this, too. The big difference (apart from the absence of dough): He *loves* it. Happiest he has ever been. He hasn't sold anything and probably never will, but the demand from his family and friends will see him through. Happy man.

Two other pals—both very focused indeed, during their professional lives—have become painters. Not the best painters in the history of the world but very good. *Very* good. And *so* into it. Happy men and women.

If you are still working, hang on hard to the pleasures of your creative side. Even if you can't afford to make it the center of your life right now, keep it alive and vibrant. You still improve the chances that there will be something there later on, when *maybe* it will become the most important thing in your life. Teach a little on the side. Do some amateur sculpting. Keep up the sports you love. Build a wooden boat. Keep that side of your brain alive.

Let's be real here, for a minute. Because we were all such dopes about money, when we had it, most of us are going to have to work a fair amount, almost all the way out—for money. And sure enough, some of us are going to have to do whatever work we can get. But, if there is any give in your situation, it sure makes sense to pick the next job on the basis of doing what you love.

Get Over Yourself, At Least Your False Self

We are taught, if we do well, to be crazy about ourselves. It is one of the weird luxuries of success. Here is *some key advice* for retirement: Get over yourself. Your ego-crazed self, anyhow. I am not much given to worrying about former CEOs, but they often have the hardest time. CEOs—like beautiful women—always fear that you are paying attention to them because you want something. And that is often true, as CEOs often learn the second they step down. The phone does not ring, the invitations do not pour in, and they are not as funny. The classic line is about the guy who gets up the next day and climbs into the backseat of the car. Only there's no driver.

Some of the most insufferable, most boring, and most miserable people on earth come together in my beloved Aspen. Former giants of industry, finance, or the movies, they build these massive houses, strut out of them in the morning, and wait for someone to give a shit. Which no one does. Which makes them behave even worse. One of the great tests of real character, it seems to me, is being able to adjust to a change of station in life—to be satisfied with who you are, not your office. Not a problem for most of us, we weren't that huge in the first place. But the generalizations still stand: Get real, get personal, and get over yourself. Sooner would be better. "Coming! In the Third Act! *You* played by *You!*" Ta-dah! Gonna be great.

Take Control

Here is some nice advice I got from a recently retired computer guy who came to one of our Aspen retreats. He was obviously doing well and I asked him his secret. "Perfectly clear," he said. *"You've got to take control of all the major steps in your life.* Retirement or what you call the Third Act—is sure as hell one of them. Don't want to *drift* into retirement . . . *drift* into the next job or location or whatever it is. You are going to be doing some of these things for the rest of your life. You have to take those decisions seriously. *Gotta take charge. Gotta go for it! This is serious.*"

I loved the sound of that, coaxed him to expand.

"Think about it," he said. "When you make up your mind to do something important in life—whether it's getting in shape or changing careers—you want it to be *yours.* You want to *own* it. You don't want your wife or your boss to push you into it. If it's their idea, you'll sulk all the way through and have no fun. Gotta own it or it won't feel good."

"And retirement's like that?"

"Of course retirement's like that," he said, a little impatiently. "Lot of people, at the end of their first careers, they're numb—go wandering off as if they'd been thrown out of the club or something. As if they'd been told they're not wanted around here anymore. Get the hell out. And of course that's true, really, if you wait long enough. Me, I'd rather think about it in advance, make up *my own mind* and *step out there*, long before they want me gone. I don't want to be like some jerk, his girl's thrown his shit out the window and he's got no place to go. Your attitude is completely different if it's your idea. And you have a prayer, at least, of being happy."

My favorite part of his story came *after* his great second career. He lived with his wife out in Michigan someplace—perfectly happy, you know. But his second career was winding down, and they wanted to do something new. So—with absolutely no connections, no job, nothing—they moved to New York City. He's older now so he wanted to work less. But he didn't want to be idle. So he made *living in New York* his *job.* They go to new restaurants all the time, as if they were reviewers. They haunt museums and art galleries. See a lot of plays. And they walk all over town, including the nontourist parts. They make *living in New York* their job. I admire that *so* much. Clever idea. Hilary and I have tried it a bit, and it's more of a challenge than you think. A sweet one, though.

The Gifts of Women

Women have more of a flair for the Third Act than men. Not entirely clear why, but there is no question about it. Perhaps because they have been experts at change all their lives: jobs, kids, marriages and divorces, menopause and beyond. The prospect of the Third Act and profound change scares the hell out of a lot of men. Women, not a bit. A generalization but strikingly true. Time and again you see women *surge* in their fifties and sixties. Maybe it's because they have always been better at the limbic life, which becomes dominant in the Third Act. Whatever, they have a flair. And live four years longer than men. Watch 'em, boys. See if you can learn something.

Get Your Lines Out Early

There are two things that almost everyone is completely stupid about. One, they spend dough all their lives as if they were always going to be earning what they earn today, a deeply mistaken idea for everyone. And two, they spend almost no time while they are working at their first career planning for the next one. On the business of planning the Third Act: For God's sake, *do it*. Think what you may want to do. Look into what may and may not be possible. And get your lines out early. Connect with people who are doing what you might like to do. Scheme a bit. But be aggressive about it. As if, for God's sake, it *mattered*. Which it so profoundly does.

Keeping Your Lines Out All Your Life

Sooner or later in this life, you are almost certainly going to conclude that family and friends count for far more than work, to which you give so much. That is an obvious truth but one upon which we do not act vigorously enough. Losing track of or connection with family and real pals is a dreadful idea. A tragedy, in fact. The obvious advice: Cherish your family. Treasure your friends. If you're sore at this one or that for some reason, see if you can't get over it. I tickled Hilly the other day by saying of some difficult old pal of mine: "I cherish his love more than I resent his betrayals." A good line and, much of the time, good policy. Relationships require care and feeding, or they'll go away. They will rot, like the signaling systems you ignore. *Everything you care about requires care.* Including your friends and family.

Ranie and the Great Kedge

We have talked about *kedges* from time to time. One of the very best things you can do—at the outset of the Third Act and regularly thereafter—is set yourself some great goals, some great *kedges* to help move you into the great shifts that are going to be necessary in the Third Act, and to motivate you for and to shape your future. I have no specific advice but the general thesis is sound.

My beloved daughter Ranie recently turned fifty. Her two girls—to whom she had devoted her whole life—were going away to college or were already gone. She had a good marriage but she had to re-pot herself for her next act. And she was stuck about what to do. She had gotten overweight at some point and came out to one of our Aspen retreat weeks. She got tight with Riggs, he set her feet on what turned out to be a thirty-five-pound weight loss program and her optimism perked right up. Excellent. But that's not the story.

Emboldened by that success, she began casting about for a damn good *kedge.* Ranie lives north of San Francisco and had become something of an open water swimmer, in freezing, wind-tossed San Francisco Bay. She liked it and had a flair for it. Not fast but very steady. And brave as a lion.

So she decided to swim the English Channel. Fewer people have swum the channel (under 1,400) than have climbed Mount Everest because it is so much harder. Thousands set out, again and again, and are turned back by hypothermia (you do not wear a wet suit) or the tides or storms. Ranie trained long and relentlessly and—very long story short—she simply did it. In some of the worst weather of any successful swim (rain, wind, and up to five-foot waves) she simply did it. It took almost nineteen hours, in the fifty-eight-degree water; she was taking on water in those waves, every third stroke. She thought often about quitting. And did not. For almost nineteen hours. Until she walked ashore in France. I am her father, of course, and do not have to be objective. But I thought it was one of the bravest things I had ever seen. I am a bit of a swimmer, I have some notion of open water. But *this!* I thought it was incomprehensibly hard. And brave. And she just kept on going. And did it.

A kedge doesn't have to be quite as extreme as Ranie's. Hers was one tick this side of crazy, but a good one can make some interesting changes *forever* in your life. Ranie is simply a different person. So if you're a hair overweight, lose it; get in shape; do a serious kedge. And *coast* into this Third Act, of which you are the star.

Full House

Old pals of ours from down South found themselves facing some serious changes in their lives, changes that suggested it made sense for them to move up North for a year. They weren't going to sell the big house down South, but they were thinking about renting. Maybe up our way, in the Berkshires. They are close friends, they have perfect manners (we look like thugs by comparison), and their two little boys, five and seven years old, are heaven. We said forget about renting. We have lots of space; move in with us for a year. Which, after a lot of persuasion, they did. The two parents, the two little boys, and two big dogs. And it has been a sheer pleasure ever since. Friends of both of ours tend to think it's a little weird, but not a bit of it. The kids are thriving in a local school, and none of us has had a cross word.

And guess what: Our house—which was a bit big and empty—is a limbic stew these days. Full of noise and kids and dogs (our dog, Olive, had the hardest adjustment, but *she* has become a much better dog, of all things). A privilege, believe me. I admit that there are not many people you could do it with, but we've done amazingly well.

I grew up in a big farmhouse like that, full of family and friends and guest families who came to stay for a year with their children and dogs. Two grandmothers for years. Maybe it was hard on the grown-ups some of the time; I don't know. But it was an unmixed joy for us kids, and it looked like fun for my parents. Arrangements like that used to be a fairly common experience, back in the Depression and before, when we weren't all quite so rich. That shouldn't be the deciding factor.

If you have a little yen for that life, and a big house and some truly solid pals who could use a place to rest for a bit, go for it. It can be *sweet*!

The Old Girl on 57th Street with the Four-Footed Cane

Remember the old girl on the sidewalk, with the four-footed rubber-tipped cane? My next-door neighbor who had broken her hip badly and was taking those tiny steps, looking down? Scared to death. She was well into her eighties, she looked bad, and I at least was afraid she was dying. So sad: She had a great sense of humor—edgy and fun. And was still a beauty, for all that her hip was messed up. It was, you will remember, a glass box story. Her glass box was closing in.

Didn't happen. And not because she started eating kale or lifting weights either. One day an old admirer came to the door. Dapper gent, full of life and charm, a guy who had always loved her but it hadn't worked out. So here he was—too late. Or so you might assume. She came to the door, looking like hell I imagine. Saw who it was and said, "Excuse me. Do come in and sit down, I'll just be a minute." She quickly washed her face, put on some makeup, threw the four-legged cane under the bed, and *swanned* back into the living room, this beautiful and wonderful creature from out of their past. How she pulled that off, I cannot imagine, but she did. He was charmed, of course; she had been charming men since she was ten. And their lives together began.

Her hip, which had been rotting away for months, healed miraculously overnight. Her health—and delicious sense of humor—was restored, and soon she was walking down the street, where she had been but a ghost a month before, like springtime. They were married a year later and lived happily ever after. We see them all the time, and it is a joy. We were at the wedding. Great event. One of her sons gave her away. I think he was sixty-five.

What happened to her bad hip? I have no idea. Except for this: We are designed to roll about with one another. My beloved neighbor was back in the pack and her coat was glossy in no time and her nose was wet. And her sense of humor was, once again, delicious and rough. And her hip simply got better. A limbic miracle.

The lesson here is slightly obvious. We are mammals. We are designed to play together in packs and herds. And marriages. Marriages are not the only way to go, God knows. Plenty of us do fine without. Good friends are a close substitute, if you have a flair for friendship. A damn good dog will work miracles. But marriage is not so dumb either. If you just happen to have one that can bear the strain and drama of this Third Act, you're lucky. Me, too.

The Recap: The Three-Legged Stool

The good life is a three-legged stool: exercise, nutrition, caring. Exercise is the great flywheel. The *great* flywheel. Nutrition comes a close second, the building block of life—you'd be nuts not to get your butt down off that Mountain of Slop and Despair as fast as ever you can. But the third leg—of which we speak the least—may be the most important of the three: Care, connect, and commit. We are mammals in the end. We are designed and built to be closely connected. And to care like crazy about one another.

The possibility that you will have the energy, optimism, drive, and attractiveness to make real connections and care in the Third Act will be massively improved by a serious commitment to exercise and sane eating. They are the foundation on which everything is built. But success in the Great Play of your life may very well turn, in the end, on your flair for giving a damn about someone or something else. And connecting and committing to them like crazy. We are mammals; snuggle up.

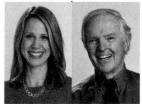

CHAPTER TWENTY-FIVE

A Day in the Life: Victory Lap

From Chris

To help us all celebrate having finished this book, Jen and her family—Chris and the two kids, Tess, six, and Austin, three—drove out to the Berkshires to bike a little, row, and have some decent meals. We had a big gang here last night for supper, after a day of hectic activity. It was a little more work, a bit more intense, and a lot more fun than any of us had anticipated. It's a little like the life we are trying to get you to try: a little harder and more intense and more fun than any of us had imagined.

I got more out of the last two years than Jen. I look adorable, for one thing. Well, adorable is strong, but I look noticeably better without that fifteen pounds. People mention it. And Jen was absolutely right, that first day, about *feeling* better. Not lugging those fifteen pounds around makes life so much easier. Which is to say, easier on your joints—as advertised. And easier on your mobility and flexibility in general. I am an extremely old boy, but my biking and skiing are both better than they were two years ago when I began. A miracle at my age. I would not go so far as to say that I am "younger" all over again. That's not true. But I sure do have a ton of energy, I feel more or less terrific *all the time*, and I can *do* things I care about more and better than when we began. That's *something!*

But the real miracle for me is that Jen's regimen really took hold. It is permanent. Talk about your old dog and the new tricks: We just plain eat differently today. We really do eat a huge amount of good vegetables and whole grains. We really do skip—almost completely—the Dead Foods and fried stuff. Almost no beef and not such an awful lot of other meat. I am still a bit of a fool about butter. And I am never going to have less than two glasses of wine a night—and the occasional martini. But lots of things have all but disappeared from our lives. Pizza, for instance. I miss it slightly, but we rarely even *think* about that anymore. Burgers are mostly gone, one or two a month instead of several a week. Cheese in general is gone. That is a real loss, but Jen's stories about the workings of solid fat were too powerful; only butter survived them.

One of the biggest and easiest changes: We eat almost nothing but whole grains now: lots of brown rice, farro, and quinoa. Lots of whole oats at breakfast and lots of whole-grain bread. For me, this change has been all pleasure and no strain. The whole grains taste better. Quite a lot better in most cases. *Except* for French baguettes. I am still an utter fool for a good baguette with butter. Or cheese. If cheese and butter take a few months off my life? Hey, it's a reasonable deal. Same with maple syrup. And excessive popcorn. Gotta have popcorn, most days. Which would be fine, apparently, if it was not cooked in oil. Which, of course, it is.

A huge change: I sleep better. During the writing of the book, my sleeping wasn't so great. I carried the job pretty heavily for a while, and I tossed and turned way too much. But now—with the book in hand and the new regimen coming into its own—I am sleeping much, much better. That's a joy. A *real* joy. Hate to tell you, but less booze is part of that. And less meat, I suspect. Both are enemies of sleep.

It is impossible to unbundle the effect of being a little lighter and eating very differently. I don't know which gets credit for what. What I *feel and see* is the weight loss; I just plain *love* that and tend to credit it with the general improvement in achiness and everything else. But that may be wrong. Jen says that having a much higher density of nutrients in my system may have a much greater impact. Whatever, I don't need to worry about sorting it out: The combined effect is sweet indeed. And it is clear that both changes are permanent. We eat differently. And it is not a diet, not a way to lose weight. It is just how we eat now, and we prefer it. We really, really do. Hard to believe if you haven't been there, but it's true. What we didn't notice before was that eating garbage made us *feel* crappy, much of the time. When we dip into garbage on occasion now, we *really* notice it. Eating garbage makes you feel *awful*. You just don't notice it until you stop.

This change is *realistic*. The Great American Diet has not been around forever. It is not deep in our DNA. It is just something we have been *sold* by people who had a tremendous amount to gain by selling it to us. When we mostly dropped it, we did not miss it much at all. Well, twinges, but surprisingly minor. This change is forever, too. The worst stuff—which looked wonderful to us two years ago—looks more or less disgusting now. Which it *is*, of course. Helps to know that. The secret ingredient in this book is knowledge. We always knew that intuitively, Jen and I, but it turns out to be true. There are things in here that you cannot unlearn: the basic notion of Dead Food, for example. The "open sewer" around your gut for another. The rats at night. Once you *know* what is going on inside, there are things you just won't do anymore.

From Jen

Chris is lucky, in a way: He gets to see and feel changes. And I am lucky, too, because even though I have been on this regimen for a long time, I can now see how invaluable telling others about the science behind exercise, nutrition, and weight control is. What I did get was a revelation and some insights. Writing a popular book—even a fairly sophisticated one—is so different from anything I've ever done. In the early days, I was astonished at just how difficult it is to take complex scientific information and put it into comprehensible and useful form for the educated layperson. That was hard, and Chris suffered a lot of it with me. Helped a lot, too. I am sure we could have gotten impatient and furious with each other. Instead, we came to rely on and help and trust each other to an extent that was new for me. A nice sample of that limbic life that Chris just wrote about.

But the consequences of going through that process were interesting. I began to see my own profession—and the worlds of nutrition science and exercise—in a much broader context, and they became more rather than less important to me. People like me tend to live and work focusing on one scientific question at a time. We are rarely given the opportunity to put important findings into a broader context, beyond academic meetings and seminars. Spending this time thinking about people who are somewhat overweight—or obese in too many cases—and in bad shape, but who want to change, has both energized me and given me new focus.

Over the years, my sense of urgency about the obesity epidemic, especially the childhood obesity epidemic, has grown sharply. I am always thrilled to find new ways to utilize my expertise on this front. And I am even more impatient with junk science and false advertising than I was at the beginning. That whole business is such an outrage.

And having been forced to articulate what have always been my views about exercise has made me a near fanatic on that subject. I think we have gotten it fundamentally wrong in so many of our efforts to deal with obesity when we do not put physical activity front and center. I have always believed—intuitively and scientifically—that exercise was the *flywheel*, as we say, of weight loss and the good life. No one knows better than I that we have to change the way we eat, too. But I think it is nuts not to put exercise at the center of our lifestyle efforts, as we have done in the book. This *is* the right emphasis. This *will* work. I think you'll see that sometime soon.

Also, I love the idea that we have been able to be so blunt about the utter necessity of fundamental change. So often, in my field, professionals mince their words, both about the bad forces that are making a mess of American life and about the need for fundamental change to promote the good life. We cannot solve the obesity epidemic by working out one day a week. Or cutting back on fast food here and there. *Fundamental change* is what it is going to take, and I love the idea of being out there and saying that, loudly. We need to make fundamental changes in this country in the way we eat and the way we move. Period. I *know* it will work for some people. I *hope* it will work for a lot of you. A hundred million would be good. We have to start somewhere.

From Chris

I passionately agree with all that. But I am the "living the life" guy in the book. So let me tell you just a little about this day with Jen and her family, and the pleasure it was. First we took a hell of a bike ride. Back up Bash Bish Falls, in fact. Not the full fifty miles, but I dragged Jen up the mighty hill. (No surprise: She made it handily, even though she is not a regular cyclist; she says she wanted to quit a couple of times but was not willing to give me the satisfaction.) We went by my old house again, talked about different lives in different eras. Black ice. That interested her—the layering of lives, over time.

Not going to repeat myself, but let me say what a pleasure it is to still be biking *up the waterfall* at my tender age. Instead of flying over it. Jen has helped a lot with that. This was an easier climb than the one I did up the same hill a year ago.

We did not stop and see Ted. Not enough time. But we did pay our respects to Jack. Reported on our success, frankly. Then blew him the traditional kiss—both of us this time: Jack loved getting kissed by strange girls. Then home to cook dinner for a dozen or so of us. The meal was that big shrimp and veg pasta dish you've already read about. The only difference was the cast.

The next morning, we were down at the lake by six-thirty to go for a short row. The fact that I am still rowing at my age is like a dog walking on its hind legs: It is not a matter of being graceful; it is doing it at all that's the miracle. Watching Jen, however, was the full-blown miracle. She is *so* strong, *so* graceful. Her balance was so perfect, the boat might as well have been on *rails of steel*. And the power? Oh, boy! I have hung around rowers and rowing for a while now, and I can tell. The swirls from her strokes, flying toward the stern: Something! She looked exactly like what she is: an all-American rower who has stayed in absolutely superb shape. A joy to see. Check the website; you can see her do it. Me too, but please, no insidious comparisons. Remember, we have a dog here who is walking on his hind legs.

From Jen

Thanks, but Chris is a better rower than he says. He's been rowing for over fifty years, and it shows in the set of the boat, the evenness of the stroke. It's a pity rowing isn't a more widely practiced sport: It is *so* great for you. And you can do it forever.

From Chris

Yeah, well, thanks a lot. But as practiced by Jen, it is simply a different sport. Such a treat to watch. Okay, Jen, how do we leave 'em?

From Jen

The way we began, I guess—with advice. Change the way you *eat*, eat better and eat less. And change the way you *move*, and move more—then you can have a radically better life. You can be biking and rowing and *thinking and acting* like Chris, at almost eighty. And—I strongly suspect—for a long time after eighty. And having *fun*. His life, on the brink of eighty, is about a hundred times more fun than most people's lives. And that doesn't just happen, believe me. You have to work for that. Exercise, nutrition, commitment. Try it.

From Chris

Our life *is* a pleasure, Hilary's and mine, and it has been for a while. But writing—and eventually living—this book with Jen has been a major part of it lately. This was a tough project at times. And Jen was always optimistic, upbeat, and hardworking. All that made *such* a difference. She is as solid as she is smart, and that's saying a lot. And we did have fun, didn't we?

From Jen

We sure did. I hope it will be infectious and that you'll try the regimen. We think that it'll be fun, too. It will absolutely change your life.

From Chris

There you go. Let's go get our bikes and do Bash Bish again. Last one up the waterfall is a rotten egg!

Jen's Rules

1. Make up your mind: Set your goal and go for it.

2. Exercise for forty-five to sixty minutes a day, six days a week, for the rest of your life.

3. Eat less and be mindful.

4. Don't eat Dead Food.

5. Eat plenty of produce—half your diet should be vegetables and fruit.

6. Eat healthy fats in moderation and avoid saturated and trans fats.

7. Eat less meat and make it lean.

8. Don't drink your calories.

9. Don't skip meals.

10. Embrace change—in your new body and health.

Other Stuff

THINNERTHISYEAR.COM
YOUNGERNEXTYEAR.COM

This book spills over, I'm afraid. There's so darn much that we just can't fit it all in. And there are important things which even the very best books just can't do. Think about strength training, for example. Eventually you want to see the guy *doing it. Moving.* Maybe taking you beyond the Sacred 25.

Then there's *food.* Wouldn't it be kind of neat to see a human being cooking up a storm? Demonstrating some of this stuff in the kitchen . . . making it real?

And how about updates and warnings and "think pieces"? Nutrition in particular is a field where the legitimate science is jumping out of the labs like rabbits. How do you keep up?

Most important of all, how about *community*? How the devil do you find someone to *do this stuff with*? We keep saying that this great effort is best done in company . . . best done in the "limbic stew." But how do you do that? Suppose your spouse doesn't give a damn. Or he or she ran off, like the girl down at Ted's Store, years ago. Your friends think you're crazy and the dog just looks at you funny . . . just rolls over and goes back to sleep. Then what? How do you find a *community of like-minded people* who are trying to *change their lives*? Like you?

We have thought about this a lot and believe we've come up with a pretty good idea. Not a perfect one, but not a bad one either. Take a look at ThinnerThisYear.com (YoungerNextYear.com takes you to the same place.) You may be skeptical about how much a website can do. Me, too, but I was wrong, I think. They can do a lot. As we learned with the beta test. It's a work in progress, but coming.

The Beta Test

When the book was almost done, we did an interesting thing. We gave rough copies to more than a hundred people and asked 'em to try it out. To see if the weight loss stuff was realistic . . . to see if the whole thing worked. As of this writing that was only six weeks ago (and the test runs for six months), so we don't know yet. But the early results are wonderful. People have lost a lot of weight; they have really gotten into the exercise. And they are having fun. How come? Well the book helps, thank God. And the magic of exercise in particular. We had that right. But the second most important thing may be the online community, the online support. Interesting.

I write letters for it, as does Jen. But the big thing is the communication among the betas themselves. Their blogs and comments. Their sense that they are doing this with people like themselves. And that they all care. We think that communities like that can matter a lot. And they're kind of fun. See what you think.

Other Stuff

The website is also a font of information and stuff to buy. An inexpensive "home gym" for example. The TRX gadgets . . . stuff like that. And, we hope, an app, just for this book, to keep track of your food and exercise. That could be truly helpful. Maybe a customized TTY heart rate monitor . . . working on that, too.

Bill Fabrocini's DVDs will be a help. They'll show people doing the Sacred 25 exercises, and Bill talking about them. (I hover in the background . . . kibitz a little). Lots of you will find them a godsend, I bet.

And for those who want to go nuts on aerobic and other training, **Riggs Klika's YNY/FIT** offers customized one-on-one training. He's a hound for this stuff and YNY/FIT is wonderful.

Aspen Total Immersion Weeks

Finally, let me give a plug to our Aspen Club/Thinner This Year/ Younger Next Year "Total Immersion Weeks." They are fun. And life-changing. I have often said that Michael Fox's Aspen Club and Spa has been the "engine room" of this book and of YNY, too. A lot of the groundwork for the exercise part of this book was done there, high in the Rockies . . . in one of the best health facilities in one of the prettiest (and healthiest) towns on earth. And some of that work was done during Total Immersion Weeks, which Michael and I (and Riggs Klika) run there. You come for a week, stay in a grand hotel, eat in the very best restaurants (but off a *Thinner* menu . . . one glass of wine) and work out in the hills and in the club and learn a ton about diet, exercise, and the good life. Bit of a life-changer, as all the participants say. It's an investment, but talk about a good kedge. Oh my.

Do take a quick look at the website. We think it completes the book in important ways. Hope so, anyway.

Index